T0226403

Advances in Palliative Medicine

Editor

KATHERINE J. GOLDBERG

VETERINARY CLINICS OF NORTH AMERICA: SMALL ANIMAL PRACTICE

www.vetsmall.theclinics.com

May 2019 • Volume 49 • Number 3

ELSEVIER

1600 John F. Kennedy Boulevard • Suite 1800 • Philadelphia, Pennsylvania, 19103-2899
http://www.vetsmall.theclinics.com

VETERINARY CLINICS OF NORTH AMERICA: SMALL ANIMAL PRACTICE Volume 49, Number 3
May 2019 ISSN 0195-5616, ISBN-13: 978-0-323-67784-4

Editor: Colleen Dietzler
Developmental Editor: Meredith Madeira

Veterinary Clinics of North America: Small Animal Practice (ISSN 0195-5616) is published bimonthly by Elsevier Inc., 360 Park Avenue South, New York, NY 10010-1710. Months of issue are January, March, May, July, September, and November. Business and Editorial Offices: 1600 John F. Kennedy Blvd., Ste. 1800, Philadelphia, PA 19103-2899. Customer Service Office: 3251 Riverport Lane, Maryland Heights, MO 63043. Periodicals postage paid at New York, NY and additional mailing offices. Subscription prices are $338.00 per year (domestic individuals), $662.00 per year (domestic institutions), $100.00 per year (domestic students/residents), $451.00 per year (Canadian individuals), $823.00 per year (Canadian institutions), $474.00 per year (international individuals), $823.00 per year (international institutions), and $220.00 per year (international and Canadian students/residents). To receive student/resident rate, orders must be accompanied by name of affiliated institution, date of term, and the *signature* of program/residency coordinator on institution letterhead. Orders will be billed at individual rate until proof of status is received. Foreign air speed delivery is included in all *Clinics* subscription prices. All prices are subject to change without notice. **POSTMASTER:** Send address changes to *Veterinary Clinics of North America: Small Animal Practice*, Elsevier Health Sciences Division, Subscription Customer Service, 3251 Riverport Lane, Maryland Heights, MO 63043. Customer Service (orders, claims, online, change of address): Elsevier Periodicals Customer Service, Elsevier Health Sciences Division Subscription **Customer Service 3251 Riverport Lane Maryland Heights, MO 63043. Tel: 1-800-654-2452 (U.S. and Canada); 314-447-8871 (outside U.S. and Canada). Fax: 314-447-8029. E-mail: journalscustomerservice-usa@elsevier.com (for print support); journalsonlinesupport-usa@elsevier.com (for online support).**

Reprints. For copies of 100 or more of articles in this publication, please contact the Commercial Reprints Department, Elsevier Inc., 360 Park Avenue South, New York, NY 10010-1710. Tel.: 212-633-3874; Fax: 212-633-3820; E-mail: reprints@elsevier.com.

Veterinary Clinics of North America: Small Animal Practice is also published in Japanese by Inter Zoo Publishing Co., Ltd., Aoyama Crystal-Bldg 5F, 3-5-12 Kitaaoyama, Minato-ku, Tokyo 107-0061, Japan.

Veterinary Clinics of North America: Small Animal Practice is covered in *Current Contents/Agriculture, Biology and Environmental Sciences, Science Citation Index, ASCA, MEDLINE/PubMed (Index Medicus), Excerpta Medica,* and *BIOSIS.*

Contributors

EDITOR

KATHERINE J. GOLDBERG, DVM, LMSW
Founder/Owner, Whole Animal Veterinary Geriatrics & Palliative Care Services, Counselor Therapist, Cornell Health, Counseling and Psychological Services, Ithaca, New York; Core Instructor, University of Tennessee Veterinary Social Work Certificate Program, Knoxville, Tennessee

AUTHORS

COURTNEY BENNETT, DVM
Owner and Veterinarian, Heart's Ease Veterinary Care, Louisville, Kentucky

GAIL A. BISHOP, BS
Argus Institute Director and Pet Hospice Advisor, Colorado State University Veterinary Teaching Hospital, Fort Collins, Colorado

JORDYN M. BOESCH, DVM
Diplomate, American College of Veterinary Anesthesia and Analgesia; Senior Lecturer, Section of Anesthesiology and Pain Medicine, Department of Clinical Sciences and Cornell University Hospital for Animals, Cornell University College of Veterinary Medicine, Ithaca, New York

SANDRA BRACKENRIDGE, LCSW, BCD
Former Associate Professor of Social Work, Texas Woman's University, Denton, Texas; Idaho State University, Pocatello, Idaho; Veterinary Social Worker, Center for Veterinary Specialty + Emergency Care, Lewisville, Texas; Social Work Consulting and Counseling, Veterinary Practices, Corinth, Texas

MARK D. CARLSON, DVM
Associate Veterinarian and Chief of Surgery, Stow Kent Animal Hospital, Kent, Ohio

NATHANIEL COOK, DVM
Owner and Veterinarian, Heart's Ease Veterinary Care, Louisville, Kentucky

EMMA S. DAVIES, BVSc, MSc
Diplomate, European College of Veterinary Neurology; Department of Clinical Sciences, College of Veterinary Medicine, Cornell University, Ithaca, New York

CURTIS WELLS DEWEY, DVM, MS, CTCVMP
Diplomate, American College of Veterinary Internal Medicine (Neurology); Diplomate, American College of Veterinary Surgeons; Department of Clinical Sciences, College of Veterinary Medicine, Cornell University, Ithaca, New York

JULIE M. DUCOTÉ, DVM, MA
Diplomate, American College of Veterinary Internal Medicine (Neurology); CEO, Staff Neurologist, Center for Veterinary Specialty + Emergency Care, Lewisville, Texas

KATHERINE J. GOLDBERG, DVM, LMSW
Founder/Owner, Whole Animal Veterinary Geriatrics & Palliative Care Services, Counselor Therapist, Cornell Health, Counseling and Psychological Services, Ithaca, New York; Core Instructor, University of Tennessee Veterinary Social Work Certificate Program, Knoxville, Tennessee

MARIA GORE, MSW
Counselor and Pet Hospice Advisor, Argus Institute, Colorado State University Veterinary Teaching Hospital, Fort Collins, Colorado

MICHAEL KISELOW, DVM
Diplomate, American College of Veterinary Internal Medicine (Oncology); Sage Centers for Veterinary Specialty and Emergency Care, Campbell, California

SUSAN E. LANA, DVM, MS
Diplomate, American College of Veterinary Internal Medicine Oncology; Professor, Clinical Sciences, Colorado State University, Fort Collins

BETH MARCHITELLI, DVM
4 Paws Farewell, Mobile Pet Hospice, Palliative Care and Home Euthanasia, Asheville, North Carolina

LISA MOSES, VMD
Diplomate, American College of Veterinary Internal Medicine (Small Animal Internal Medicine); Pain and Palliative Care Service, MSPCA-Angell Animal Medical Center, Faculty and Research Fellow, Center for Bioethics, Harvard Medical School, Bioethics Scholar and Chair, Animal Ethics Study Group, Boston, Massachusetts; Bioethics Scholar, Yale Center for Interdisciplinary Bioethics, New Haven, Connecticut

JESSICA PIERCE, PhD
Center for Bioethics and Humanities, University of Colorado Anschutz Medical School, Aurora, Colorado

TAMARA SHEARER, DVM, CCRP, CVPP, CVA, CHPV, CTPEP
Smoky Mountain Integrative Veterinary Clinic, Sylva, North Carolina; The Chi Institute, Reddick, Florida

ANTHONY J. SMITH, DVM, MBA
IAAHPC Certified Hospice and Palliative Care Veterinarian, Founder, Owner, Rainbow Bridge Veterinary Services, Hercules, California

MARY BETH SPITZNAGEL, PhD
Associate Professor, Department of Psychological Sciences, Kent State University, Kent, Ohio

ELIZABETH B. STRAND, PhD, MSSW
Director, Veterinary Social Work Program, Clinical Associate Professor, University of Tennessee, College of Veterinary Medicine, College of Social Work, Knoxville, Tennessee

JOSEPH J. WAKSHLAG, DVM, PhD, CVA
Diplomate, American College of Veterinary Nutrition; Diplomate, American College of Veterinary Sports Medicine and Rehabilitation; Department of Small Animal Clinical Sciences, College of Veterinary Medicine, University of Florida, Gainesville, Florida; Department of Comparative, Diagnostic and Population Medicine, Reddick, Florida

HUISHENG XIE, DVM, MS, PhD, CTCVMP
Department of Small Animal Clinical Sciences, College of Veterinary Medicine, University of Florida, Gainesville, Florida; Department of Comparative, Diagnostic and Population Medicine, Reddick, Florida

PAGE E. YAXLEY, DVM
Diplomate, American College of Veterinary Emergency and Critical Care; Assistant Professor, Small Animal Emergency and Critical Care, The Ohio State University College of Veterinary Medicine, Columbus, Ohio

Contents

This article provides a brief review of important foundational concepts and an overview of major milestones in the history of animal hospice and palliative care. This article also presents a view of future goals and challenges that lie ahead of the veterinary profession as the field of animal hospice and palliative care evolves. Some examples of topics reviewed and explored in the article include current "state of-the-art" of animal hospice, future research goals, improved veterinary college curricula, collaboration among medical disciplines, and support of the veterinary staff.

Section I: Established Programs and Curricular Initiatives

Serving clients since 2004, Colorado State University's Veterinary Teaching Hospital is the first and only program to offer a student-run pet hospice program. Under the supervision of faculty and staff advisors, student volunteers provide home hospice care to families who have a terminally ill pet. This article describes the history of the program, how it is organized, the roles and responsibilities of the students, the challenges of the program and future goals. This article seeks to serve as a follow up on the 2008 Journal of Veterinary Medical Education article on the Colorado State University pet hospice program.

In 2011, Michigan State University College of Veterinary Medicine founded the second veterinary hospice in academic practice. This program was designed to meet the growing demand for veterinary end-of-life care in the community. Veterinary Hospice Care provided patients and their families palliative care services, through utilization of an interdisciplinary team, from the time of terminal diagnosis to the time of death. Families also received dedicated emotional support. As a direct result of the hospice care service, Michigan State University veterinary students as well as in-state technical college students received an increase in end-of-life care in the curriculum.

A veterinary palliative care service was developed as a specialty service in 2006 at a large, nonprofit teaching veterinary hospital. The service

Section II: Concepts and Essential Viewpoints

Treating the animal patient as a "person" involves refining the capacity to see the patient as clearly as possible. Veterinary end-of-life care can usefully engage with the science of animal emotion and cognition to help bring the patient into 3-D. This article highlights 3 specific areas in which engagement with the ethology literature and more careful attention to the subjective experiences of animals could improve end-of-life care: (1) interpretation and management of pain, (2) assessments of quality of life, and (3) attention to the autonomy of animal patients.

This article describes veterinary client caregiver burden, including how it differs from other key client experiences in the palliative care setting. Caregiver burden in human relationships is reviewed. Research examining veterinary client caregiver burden in the context of serious illness (or pet caregiver burden), including the link between pet caregiver burden and client psychosocial well-being, is summarized. Risk factors for development of pet caregiver burden are discussed in the context of beginning to address how it might be reduced or prevented. Finally, suggestions are provided for veterinarians working with clients facing these issues in a palliative care setting.

Section III: Advances and Information to Guide Clinicians

One of the most important goals of palliative medicine and hospice care is pain relief. Although great strides have been made in veterinary analgesia, severe pain, especially at home, is still difficult to control. Pain control in the context of palliative medicine and hospice care is far more advanced in human medicine. Many modalities used in chronically or terminally ill humans might be adapted to animals to better manage severe pain. This article discusses drugs and procedures used to control pain in humans that are relatively nascent or unavailable in veterinary medicine and deserve further attention.

Most neurologic diseases are incurable. Palliative care is vital in the treatment of companion animals with serious or chronic neurologic disease. A Neuropalliative Care Core Skill Set includes multifaceted communication competencies and symptom management. Because some of the most common clinical signs of neurologic disease are also associated with stress of caregiving, veterinarians should understand their clients' unique potential for caregiver burden. Acknowledging caregiver burden in their clients, means that veterinarians treating patients with neurologic disease must be proactive in building their own resilience to the occupational

palliative medicine, hospice, and end-of-life care. The characteristics of, and unique considerations associated with, this practice's patient population are discussed. Demand for hospice and palliative care services is increasing even though these fields are in the early stages of growth and development, and availability of services is limited. Research is an essential step toward improving care provision and evaluating the value of hospice and palliative care services in terms of patient comfort, quality of life, and survival time.

VETERINARY CLINICS OF NORTH AMERICA: SMALL ANIMAL PRACTICE

SERIES OF RELATED INTEREST

Veterinary Clinics of North America: Exotic Animal Practice
https://www.vetexotic.theclinics.com/

THE CLINICS ARE NOW AVAILABLE ONLINE!
Access your subscription at:
www.theclinics.com

Preface

Advances in Palliative Medicine

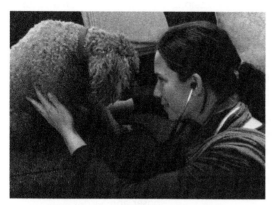

Katherine J. Goldberg, DVM, LMSW
Editor

The seemingly easiest and most sensible rule for doctors to follow is: always fight. Always look for what more you can do…But our fight is not always to do more. It is to do right by our patients, even though what is right is not always clear.
—*Atul Gawande, MD, MPH*

It is with great joy and gratitude that I introduce this issue to you. It is a compilation of the most current advances in palliative medicine for companion animals and represents many years of clinical service, innovation, and professional and personal growth of its contributing authors. If there is a unifying theme, it is: **rigor**. A commitment to academic rigor in this project has been a guiding principle from its earliest development, with the goal of adequately presenting palliative medicine in its truest form. From there, translation into a veterinary context may be considered: what has been done already, and what might be done in the future. I am pleased to say that the issue accomplishes what it set out to do, thanks to its extraordinary group of authors.

It describes each hospice program which has been developed in a veterinary teaching institution, a formal palliative care curricular intervention, a palliative care service within a nonprofit teaching hospital, and a multidoctor mobile palliative care practice. As such, it reflects the current "state-of-the-art" in terms of program development and curricular initiatives, with their associated challenges as well as victories, and serves as a guide for future development of the field. It presents perspectives on clinical signs and syndromes from a palliative care perspective, altering the lens through which veterinarians might consider serious illness care for their patients. It presents conceptual material which is the very foundation of veterinary palliative medicine provision, and

Vet Clin Small Anim 49 (2019) xiii–xv
https://doi.org/10.1016/j.cvsm.2019.02.001
0195-5616/19/© 2019 Published by Elsevier Inc.

vetsmall.theclinics.com

finally, it provides information such as tools for conflict management to help clinicians better understand and address challenges inherent in this work. Lisa Moses' article, "Overcoming Obstacles to Palliative Care: Lessons to Learn from Our Physician Counterparts," is the only published work of its kind. I am immensely grateful to the physicians, pioneers in palliative care and experts in the field, who shared their wisdom and advice for the betterment of our veterinary profession. The inclusion of such a collaboration in this issue is extraordinary.

The history of palliative medicine within the veterinary profession, like most knowledge-building endeavors, has had its share of obstacles and confusion. Different ideas about what this field should look like, "What is the work that we are actually trying to do?," have emerged. Of primary importance to me is the ethical defensibility of this work, both clinically (prioritizing animal welfare) and professionally (maintaining sound judgment, utilizing evidence-based interventions where they exist, and recognizing limits). Accurate characterization of services as well as discernment between what level of care may be expected from primary care veterinarians, boarded specialists, and other providers are important, given the potential for misalignment between client expectations, marketing of services, and delivery of services, particularly when clients are vulnerable. For example, mobile euthanasia services have dominated the end-of-life care market in veterinary medicine to date; however, these are neither hospice nor palliative care services per se. In a veterinary setting, palliative care may be provided to stable patients of any age as well as seriously and chronically ill patients. Hospice care is delivered as death approaches (ie, palliative care at the end of life). Given the legal availability of euthanasia for animals, delineating "hospice" from palliative care and/or determining which illnesses are "terminal" in patients whose lives can be ended at any time, is murky at best. It is for these reasons that thoughtful and rigorous discourse is critical. To assist with this discourse, and place this issue in context, the following definitions are provided:

Palliative care, which may be provided to patients of any age, at any time over the course of an illness, is a growing medical specialty that attends to suffering resulting from both serious illness and its treatment. It provides relief from the symptoms, pain, and stress of serious illness as well as emotional support and help in navigating the health care system for patients and families. While palliative care is commonly associated with hospice, these terms are not synonymous.

Hospice is the philosophy of care that regards death as a natural process, prioritizes comfort and quality of life over quantity of life as death draws near, and supports the cultural and spiritual aspects of dying.

While veterinarians have historically provided many of the defining elements of hospice and palliative care, their evolution as distinct areas of veterinary practice is a relatively recent phenomenon. Palliative care as a discipline within veterinary medicine is still emerging. However, principles and philosophy of care are identical to those in human medicine; several of these principles are outlined in the pages that follow. Many veterinarians are already providing palliative care on a regular basis for their patients and clients and may choose to further develop this area of their practice. Others are cultivating independent practices or services within larger hospital systems dedicated solely to palliative medicine.

Reminiscent of its trajectory within human medicine, this work is embraced by some in the established veterinary profession as a necessary and legitimate area of care and rejected by others. It is my belief that this is in large part due to confusion and misperceptions around what palliative medicine is, as well as a lack of academic rigor in some end-of-life care practices within the "animal hospice" movement. It is with the goals of mitigating these misperceptions and building the literature in meaningful ways that this issue has come to be. I am grateful to Tami Shearer, guest editor of the 2011 *Veterinary Clinics of North America: Small Animal Practice*, Palliative Medicine and Hospice Care, for sharing her perspective and historical context. Her contribution to this issue reflects our shared values of collaboration, integrity, and advancement of the field, as she bridges the 2011 issue with this one.

The focus and framework of the current issue are the following: (1) Data from established programs, past and present; (2) Fundamental concepts not previously explored in the veterinary literature; and (3) Advances and information to guide clinicians. Of note, and unique among veterinary publications in this area, it draws upon the experience of veterinary specialists as well as concepts and collaborations from palliative care in human medicine. Importantly, it is written by an interprofessional, interdisciplinary team. Veterinarians, social workers, ethicists, and others have contributed their expertise. In this way, the team of authors reflects the interdisciplinary nature of palliative care teams themselves.

The insights, perspectives, and tools described by each author are too numerous to mention individually here, but their impacts are tremendous. My hope is that readers will be informed, inspired, and challenged by this issue, and patients, clients, and clinicians will reap the benefits. To each and every contributing author: thank you endlessly for your hard work and dedication to this project, for building knowledge, and for contributing to the field. You have not only created an essential publication but also pushed the edge of forward momentum toward new ways of supporting human-animal relationships. I am forever grateful.

Do not go where the path may lead, go instead where there is no path and leave a trail.

—*Ralph Waldo Emerson*

Katherine J. Goldberg, DVM, LMSW
Whole Animal Veterinary Geriatrics & Palliative Care Services
Ithaca, New York
Cornell Health, Counseling and Psychological Services
Ithaca, New York
University of Tennessee Veterinary Social Work Certificate Program
Knoxville, TN

E-mail address:
kgoldberg@wholeanimalvet.com

Where Have We Been, Where Are We Going
Continuity from 2011

Tamara Shearer, DVM, CCRP, CVPP, CVA, CHPV, CTPEP

KEYWORDS

- Pet hospice • Palliative • End-of-life care • Animal hospice research
- Interdisciplinary team

KEY POINTS

- The formal history of animal hospice and palliative care began in the 1990s.
- The current state of affairs in animal hospice and palliative care includes hospice guidelines and emerging research.
- The future goals in the field of animal hospice and palliative care include consistent teaching of the topics in veterinary college curricula, moving the profession toward a specialty and using an interdisciplinary team.

INTRODUCTION

This is "where we have been": more than 8 years ago, the May 2011 *Veterinary Clinics of North America: Small Animal Practice* was the most extensive professional publication exploring veterinary palliative medicine and hospice care to date. The Elsevier team recognized the importance of sharing critical information with the veterinary profession about a topic that was just emerging. This author was honored to be the Guest Editor of that issue and to use her experiences to present vital information that might shape the future of veterinary hospice and palliative care as it was known at that time. Ultimately, the decision was made to include 14 articles and 3 case studies in that issue to turn information into usable knowledge. Topics ranged from hospice and palliative care protocols and symptom management to safety and legal concerns. Those articles were written by a panel of gifted professionals and me; it was a collaboration and compilation of what the profession had learned over the years from other disciplines, including human hospice, pain management, physical therapy and rehabilitation, oncology, ethics, and behavior. The current Guest Editor, Dr Katherine

Disclosure statement: The author has nothing to disclose.
Smoky Mountain Integrative Veterinary Clinic, 1054 Haywood Road, Suite 3, Sylva, NC 28779, USA
E-mail address: tshearer5@frontier.com

Goldberg, is taking us to "where we need to go." She is the guardian to oversee that the profession moves to a more advanced level of care for hospice and palliative care patients. This article provides a brief review of important foundational concepts as well as a view of future goals that lie ahead of the veterinary profession as the field of animal hospice and palliative care evolves.

WHERE HAVE WE BEEN: A SUMMARY OF HISTORY

Long before the formal concept of hospice had evolved and before the modern animal hospice movement, some veterinarians were already practicing the philosophy of hospice and palliative care. There is historic evidence of veterinarians and pet owners helping maintain quality of life for patients who otherwise would have died or been euthanized. One example of palliative care was captured in a photograph of an aged dog on April 7, 1934. Sparky, a 14-year-old dog, was hit by a car and fractured his right rear leg. His veterinarian amputated the injured leg and then devised a prosthetic limb (**Fig. 1**). In 1938, a dog named Pete received palliative care for a broken back with the help of a homemade cart for his paralysis (**Fig. 2**). It was likely that in most situations both dogs would have been euthanized, but with supportive treatment, they regained a good quality of life that likely required ongoing care. These examples align with the concept of hospice and palliative care, but before the 1990s, the concept of modern hospice and palliative care had not yet evolved in veterinary medicine.

In the 2011 *Veterinary Clinics of North America: Small Animal Practice* issue, Dr Kathryn Marocchino, PhD reviewed the history of human hospice and compiled the first, and most complete, history of early animal hospice.[1] More recently, "Veterinary Hospice and Palliative Care: A Comprehensive Review of the Literature," not only is the first literature review but also serves as a detailed history of veterinary hospice publications.[2] The following is a brief summary of major hospice developments in the veterinary profession. Major milestones from 1995 to 2005 are summarized in **Boxes 1** and **2**, which review some of the early events and acknowledges pioneers like Drs Guy Hancock, Eric Clough, and Alice Villalobos.

The catalyst that inspired many early veterinarians to investigate hospice care was the Nikki Hospice Foundation for Pets (NHFP). It was the first organization to provide

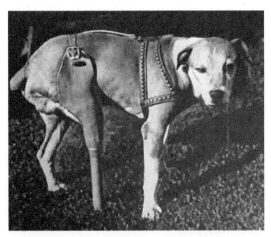

Fig. 1. Sparky: April 7, 1934 modeling his prosthetic limb. (*Courtesy of* Tamara Shearer, DVM, CCRP, CVPP, CVA, CHPV, CTPEP, Sylva, NC.)

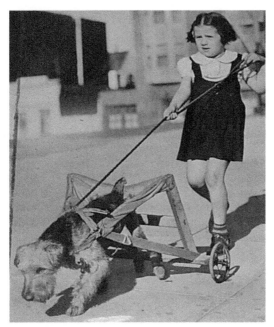

Fig. 2. Pete and Martha: March 30, 1938 using a homemade cart for mobility. (*Courtesy of* Tamara Shearer, DVM, CCRP, CVPP, CVA, CHPV, CTPEP, Sylva, NC.)

assistance and encouragement to anyone seeking information about pet hospice care. In addition to many educational projects, NHFP's founder, Kathryn Marocchino, PhD, worked tirelessly to organize the First International Pet Hospice Symposium, held at UC Davis School of Veterinary Medicine in April 2008 with the assistance of the Assisi International Animal Institute. After NHFP launched their symposium, other major conferences soon embraced lectures covering hospice topics in their annual meetings. In October 2008, the Central Veterinary Conference (now "Fetch: DVM360") in San Diego and the 2010 American Veterinary Medical Association

---

Box 1
Summary of animal hospice milestones 1995 through 2000

1995: "Hospice Concept for Animals" presented at the 10th Annual Delta Society Meeting by veterinarians Guy Hancock and James Harris with Bonnie Madder, MS.

1996: NHFP, founded by Dr Kathryn Marocchino, PhD. The first animal hospice resource for pet owners and veterinarians.

1997: *Veterinary Economics* printed one of the first articles on veterinary hospice, featuring Dr Eric Clough. "Hospice Concepts and Geriatric Animal Medicine" was presented at the North American Veterinary Conference (NAVC) and the American College of Veterinary Internal Medicine (ACVIM) by Dr Guy Hancock.

1998: Hospice lectures continue at the ACVIM, AVMA, and Annual Symposium on Advances in Clinical Medicine at UC Davis College of Veterinary Medicine.

1999: NHFP developed the first guidelines for animal hospice care.

2000: Pawspice was introduced by Dr Alice Villalobos. *Journal of the American Veterinary Medical Association* featured an article on Pawspice.

Box 2
Summary of animal hospice milestones 2001 through 2005

2001: AVMA developed hospice care guidelines.

2002: "Hospice Concept for Animals" NAVC Technician Master Class taught by Dr Guy Hancock.

2003: Argus Institute for Families and Veterinary Medicine and Colorado State University College of Veterinary Medicine started Colorado State University Pet Hospice. Pet Hospice and Education Center founded by Dr Tami Shearer opened in Columbus, Ohio.

2004: Hancock, McMillan, and Ellenbogan authored "Owner Services and Hospice Care" in *Geriatrics and Gerontology of the Dog and Cat. Washington Post* and *Bark Magazine* are featuring animal hospice articles.

2005: Leaders in hospice care continue to lecture at national meetings. AAHA Senior Care Guidelines are released.

(AVMA) conference in Atlanta offered day-long hospice tracts organized by the author. These early conferences and organizations motivated more veterinarians to embrace the philosophy of these disciplines in private practice. By the mid 2000s, some veterinary businesses had started to cater to hospice patients; others provided mobile euthanasia services. Business consultants began to advise practice owners on hospice care provision. (For a more detailed early history, refer to Marocchino[1] and Goldberg.[2])

With momentum from the First International Pet Hospice Symposium, a small interdisciplinary group of veterinarians and other professionals launched the International Association of Animal Hospice and Palliative Care (IAAHPC) as a new organization in 2009. Dr Amir Shanan was its first president, and Dr Anthony J. Smith was its vice president; other nonveterinarian board member pioneers included Gail Pope, Robyn Kesnow, and Coleen Ellis. Like the NHFP, the IAAHPC includes anyone who has an interest in hospice care. The Veterinary Society for Hospice and Palliative Care (VSHPC) is currently the only organization that was created solely for veterinarians interested in the practice of veterinary hospice and palliative medicine, with a focus on building knowledge through research and a long view toward development of hospice and palliative care as a recognized specialty. The VSHPC was conceived of and cofounded in 2012 by Drs Page Yaxley and Katherine Goldberg, and with founding board members, Drs Michael Kiselow and Catie McDonald, its current LISTSERV launched in 2013.

WHERE HAVE WE BEEN: HOSPICE CARE BASICS

For 2 decades, pet owners and even veterinary professionals have been seeking hospice and palliative care for their pets because of good experiences with human hospice care. Two important concepts were defined in the *Veterinary Clinics of North America: Small Animal Practice* 2011 issue that has served as a starting point for veterinarians to apply the philosophy of hospice and palliative care: (1) criteria for hospice care program patients and (2) the 5-step strategy for palliative and hospice care. These concepts are reviewed in later discussion.

Early Hospice and Palliative Care Foundation Concepts from 2011

Concept 1: patient qualifications for hospice and palliative care
The 2011 issue defined which patients benefit from hospice care.[3] If possible, hospice and palliative care for animals should begin as soon as possible after a serious

> **Box 3**
> **Hospice and palliative care indications**
>
> *Circumstances that warrant palliative or hospice care:*
>
> A decision not to pursue curative treatment
>
> A diagnosis of a life-limiting illness
>
> Symptoms of a chronic illness that interferes with the pet's routine
>
> Curative treatment has failed
>
> A pet requires long-term intensive care
>
> A pet has a progressive illness or trauma with associated health complications

condition is identified before any clinical signs develop. Patients who benefit from hospice and palliative care include patients for whom curative treatment is declined, a diagnosis of a life-limiting illness, patient's routine is altered by symptoms of a chronic illness, curative treatment has failed, a patient requires long-term intensive care, or the patient has a progressive illness or trauma with associated health complications (**Box 3**).

Concept 2: five-step protocol for comprehensive palliative and hospice care

The 2011 publication emphasized the use of a standard protocol to help guide veterinarians through the care of a chronically or terminally ill pet. The 5-step strategy for comprehensive palliative and hospice care was developed by the author to allow the veterinarian and staff to feel confident that no part of the patient's care had been neglected and to allow for care to be applied on a case-by-case basis (**Box 4**).[3] Each step in this protocol is of equal importance. The first step that sets the foundation for hospice care is to evaluate the pet owner's needs, beliefs, and goals for the pet. Step 2 involves the education of the pet owner about the disease process. The next step involves developing a personalized plan for the pet and the owner drawing on information gathered from step 1. In step 4, pet owners are taught the techniques needed to support the pet. The final step is to provide emotional support during the entire care process, including support before, during, and after the death of the pet.

There are many benefits for practitioners that warrant investing the time required to follow the 5-Step Protocol. It not only influences how a patient is treated but also improves the client-patient-doctor relationship through better communication. It helps define what diagnostics are used to obtain additional information, and which treatments will support the patient. It also improves the efficiency of care when there are

> **Box 4**
> **Hospice and palliative care protocol**
>
> *Five-step strategy for comprehensive palliative and hospice care*
>
> Step 1: Evaluation of the pet owner's needs, beliefs, and goals for the pet (psychosocial needs)
>
> Step 2: Education about the disease process
>
> Step 3: Development of a personalized plan for the pet and pet owner
>
> Step 4: Application of palliative or hospice care techniques
>
> Step 5: Emotional support during the care process and after the death of the pet

---

Box 5
Benefits of applying the 5-step protocol

Benefits of evaluating the caretaker's psychosocial needs

Improves client-patient-doctor relationship

Influences how a problem is treated

Influences the selection of diagnostics

Improves the efficiency of care when there are time-sensitive issues

Strengthens communication

Helps put the caretaker at ease

Enhances trust and respect for veterinarian's recommendations

Lessens the emotional side effects for the family

Minimizes conflict between veterinarian, family, and family members

---

time-sensitive issues. All of this helps to put the caretaker at ease, enhances trust between client and veterinarian, and cultivates respect for the veterinarian's recommendations through a shared decision-making process. The 5-Step Protocol lessens the emotional side effects for the family and may minimize conflict between veterinarian, family, and family members (**Box 5**).

Defining Common Terms Used in Animal Hospice and Palliative Care

Early on, standardization of terms commonly used in hospice care has helped to improve communication among hospice care providers. Defining concepts such as "natural death" versus "hospice-assisted natural death" helps prevent confusion in discussions with other practitioners and pet owners. A review of a few of these terms is described here.

Palliative care
Palliative care addresses the treatment of pain and other clinical signs to achieve the best quality of life regardless of disease outcome.

Hospice care
Hospice is a specialized form of palliative care that focuses on caring for patients in the end stages of an illness, near death. It relies on a philosophy of care that embraces death as a normal process.

Natural death
A natural death is dying that occurs in its own time without intervention.

Hospice-assisted natural death
This type of dying is supported with interventions to prevent or minimize the adverse clinical manifestations of the disease process or processes that are causing death.

WHERE ARE WE NOW: CURRENT STATE-OF-THE-ART

One only needs to search the Internet to appreciate the current level of interest in hospice and palliative care for animals. The topics covered in later discussion serve as a summary of only a few examples of the current state-of-the-art. First, a scholarly literature is finally emerging in the field of animal hospice. There are new drugs, supplements, and supportive care products for patients. An Internet search will also reveal many more veterinary practitioners who embrace the philosophy of hospice care compared with 10 years ago. For veterinarians who want to learn more about hospice and palliative care, there are continuing education courses for veterinarians to hone their skills, ranging from 8 hours to 110 hours of lectures.[4,5]

Current Research

One example of the professional literature is Goldberg's 2016 "Veterinary Hospice and Palliative Care: A Comprehensive Review of the Literature."[5] This review established the "state of the art" for the disciplines of animal hospice and palliative care, and concluded that they are currently hindered by an inadequate amount of research to give credibility to the field and guide practice. Although it was not setting out to answer a specific research question, it was one of the first steps in building the field of hospice care in veterinary medicine and provided a nice adjunct to the history of veterinary hospice. Five types of literature were evaluated, including peer-reviewed articles, refereed works that were subject to editorial review, non-peer-reviewed sections of a peer-reviewed publication, veterinary magazines or publications, and lay magazines and newspapers.

Next, a pilot study was performed in 2015 by Dr Beth Marchitelli and the author evaluating euthanasia versus hospice-assisted natural death, related to patient diagnosis and symptom burden.[6] Preliminary data demonstrate contrasting results compared with the 2011 study by Fleming and colleagues[7] of mortality in dogs in North American veterinary teaching hospitals between 1984 and 2004. In the Marchitelli and Shearer study, the cause of death or choice of euthanasia was evaluated in a mobile practice focused solely on hospice care and was compared with a stationary practice providing integrative care, including acupuncture and physical medicine, for hospice and palliative care patients. It was not surprising that the top 5 causes of death were different between the 3 study groups (mobile practice, brick and mortar practice, and teaching hospital), especially when patients receive hospice or palliative care at their end of life. For example, the Marchitelli and Shearer data showed that death from musculoskeletal changes dropped from second in the Fleming study (teaching hospital) to eighth in frequency in the brick and mortar practice providing physical medicine.

Kathmann and colleagues[8] showed that physiotherapy is an important tool for maintaining mobility in dogs with degenerative myelopathy; affected dogs who received physiotherapy remained ambulatory longer than a control group in their study. More research is needed to determine if supportive care at end of life can change the cause of death.

Current, New, and Improved Pharmaceuticals and Supportive Devices

New pharmaceuticals are becoming available to better fit the needs of symptom management for an aging population and for hospice or palliative care patients. The following are 3 examples: First, Galliprant (grapiprant) is a non-Cox inhibitor that is indicated for use in patients who do not tolerate other nonsteroidal anti-inflammatory drugs.[9] It is a piprant that is a prostaglandin receptor inhibitor that blocks the EP4 receptor, a primary mediator for osteoarthritis. Next, Entyce (capromorelin) is an appetite stimulant that acts as a ghrelin receptor agonist.[10] It binds to receptors in the brain and signals appetite stimulation in the hypothalamus. It also binds to pituitary growth hormone secretagogue receptor to increase growth hormone production. Finally, new formulations of existing drugs are emerging. Transdermal mirtazapine for cats, Mirataz by KindredBio, is the first and currently the only Food and Drug Administration–approved medication for weight loss in cats. It provides a reliable, noninvasive transdermal delivery of mirtazapine that is documented in measured plasma levels.[11] This product may be beneficial for cats who do not tolerate oral administration of drugs.

Less than 2 decades ago, some assistive devices and commercial hygiene products did not exist or were difficult to locate. Improvement in availability of these products makes nursing care easier and can now offer immediate relief for the hospice pet and the owner without having to do an extensive search for the items. In the past, many support tools had to be fabricated from human products, like modifying baby diapers to fit pets and using log carriers as slings to enhance mobility. Stores and Web sites provide better access to products that support the care of debilitated pets that are ergonomic and affordable. Examples of some of these items include pet diapers that come in various sizes including male wraps, hind limb slings, forelimb slings, dynamic braces, protective wear, and toe grips (**Fig. 3**).

New Techniques

Techniques and procedures refined by research within both human and veterinary medicine are currently improving quality of life for veterinary hospice patients. Two examples are nebulization for temporary relief of respiratory distress and the use of palliative sedation. In general, the nebulization of saline, furosemide, and magnesium sulfate may provide comfort to the veterinary patient in respiratory distress by resetting the receptors in the airways.[12,13] The use of palliative sedation for veterinary patients was a concept and technique borrowed from human hospice. Patients who are

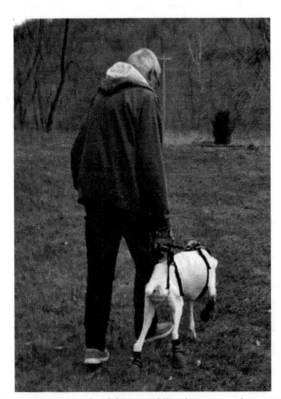

Fig. 3. Patient Harper wearing a dog-lifting mobility harness and protective boots. (*Courtesy of* Tamara Shearer, DVM, CCRP, CVPP, CVA, CHPV, CTPEP, Sylva, NC.)

not responding to medical management of their condition and are in distress while conscious may benefit from palliative sedation, using a combination of sedating drugs and anesthetics to provide various depths of sedation until death occurs or a decision can be made about care options.[14]

Physical medicine techniques are also being used to support patients who might otherwise be euthanized. A poster presentation, "Euthanasia Diversion by Use of Extracorporeal Shockwave Therapy (ESWT) to Improve Mobility and Decrease Pain in a Treeing Walker Hunting Dog," was presented at the 10th Annual International Symposium on Veterinary Rehabilitation and Physical Therapy. This case study evaluated the benefits of ESWT for a severely debilitated patient with elbow osteoarthritis that was going to be euthanized. Upon presentation, the dog had a lameness score of 3/5 on a 0 to 5 lameness scale, pain score of 8/10 on a 1 to 10 numeric visual analog scale, and poor quality of life score of 275/500 based on the Xie Quality of Life Scale.[15–17] At the end of the series of treatments, the lameness score improved to 1/5, quality of life improved, and the pain scale decreased to 2/10. Based on this case study, ESWT may be considered another treatment option over euthanasia for clients who have a desire to palliate a painful lameness.[18,19]

Ongoing research and overall acceptance of acupuncture and other traditional Chinese veterinary medicine (TCVM) modalities, like food therapy, Tui-na (Chinese manual therapy), and herbal therapies, are emerging as noninvasive tools to help hospice and palliative care patients. Clients often seek this type of integrative therapy to support quality of life for their pets (**Fig. 4**).

Hospice Guidelines

Guidelines or position statements for hospice and palliative care have been created by various organizations to give veterinarians a basic framework for providing these services. Besides the early NHFP already discussed and the AVMA, which established inaugural guidelines in 2001, the first veterinary organization to recognize the need for a position statement was the American Association of Feline Practitioners in 2010.[20–22] The most recent guidelines are the IAAHPC/American Animal Hospital Association (AAHA) End of Life Care Guidelines, published in 2016, which contain some of the previously described foundational hospice principles originally published by the author.[23]

Continuing Education

Besides information at conferences discussed earlier, there are continuing education courses for veterinarians to hone their skills ranging from short courses to certificate and certification programs. These courses mirror the steps that the veterinary

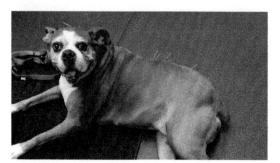

Fig. 4. Patient receiving an acupuncture treatment. (*Courtesy of* Tamara Shearer, DVM, CCRP, CVPP, CVA, CHPV, CTPEP, Sylva, NC.)

rehabilitation and sports medicine special interest group took before becoming recognized as a specialty college by the AVMA. A history of these programs is provided here. First, Dr Ella Bittel is credited for the original short course offered to veterinarians, staff, and lay people on the topic of animal hospice care.[1] Her program, Spirits in Transition, made its debut in 2006. The second organization to develop a certification curriculum was the AAHA. They offer an online, 6-module certificate course in hospice and palliative care that is open to veterinarians and staff members. IAAHPC certification was first offered in 2016 to 2017 and is currently in its third cycle of participants. The curriculum includes more than 100 hours of continuing education and requires that students demonstrate knowledge, skill, and the ability to apply what they have learned through testing and submission of case studies. IAAHPC certification is open to veterinarians and registered veterinary technicians, and a certificate has recently been developed for social workers. A related training program, the Companion Animal Euthanasia Training Academy, was founded by Dr Kathy Cooney in 2016 and teaches skills to help make euthanasia a peaceful event. It offers training to veterinarians, veterinary students, veterinary technicians as well as shelter staff and grief counselors. Finally, in 2018, the Chi Institute developed a unique certificate program that is integrative, teaching both Western and Eastern medicine to improve hospice care. It is restricted to veterinarians only and those who have had prerequisite experience in acupuncture, herbal formulas, Tui-na, or food therapy. It is important to note that the AVMA does not recognize "certified" veterinarians in any field as "specialists," nor is any area of medicine recognized as a veterinary specialty without American Board of Veterinary Specialties designation.

WHERE ARE WE GOING: FUTURE EVOLUTION OF HOSPICE

Like other disciplines of medicine, veterinary hospice and palliative care are in a process of continual change as advances in science, communication, and care methods evolve. The following list of goals should be considered by the profession to move hospice and palliative care for animals to the next level.

Veterinary Research and Exploration of New Fundamental Concepts

Scientific research and writing is important for the evolution of hospice and palliative care. The goal is to present data and ideas with a level of detail that allows a reader to evaluate the validity of the results based on facts and to draw conclusions that are based on science. It provides a platform to disseminate information to larger communities by reporting results in scientific journals. It also aids in formation of collaborations among professional groups and provides reliable information for the public.

In human medicine, the National Hospice and Palliative Care Organization issues an annual publication of "Facts and Figures." The document reviews hospice patient characteristics, the location and level of care, Medicare spending, hospice provider characteristics, volunteer services, and bereavement services. Some of the information gathered includes the amount of time patients spend in hospice care. For example, almost 30% of human patients were enrolled in hospice care for 1 to 7 days, but patients with dementia spent the longest time enrolled in hospice (104 days).[24] Collection of data from veterinary hospice and palliative care practices that includes diagnosis, prognostic information and duration of care, cause of death, and communication records will help build a better understanding of areas that need further attention in veterinary medicine and may prove invaluable to clinicians seeking to provide better care.

College Curricula

In 2010, Dickinson and colleagues[25] presented data that assessed the current state of end-of-life training in 28 US veterinary colleges. The study concluded that 96% of the schools had "offerings" on various end-of-life topics and that 80% of the student body was exposed to those offerings. Goldberg[2] asserted that these data likely overestimated the amount of attention given to end-of-life topics in veterinary teaching institutions and called for additional details regarding what is considered an end-of-life topic offering.[2] More data and research are needed to determine exactly what topics, references, and techniques are being taught and to accurately assess the amount of time spent on end-of-life education in veterinary colleges. An important goal is to establish standard competencies in palliative medicine and end-of-life topics within veterinary teaching institutions, ideally as part of Association of American Veterinary Medical Colleges accreditation (Katherine J. Goldberg, personal communication, 2018).

More universities should also consider integrating hospice care into their veterinary teaching hospitals. There are 2 academic models to date: Colorado State University's Pet Hospice Program, founded in 2003 and still operating, and Veterinary Hospice Care at Michigan State University, which operated from 2011 to 2014. These programs are both described in this issue.

Embracing an Interdisciplinary Team

Interdisciplinary care teams have been underutilized in veterinary medicine to date. A team approach would play an important role in veterinary hospice and palliative care, particularly for sharing care responsibilities so the entire burden does not fall on one individual (typically the veterinarian). Even though the veterinarian must oversee the medical aspects of care, the creative use of other professionals can enhance patient care and client experience and support the veterinary care team as well. The integration of social workers and other mental health professionals, volunteers, grief and bereavement support staff, chaplains, and pet death industry professionals has the potential to optimize quality of care and lessen the emotional burden of care for veterinarians. Creative practice management solutions, that address financial constraints and education about the importance of a "team" approach, needs to be developed to overcome obstacles that prevent small practices from using an interdisciplinary team.

Collaboration Between Professional Disciplines

Even though the ability to relieve suffering and improve quality of life has never been more powerful, it is important to assure that new advances aligned with the field of hospice care are not overlooked. Collaboration between veterinary and human medicine may provide insight and elevate the level of medicine for animal hospice patients. Gawande and colleagues[26] discuss lethal injection and use of paralytics, for example. In that study, a consensus among human experts was that paralytic/neuromuscular blocking agents should be avoided in capital punishment due to possible masking of discomfort during dying. Meanwhile, human euthanasia practices in The Netherlands routinely use these agents. Beth Marchitelli's article, "An Objective Exploration of Euthanasia and Adverse Events," discusses neuromuscular blocking agents in human and veterinary euthanasia in this issue and highlights the complexity of reconciling some of these issues. Veterinarians should consider embracing knowledge from different disciplines within and outside veterinary medicine.

Hospice and Palliative Care as a Veterinary Specialty

The stage is being set for the proactive planning for a veterinary specialty following the path of newer specialties like dentistry and sports medicine. Currently, there are 22 specialties recognized by the AVMA. Recognition by the AVMA is a rigorous process and requires collaboration among individuals recognized in the field as experts and sound research to document the need for such a specialty.

Mindfulness of the Professional's Mental Health

An important part of the hospice philosophy is to understand the resources available to provide support to caregivers throughout the disease process. Veterinarians and staff need to take care of themselves in order to maintain good mental and physical health while providing hospice and palliative care to patients. Psychologist Dr Azaria Akashi published "Ten Tips for Veterinarians Dealing with Terminally Ill Patients" in the 2011 *Veterinary Clinics of North America: Small Animal Practice* to help support the physical and emotional needs of veterinarians.[27] More needs to be done to make sure that veterinarians who work closely with end-of-life patients and their families have the resources they need to stay mentally and physically healthy.

One tool introduced by the author is the utilization of the Critical Incident Stress Management (CISM) concept at the Western States Veterinary Conference and at the Chi Institute to help support the veterinary profession.[28,29] CISM for human medicine may apply to situations encountered in veterinary medicine and help to support the veterinary team. CISM was developed to offset negative consequences of traumatic and medical events. This concept, first used in Disaster Management, has also been adopted by other professional groups, including the American Association of Nurse Anesthetists, to help cope with loss.[30] Parts of the protocol certainly can be applied to the work done with animals. The goal of CISM is to maintain or restore the individuals involved in a critical incident to their baseline state of health by alleviating the severe effects of traumatic stress. Just a few examples of critical incidences in veterinary medicine include euthanasia of a pet, noncompliance by the pet owner, and financial constraints that negatively affect treatment choices and outcome. Over time, these incidences may exhaust one's usual coping mechanisms, resulting in distress and loss of adaptive functioning. Early support of veterinary care teams for hospice and palliative care patients may minimize the stress associated with those services and potentially mitigate other well-being concerns, such as depression, anxiety, physical manifestations of stress, and substance use.

SUMMARY

Animal hospice and palliative care will continue to evolve. The practice of hospice and palliative care requires a heightened level of commitment and devotion to using every possible care option because of the intensity of patient caseload. Better communication, solid research, discovery of newer drugs, evolving techniques, and creative ideas will continually replace those of the past and address challenges that previously lacked good solutions. Hospice and palliative care currently supports clients and prioritizes patient comfort until the time of natural death, hospice-assisted death, or euthanasia. The *future* of hospice and palliative care will provide not only these supports but also curricular interventions in veterinary teaching institutions, and postgraduate training opportunities, as well as the structure and culture change necessary for veterinary care teams to receive the support they need to do this work.

REFERENCES

1. Marocchino KD. In the shadow of a rainbow: the history of animal hospice. Vet Clin North Am Small Anim Pract 2011;41:447–98.
2. Goldberg KJ. Veterinary hospice and palliative care: a comprehensive review of the literature. Vet Rec 2016;15:369–74.
3. Shearer TS. Pet hospice and palliative care protocols. Vet Clin North Am Small Anim Pract 2011;41:507–8.
4. American Animal Hospital Association. Animal hospice and palliative care certificate program. Available at: https://www.aaha.org/professional/education/animal_hospice_palliative_care_certificate_program.aspx. Accessed October 10, 2018.
5. International Association for Animal Hospice and Palliative Care. Animal hospice and palliative care certification program. Available at: https://www.iaahpc.org/certification.html. Accessed October 10, 2018.
6. Shearer TS. Prevalence of diseases, causes of death, and common disease trajectories in hospice and palliative care patients. In: Shanan A, Pierce J, Shearer T, editors. Hospice and palliative care for companion animals. Hoboken (NJ): Wiley Blackwell; 2017. p. 84–5.
7. Fleming J, Creevy KE, Promislow DE. Mortality in North America dogs from 1984 to 2004: an investigation into age, size, and breed related cause of death. J Vet Intern Med 2011;25:187–98.
8. Kathmann I, Cizinaukas S, Doherr MG, et al. Daily controlled physiotherapy increases survival time in dogs with suspected degenerative myelopathy. J Vet Intern Med 2006;20:927–32.
9. Kirby Shaw K, Rausch-Derra LC, Rhodes L. Grapriprant: an EP4 prostaglandin receptor antagonist and novel therapy for pain and inflammation. Vet Med Sci 2016;2:3–9.
10. Zollers B, Wofford JA, Heinen E, et al. A prospective, randomized masked, placebo-controlled clinical study on carpromorelin in dogs with reduced appetite. J Vet Intern Med 2016;30:1851–7.
11. Buhles W, Quimby JM, Labelle D, et al. Single and multiple dose pharmacokinetics of a novel mirtazapine transdermal ointment in cats. J Vet Pharmacol Ther 2018;41:644–51.
12. Mellema M. The neurophysiology of dyspnea. J Vet Emerg Crit Care 2008;18:561–71.
13. Cox S. Pharmacology interventions for symptom management. In: Shanan A, Pierce J, Shearer T, editors. Hospice and palliative care for companion animals. Hoboken (NJ): Wiley Blackwell; 2017. p. 174–6.
14. Quill T, Holloway R, Shah M, et al. Primer of palliative care. 5th edition. Glenview (IL): American Academy of Hospice and Palliative Care; 2010. p. 160.
15. Millis D, Mankin J. Orthopedic and neurologic evaluation. In: Millis D, Levine D, editors. Canine rehabilitation and physical therapy. 2nd edition. Philadelphia: Elsevier; 2014. p. 182.
16. Wiese AJ. Assessing pain: pain behaviors. In: Gaynor J, Muir W, editors. Handbook of veterinary pain management. 3rd edition. St Louis (MO): Elsevier; 2015. p. 84.
17. Xie H. 3 steps of palliative and end-of-life care. In: TCVM palliative care and end-of-life care lecture notes. Reddick (FL): Chi Institute; 2018. p. 264.

18. Durant A, Millis D. Applications of extracorporeal shockwave in small animal rehabilitation. In: Millis D, Levine D, editors. Canine rehabilitation and physical therapy. 2nd edition. Philadelphia: Elsevier; 2014. p. 381–9.

19. Shearer TS. Euthanasia diversion by use of extracorporeal shockwave therapy to improve mobility and decrease pain in a treeing walker hunting dog. IAVRPT Proceedings 2008;477.

20. Clough E, Clough J. The NHFP guidelines for veterinary hospice care. Available at: www.pethospice.org. Accessed September 1, 2018.

21. AVMA. Guidelines for veterinary hospice. Available at: https://ebusiness.avma. org/files/productdownloads/hospice.pdf. Accessed September 3, 2018.

22. Thayer V, Monroe P, Smith R, et al. AAFP position statement, hospice care for cats. Available at: https://www.catvets.com/public/PDFs/PositionStatements/ HospiceCare.pdf. Accessed September 2, 2018.

23. IAAHPC/AAHA end-of-life care guidelines for dogs and cats. Available at: https:// www.aaha.org/graphics/original/professional/resources/guidelines/eolc/iteolc_toolkit. pdf. Accessed September 3, 2018.

24. National Hospice and Palliative Care Organization. Facts and figures, hospice care in America. 2017. Available at: https://www.nhpco.org/sites/default/files/ public/Statistics_Research/2017_Facts_Figures.pdf. Accessed September 7, 2018.

25. Dickinson GE, Roof PD, Roof KW. End-of-life issues in United States Veterinary Medicine Schools. Soc Anim 2010;18:152–62.

26. Gawande A, Denno D, Truog R, et al. Physicians and execution-highlights from a discussion of lethal injection. N Engl J Med 2008;358:448–51.

27. Akashi A. Ten tips for veterinarians dealing with terminally ill patients. Vet Clin North Am Small Anim Pract 2011;41:647–9.

28. Shearer T. Preserving Jing, support of the veterinarian and caretaker involved in end-of-life care. In: TCVM palliative care and end-of-life care lecture notes. 2018. p. 340–54.

29. Shearer T. Use of critical incident stress management concept to help support staff. In: WVC Proceedings, 90th Annual Conference. Las Vegas (NV), March 5, 2018.

30. American Association of Nurse Anesthetists. Guidelines for critical incidence stress management. Available at: https://www.aana.com/docs/default-source/practice-aana-com-web-documents-(all)/guidelines-for-critical-incident-stress-management. pdf?sfvrsn=ba0049b1_2. Accessed September 1, 2018.

Section I: Established Programs and Curricular Initiatives

Colorado State University, Pet Hospice Program

Maria Gore, MSW[a], Susan E. Lana, DVM, MS[b], Gail A. Bishop, BS[c],*

KEYWORDS

- Pet hospice • Veterinarians • Veterinary medicine • Companion animals
- University student programs

KEY POINTS

- The Pet Hospice Program at Colorado State University has been successful in providing a learning opportunity for professional veterinary medicine (PVM) students, a valuable service to area families, an option for referring veterinarians, and a national resource.
- The program will undoubtedly continue to grow and be a model for pet hospice programs within other veterinary professional schools.
- With families requesting pet hospice services now more than ever and veterinarians and PVM students more interested in this emerging field, this program will continue to promote and preserve quality of life of pets and their families within the comfort of their homes.

INTRODUCTION

This article serves as a follow-up to the 2008 *Journal of Veterinary Medical Education* article on the Colorado State University (CSU) Pet Hospice Program.[1] The CSU program is referred to as the model for establishing similar programs at other veterinary teaching hospitals and is an important part of the history of end-of-life care programs for animals.[1] The concept of hospice care for companion animals is slowly becoming more common in the veterinary profession and pet-owning public. Because pets are now considered to be part of the family, it is to be expected that people who have experienced compassionate care with human hospice are now attracted to and requesting the same type of care for their pets.[2–4]

Pet hospice has been referred to as a proactive response from the veterinary profession to the shifting expectations of a pet-owner population that increasingly desires the best possible care for their animal companions.[5] Advanced medical options and treatments once considered implausible for animals have now become standard in the veterinary profession, and with these advancements comes the need for

Disclosure: The authors have nothing to disclose.
[a] Argus Institute, Colorado State University Veterinary Teaching Hospital, Fort Collins, CO 80523, USA; [b] Clinical Sciences, Colorado State University, Ft Collins 80523, CO, USA; [c] CSU Veterinary Teaching Hospital, Colorado State University, Fort Collins, CO 80523, USA
* Corresponding author.
E-mail address: Gail.Bishop@colostate.edu

compassionate end-of-life care options for animals.[6] In response to the increasing demand for pet hospice services, several organizations within the veterinary profession have created hospice care guidelines, including the American Veterinary Medical Association, the American Animal Hospital Association, and the International Association of Animal Hospice and Palliative Care (IAAHPC). Despite significant interest in pet hospice from the general public, along with the steps being taken by recognized organizations within the veterinary profession to establish standards of care, there is still a lack of research and critical review of established pet hospice programs.[6]

History of the Program

CSU's Pet Hospice Program was the first pet hospice program established at a veterinary teaching hospital. The program is managed by volunteers who are professional veterinary medicine (PVM) students with the assistance of 3 faculty and staff advisors that include 1 doctor of veterinary medicine (DVM), 1 social worker, and the director of the CSU Argus Institute, a client support program at CSU's Veterinary Teaching Hospital (VTH).

Veterinarians Charles Johnson and Jack Label initiated the creation of the program's development task force in 2002 by gathering a diverse selection of professionals, including veterinarians, a professional from a local human hospice organization, a representative from the veterinary technician degree program, and the director of the Argus Institute. This task force met from 2002 through the launching of the program in 2004 to develop the goals, objectives, and structure of the program. The task force was also responsible for gaining the support of administrators in the veterinary college and teaching hospital, as well as obtaining the initial funds of $3000 needed to start the program. These expenses included costs for marketing (brochures and newspaper advertisements), a telephone, professional training for PVM student volunteers, professional liability insurance, and office and general supplies.

Since its inception, the CSU Pet Hospice Program has served 240 families and trained more than 250 veterinary students. The mission of the program is to provide compassionate end-of-life care for pets, and emotional support and education for their families. The core objectives of the program at the time of establishment included (1) to provide medical and supportive care to terminally ill pets in a home setting; (2) to offer owners emotional support and grief education to cope with the impending loss of their pets; (3) to assist referring veterinarians in providing palliative care for their patients; and (4) to educate veterinary students in providing end-of-life care for companion animals and their families. This article discusses these original objectives in relation to the current program operation and future objectives of the program.

Current Program

The current program consists of the faculty/staff advisors and PVM student volunteers who serve either as pet hospice managers, case coordinators, or case volunteers. These specific roles are described later. All volunteers have opportunities to participate in hospice cases.

Pet Hospice Managers

Pet hospice managers are PVM student volunteers. Pet hospice managers are either in their second or third year of the 4-year professional program. The managers are selected during their first year via an application and interview process, and they make a 2-year commitment to the program. The tasks of the managers have been modified throughout the course of the program and current duties are shown in **Table 1**.

Table 1
Roles and responsibilities of Colorado State University Pet Hospice program participants

Role	Responsibilities	Member
Advisors	• Oversee all activities of the program • Fund raising • Promotional activities and marketing • Liaison with VTH and college administration • Provide training as subject matter experts • Provide direct services if needed • Provide emotional support and debrief patients with student volunteers • Interview and select new managers	Faculty clinician Director of the Argus Institute Social worker/councilor
Managers	• Participate in all program activities • Create and maintain on-call schedule • Promote Pet Hospice within the college at DVM student events; plan and participate in volunteer recruitment • Attend and plan monthly leadership team meetings • Follow case flow and offer assistance if needed • Serve as case coordinators as needed, serve as case volunteers as needed • Oversee all communication and case documentation on a rotating basis • Maintain online database • Assist in development of training materials and programs • Attend and represent CSU at the annual IAAHPC Conference	DVM student volunteers who are interested in a leadership role in the program. Two to 5 managers serve at any given time, typically 1 from each DVM class; they are in the position for 2 y
Case coordinators	• Rotate coverage of the Pet Hospice referral and information phone and email • Initiate contact with pet owners or rDVMs who are seeking services • Assign volunteers to the case • Arrange initial visit with the client • Participate as a case volunteer	Volunteers who are interested in a higher level of involvement with the Pet Hospice Program
Case volunteer	• Provide direct services to the pet owners and patients • Attend training sessions • Participate in community promotional and support opportunities (annual VTH open house and pet memorial)	• DVM students typically in the first, second, and third years • Occasional prevet student club member

Abbreviation: rDVM, referring DVM.

Faculty/Staff Advisors

The 3 faculty/staff advisors oversee the PVM student volunteers in all activities. Additional tasks of the advisors include fundraising activities, marketing and promotion, debriefing cases, acting as a liaison with the VTH and college administration, training volunteers as needed, and assisting with direct services.

Case Coordinators

Case coordinators are PVM student volunteers who are selected by the pet hospice managers and participate in additional training. The responsibilities of the case coordinators include responding to calls on the pet hospice referral and information phone. Coordinators have a rotating schedule for phone coverage. They respond to all inquiries received via the phone, assess whether incoming referrals meet the criteria for pet hospice services, and work to establish the pet's core hospice team before passing the case over to a pet hospice manager.

Case Volunteers

Case volunteers are those volunteers who wish to work cases but not take on a leadership role in the program, such as a pet hospice manager or case coordinator. Two or 3 volunteers are assigned to each pet hospice case and that volunteer team is consistent throughout the duration of the case.

Recruitment and training of volunteers

PVM student volunteers are recruited once per year during the fall semester. The managers, with the assistance of one of the program advisors, hold an information session open to all interested PVM students. For those students who are interested in volunteering, an orientation is held in the fall, in which students learn about the hospice philosophy; gain communication skills for discussing end-of-life issues; and are oriented to the policies, procedures, and protocols of the program. Following the orientation, the volunteers participate in 4 training sessions annually. Training is provided by clinicians, technicians, and staff of the VTH, and community veterinarians. The following topics have been offered for these training sessions and are selected by the managers based on feedback from the volunteers.

- Basic communication skills
- Role playing
- Supporting grieving clients
- Pain assessment
- Hospice physical examination wet laboratory
- End-of-life conversations
- Natural death for pets
- Quality-of-life assessment
- Compassion fatigue and self-care
- Alternative methods of pain relief
- Cancer in our pets
- Our aging animals
- Nutrition for aging pets

The format for training is variable depending on the topic. Lectures followed by skills laboratories or role-playing activities are typical. On occasion the training is offered to all PVM students for topics of wide interest, such as natural death, nutrition, or pain assessment.

Case Management

Pet hospice cases are either self-referred by the pet owners or are referred by a DVM. The criteria for a pet to be eligible for services provided by the CSU Pet Hospice Program are a prognosis of 3 months or less to live, receiving care from a veterinarian, and live within 30 minutes of the CSU VTH.

The case coordinator obtains information from both the pet owner and the referring DVM (rDVM). The rDVM provides the initial case information, including the terminal diagnosis, medications the animal is receiving, and any other pertinent information about the pet. This information, along with information obtained from the pet owners, is recorded in a case intake form and filed on an electronic database that all volunteers are able to access. The rDVM remains part of the pet hospice care team, directing any changes in medical care, and maintains regular contact with the volunteers. The case coordinator works to assemble the family and pet's team members, including a case manager (who is also a pet hospice manager) and case volunteers **(Fig. 1)**, usually within the first 24 hours of receiving the referral, and the first visit is scheduled with the family at their earliest request. Typically, the team visiting the pet and the family at home consists of 2 or 3 volunteers. On average the team spends 1 to 2 hours with the family. During this visit, the volunteers do a brief physical examination of the pet and discuss the families' concerns and goals for both the pet and the family.

Hospice services in both human and veterinary medicine are representative of a period of transition between treatment and death.[1] Indicative of this time period, the

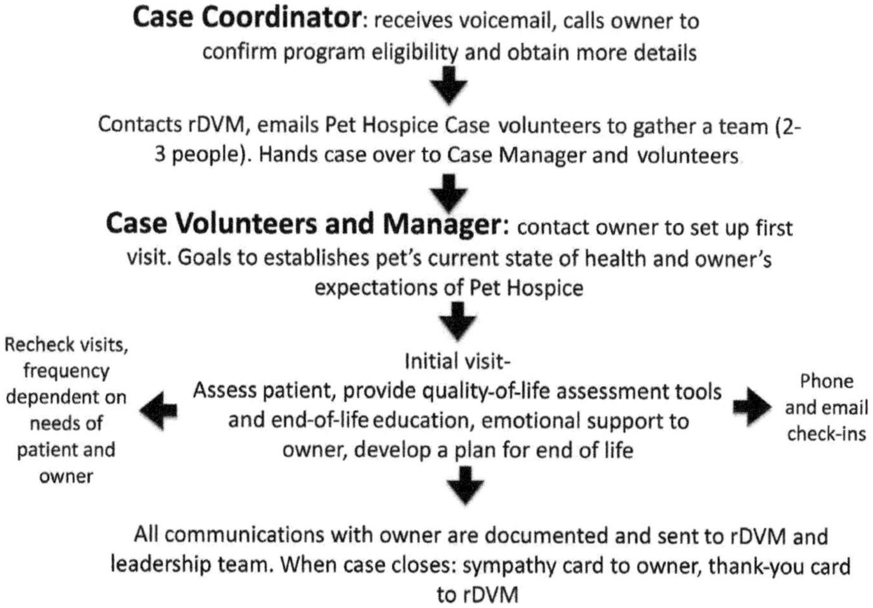

Case Coordinator: receives voicemail, calls owner to confirm program eligibility and obtain more details

⬇

Contacts rDVM, emails Pet Hospice Case volunteers to gather a team (2-3 people). Hands case over to Case Manager and volunteers

⬇

Case Volunteers and Manager: contact owner to set up first visit. Goals to establishes pet's current state of health and owner's expectations of Pet Hospice

⬇

Recheck visits, frequency dependent on needs of patient and owner ⬅ Initial visit- Assess patient, provide quality-of-life assessment tools and end-of-life education, emotional support to owner, develop a plan for end of life ➡ Phone and email check-ins

⬇

All communications with owner are documented and sent to rDVM and leadership team. When case closes: sympathy card to owner, thank-you card to rDVM

Fig. 1. Case walk-through.

family commonly is seeking education and support in assessing quality of life and making end-of life decisions. The volunteers assist in this realm by providing tools for pain assessment, suggestions for evaluating and addressing comfort for the pet, and tips to help realize comfort measures. In addition, volunteers work to create a trusting relationship with the family to support them in discussing their fears, wishes, and questions related to the impending death and loss of their pet.

All visits and communications between the family and the volunteers are summarized and sent electronically to the pet hospice advisors and the rDVM. Furthermore, summaries are documented in a secure database that the pet hospice team may access at any time.

One of the goals of the Pet Hospice Program is to assist the family in developing a plan for end of life, which can include a euthanasia plan, a natural death plan, and an emergency plan. The CSU Pet Hospice Program does not provide home euthanasia services but volunteers can be present if requested by the family. Many families who are clients of CSU choose to have their pets euthanized at the VTH and the pet hospice volunteers and/or pet hospice advisors have been present for those situations.

Following the death of the hospice patient, the volunteers send a condolence card along with a special gift of remembrance individual to the family. In addition, a thank-you card is sent to the rDVM in gratitude for the referral and opportunity to assist that family and pet. A final case summary is completed; sent to the volunteer team, pet hospice advisors, and rDVM; and uploaded to the secure database. Grief support via the counselors at the Argus Institute is offered to the family following the loss of their pet.

Program Benefits

The CSU Pet Hospice Program benefits the pets, the families, the students who volunteer, and the rDVMs that refer their clients and patients to the program. Those benefits continue to expand as the program grows. In addition, the program has an impact on the CSU VTH and the surrounding community.

At the core of the purpose and mission for pet hospice are the patients. The program seeks to improve the quality of life of the pets through assessment, preventing or relieving discomfort, and enhancing or restoring the quality of daily living for the pets. Sometimes this includes simple things such as loaning out an orthopedic bed or mobility harness for an elderly dog or cat, or suggesting area rugs to create a nonskid path in the home for pets with mobility issues, to something more direct such as teaching a family to give subcutaneous fluids so a cat does not have to make a stressful visit to the veterinary clinic 3 times a week. Similar to human hospice patients, the goal for pet hospice patients is to reduce pain and suffering and enhance and extend good quality of life. As in human hospice, although quality of life is prioritized over quantity, some patients live longer with hospice care than they would without it.

Hospice services in general are designed to cover a transition of time after the focus has shifted from cure to care.[4] Often owners report feeling confused and helpless during this time and volunteers can provide both education and support so that owners can feel empowered and involved in the care of their beloved pets.[4] One of the goals of the pet hospice volunteers is helping a family feel more at ease with the decisions they are making for their pets and the care they are providing. Volunteers provide pain scales to help assess pain and tools to help family members define quality for their particular pet. In addition, volunteers can help the family with communication dynamics such as explaining events to children and encouraging parents to find ways to involve their children at age-appropriate levels of engagement. Recognizing that caregiving for a family member has a deep impact, it can be important for volunteers to open this area for discussion and help pet owners assess their own quality of life. Often the volunteers offer tools and resources for families to decrease their levels of helplessness and improve their overall well-being. Such tools include access to a pet-sitting list for respite care, helping the family create bucket-list items, and helping them to identify and minimize regrets.

As stated previously, volunteers also aid in helping the family develop an end-of-life plan. This plan includes the standard decisions of who will perform the euthanasia, where it will take place, what body care option is desired, and who in the family wants to be present. Volunteers encourage families to think outside of the box, perhaps an out-of-town family member will need to FaceTime or one family member may want to feed the pet a favorite treat right before the euthanasia. The volunteers also aid in helping the family develop an emergency plan in case a crisis occurs. Hospice services are meant to foster an environment of trust for families adjusting to the impending loss and the grief process that will accompany the death of their beloved pet. This environment may be one of the more valuable aspects of pet hospice services because the grief associated with pet loss is still considered a disenfranchised grief, not readily acknowledged or validated by society in general.

We are so thankful that the CSU hospice team was there for us and our family throughout the entire process of losing our dog. They treated us and our beloved dog with unsurpassed care and affection, and walked us through a difficult process with kindness, love and support.

CSU hospice client

Apart from the patients and families, volunteers benefit greatly from participating in the Pet Hospice Program. Training for the program consists of in-depth communication training that goes beyond the core curriculum. They develop and expand their skills in quality-of-life and end-of-life discussions. Visiting with families in their homes takes students out of the comfort zone of the VTH and challenges them to communicate with multiple family members, including children. In addition, having access to the pet hospice advisors who have in-depth communication experience provides opportunities for students to both brainstorm and debrief communication scenarios. Student volunteers obtain skills in creating plans for care and documenting case notes. Engaging with the rDVMs allows volunteers to network and develop professional relationships with community veterinarians. Once per year, the program sponsors up to 2 pet hospice managers to attend the annual IAAHPC conference, allowing additional educational and professional networking opportunities. The training sessions, the direct care of patients at end of life, and the communication opportunities all work to expand veterinary students' professional depth and qualifications as future veterinarians. It would be beneficial at some point to conduct a qualitative study collecting data on the volunteers' perceptions of what impact participation in a pet hospice program has on their professional careers.

Through the Pet Hospice Program I found my calling as a Hospice and Palliative Care veterinarian yet what I gained from being a volunteer would help tremendously in any area of practice. I can't thank the Pet Hospice Program enough for giving me the opportunities to learn and grow through experiences I wouldn't have had at any other school."

CSU pet hospice student volunteer, 2016 College of Veterinary Medicine and Biomedical Sciences DVM graduate

In referring their clients to CSU's Pet Hospice Program, rDVMs benefit through their ability to provide a strong resource to their clients and patients for the best end-of life experience. In addition, veterinarians are able to address the care of the pets without bearing the full impact of an emotionally charged time period. Through home visits, the hospice volunteers are essentially the eyes and ears of the veterinarians and help owners convey accurate information to their medical providers. It can be difficult for veterinarians to give the attention pet owners need during this time while working within the time constraints of a busy practice.[5] Although there are no existing data to evaluate, it is hoped that, by having a resource such as CSU's Pet Hospice Program available as a referral for clients, this may aid in the prevention of burnout and compassion fatigue often reported by veterinarians.[7,8]

The College of Veterinary Medicine and Biomedical Sciences at CSU benefits in a variety of ways. By being the first teaching hospital to offer these services, CSU is considered to be an academic pioneer in this field. Students that participate in the program graduate with an increased skill set, particularly with regard to educating clients on end-of-life matters related to their pets. Furthermore, the program allows the opportunity for the college to continue to have a significant impact on the pet hospice field of interest.

The local community benefits by having a no-cost resource for end-of-life care for their pets. It is our hope that, by providing this service and associated promotional materials, we can initiate a conversation about the often taboo subjects of death and end of life.

Program Impact to Date

Since its inception, the CSU Pet Hospice Program has served 240 families and their pets and trained more than 250 student volunteers. The types of cases that are referred for hospice care include 66% neoplasia, 21% endocrine/metabolic disorders such as end-stage renal disease or liver failure, 6% degenerative neurologic or mobility issues associated with arthritis, 3% heart disease, and 4% of the cases having no documented cause of the pet's decline (**Fig. 2**). Dogs are the most frequent species seen (70%), followed by cats (20%) and 1 exotic case served (ferret). No equine patients have been referred to our program, although this service is available. The average age of our patient population entering hospice is 11.8 years, with the oldest being 20 years and the youngest being 8 months. The average feline referral is 14 years and the average canine referral is 11 years.

Veterinarians from the local community refer 66% of the cases seen, with some individual rDVMS referring between 10 and 25 cases each. Internal referral from the CSU VTH accounts for the rest of the cases at 33%. The number of visits per case ranges from 1 to 13, and visits are typically once a week or occasionally at longer intervals, with phone and email contact in between.

Support for the Program

The operating budget for the program is nominal at approximately $5000 each year because the advisors are salaried employees funded by the College of Veterinary Medicine and Biomedical Sciences with pet hospice responsibilities falling within the scope of their service/volunteer responsibilities. Historically, the program received funding from grants and grateful donors. Over the last several years the program has benefited from generous donors who have provided a significant contribution toward the annual budget of the program, which is currently at $7000. The program has also benefited from in-kind donations of supplies and comfort materials. In addition, the program seeks sponsorship for training events. Other annual expenses include

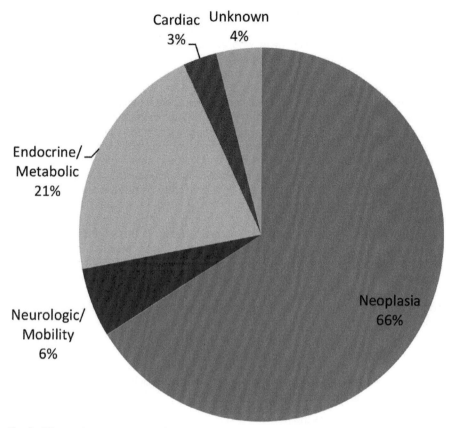

Fig. 2. Disease types represented.

recruitment, training sessions, liability insurance, telephone services, memorial gifts, promotional materials, office supplies, conference registration for advisors and/or pet hospice managers, and the related travel expense.

Marketing and advertising of the CSU Pet Hospice Program has primarily been repeat rDVMs referring their clients to the program, advertisements, and news articles in local newspapers. In addition, many families whose pets are patients of the VTH self-refer and this may in part be caused by the program brochures being abundant throughout the VTH. Argus staff members are also asked to contribute to blogs and university-accessible articles, and have been interviewed by local journalists regarding the CSU Pet Hospice Program, and undoubtedly this exposure increases awareness of the services offered.

Lessons Learned

The program has maintained and improved since the beginning, but there have also been some challenges along the way. The unpredictable case load has been a challenge in that the ratio of volunteers eager to work a case may decrease in a time period in which there are few active cases. Alternatively, the program can experience a sharp increase in cases at a time when students are not readily available; for example, during the summer months and around the holidays. The students have tight and varying class schedules and it can be difficult to schedule orientations or training sessions that present the best opportunity for recruitment and retention of volunteers. Scheduling visits with the families can be challenging when there are 2 to 3 volunteers planning to participate in a given case who are operating within their own schedule constraints as well as those of the owner.

Duration of the cases is an important consideration. Out of the 240 pet hospice cases, 211 cases lasted an average of 23 days, with only 8% of the cases lasting more than 100 days. When cases resolve too quickly, less than the average, it affects the opportunities for improving the quality of life for the patient, aiding in preparing the family for the loss, and limits the level of direct engagement the volunteers are able to experience. The short duration of these cases may be caused by referrals happening later in the pet's disease process. It is difficult to accurately gauge this, because delayed referrals to the program could be greatly influenced by the owner's reluctance to consider hospice services. One avenue to address this is networking with community veterinarians and providing more education to the general public on pet hospice services.

Another challenge that the program has encountered is that euthanasia services and direct medical care are not provided by the volunteers. Instead, the rDVM provides medical direction that the volunteers help the families fulfill, which may inhibit a comprehensive experience for both the families and the volunteers. Moreover, some of the rDVMs do not offer in-home euthanasia and families have to involve another party to what ideally should be an intimate time with a close-knit team. The program does not have the current capacity to offer medical care and euthanasia but it is worthy of consideration for future program development.

Future

As the CSU Pet Hospice Program looks for areas of growth, the key areas being considered include the following:

- Ways to better serve the patients and the families
- Ways to expand the student experience
- Ways to positively influence veterinary hospice
- Ways to continue to serve as a model for pet hospice programs in an academic setting

With privatized hospice care services increasing across the nation, it is important to explore where the CSU Pet Hospice Program can advance the educational pathway for veterinary students who wish to pursue this career path. The potential possibilities include partnering with private pet hospice practices to offer externships to pet hospice volunteers or exploring an avenue to develop an in-home euthanasia service within the CSU VTH program. Expansion of the program in these areas would serve the patients and the families well and offer the students a full exposure experience to hospice services and in-home euthanasia. In addition, the program could consider potential data collection to evaluate the broad impact on the community, the college, and the students. A project directed at evaluating levels of satisfaction felt by the rDVMs may be helpful in guiding the future of the CSU program and how best to serve the community. Furthermore, the current CSU program does not collect data on what type of support is typical for each hospice case or visit and this type of data may be beneficial to the broader field of pet hospice services.

The program will continue to offer expanded professional opportunities for the student volunteers by attending and presenting at conferences, offering local workshops, and speaking at public meetings. An increased caseload would naturally augment the direct contact portion of the student's volunteer experience and thus positively influence the future veterinarians working in pet hospice.

The Pet Hospice Program at CSU has been successful in providing a learning opportunity for PVM students, a valuable service to area families, an option for referring veterinarians, and a national resource. The program will undoubtedly continue to grow and be a model for pet hospice programs within other veterinary professional schools. With families requesting pet hospice services now more than ever and veterinarians and PVM students more interested in this emerging field, this program will continue to promote and preserve quality of life of pets and their families within the comfort of their homes.

REFERENCES

1. Bishop G, Long C, Carlsten K, et al. The Colorado State University pet hospice program: end-of-life care for pets and their families. J Vet Med Educ 2008;35(4): 487–95.
2. Gregersen S. Giving your clients the best end-of-life experience with their pets. Veterinary Nursing Journal 2016;31(8):241–4.
3. Hancock CG, McMillan FD, Ellenboger TR. Owner services and hospice care. In: Hoskins J, editor. Geriatrics and gerontology of the dog and cat. St. Louis (MO): Saunders; 2004. p. 5–17.
4. Kerrigan L. Veterinary palliative and hospice care-making the transition from 'cure' to 'care'. Vet Nurse 2013;4(6):316–21.
5. Gregersen S. Getting the best result at the end using animal hospice. Vet Nurs J 2016;31(9):271–5.
6. Goldberg K. Veterinary hospice and palliative care: a comprehensive review of the literature. Vet Rec 2016;178(15):369–74.
7. Brannick E, DeWilde C, Frey E, et al. Taking stock and making strides toward wellness in the veterinary workplace. J Am Vet Med Assoc 2015;247(7):739–41.
8. Lovell BL, Lee RT. Burnout and health promotion in veterinary medicine. Can Vet J 2013;54:790–1.

Michigan State University Veterinary Hospice Care
An Academic Hospice Practice 2011 to 2014

Page E. Yaxley, DVM

KEYWORDS

- Hospice • Palliative medicine • Veterinary • End of life • Academic practice

KEY POINTS

- Hospice care meets the needs of terminally ill veterinary patients while providing emotional support to caregivers as 1 unit of care, from diagnosis until the time of death.
- Michigan State University Veterinary Hospice Care was the second hospice practice based out of an academic institution.
- Relationship-oriented, patient-focused, goal-centered care was individually tailored for patients enrolled, led by a single veterinarian, with care supported by and provided through a team of interdisciplinary members.
- Awareness for end-of-life care, including increase in core curriculum for veterinary and veterinary technician students, was a direct result of the development of the Veterinary Hospice Care program.

INTRODUCTION

One of the most consistent relationships humans have is the one with companion animals. At least 80% of Americans say they view pets as part of their families, with the American Pet Products Association suggesting 90%, a recent Harris Poll reporting this number to be as high as 95%, and a phenomenon of pet parenting taking hold, particularly in developed nations.[1–6] A diagnosis of terminal or life-altering illness in companion animals can be overwhelming, and many owners struggle not only with the concept of euthanasia but also with when and how that will take place.[7] No doubt, they lean heavily on their veterinary care team during this time.

Veterinarians have a unique role within the allied health care professions. Similar to human physicians, veterinarians are responsible for the health and well-being of their patients. Yet veterinarians are unique in that they often also are responsible for their deaths, through euthanasia. The Accreditation Council for Graduate Medical

The author has nothing to disclose.
Small Animal Emergency and Critical Care, The Ohio State University College of Veterinary Medicine, Columbus, OH, USA
E-mail address: Yaxley.1@osu.edu

Vet Clin Small Anim 49 (2019) 351–362
https://doi.org/10.1016/j.cvsm.2019.01.003
vetsmall.theclinics.com

Education mandates core curricula on end-of-life care training for human medical residents. It has proved that educational intervention in end of life improves both patient well-being and physician longevity and success.[8] No such mandate exists, however, for educating veterinary students. End-of-life curricula are frequently addressed in as little as 1 hour during veterinary training and historically have been perceived as unimportant.[9] As such, veterinarians are often ill prepared to cope with the emotional demands associated with euthanasia or death of a patient.[10,11]

Hospice embraces the philosophy of ensuring compassionate end-of-life care, while providing comfort to the patient and emotional support and education to the family, allowing time to prepare and plan for impending death.[12] Under the Medicare hospice benefit, hospice services are provided free of charge to people facing life-ending illnesses in the United States.[13] Hospice recognizes the patient and family as the unit of care and has been proved to benefit patients by supporting their mental, physical, emotional, and spiritual needs while helping families cope with the loss of their loved ones. Increasing numbers of people are choosing to be under the care of hospice at the time of their death.[14]

Veterinary hospice is a growing trend in veterinary medicine. The American Veterinary Medical Association (AVMA), recognizing the value in end-of-life care, established guidelines for hospice practice many years ago.[15,16] Since then, these guidelines have been continuously reviewed and updated, and other organizations have developed additional standards of care.

ESTABLISHMENT OF VETERINARY HOSPICE CARE

Recognizing the growing demand for end-of-life care for the terminally ill companion animal, this author, a small animal criticalist at Michigan State University (MSU) College of Veterinary Medicine, founded the second veterinary hospice practice in academia, in 2011. The Veterinary Hospice Care (VHC) mission had 4 main goals. First, VHC would provide excellence in palliative medicine and home hospice services to meet the needs of terminally ill patients and provide emotional support to their families, as 1 unit of care. This care would bridge the gap between diagnosis of serious or terminal illness and death. Care for the hospice patient would be provided within the guidelines established by the AVMA guidelines for VHC.[15] The service would focus on relationship-oriented, patient-focused, goal-centered care, individually tailored for the patient and family. Second, VHC would provide a source of outreach, by collaborating with an interdisciplinary team, to provide understanding and awareness of end-of-life care in veterinary medicine. VHC would be a visible source of support for patients, families, and veterinary professionals alike. In providing this, VHC hoped to address and alleviate the compassion fatigue and moral distress often experienced by the veterinary care team when caring for terminally ill patients and grieving families. Care would continue for the family after the death of the patient, if chosen by the family, through the MSU Companion Animal Loss Support Group (established in 2006). Next, VHC would increase educational content in core and elective curricula to veterinary medical students and veterinary technician students, in the areas of palliative medicine and end-of-life care. Additionally, VHC would provide ongoing continuing education to members of the veterinary community through presentations in local, regional, state, national, and international conferences in veterinary medicine. Finally, VHC would build a foundation for observational, retrospective, and prospective research in palliative medicine and end-of-life care topics within the veterinary field. These 4 goals of (1) service, (2) outreach, (3) education, and (4) research mirrored the mission of the College of Veterinary Medicine at large.

The program was supported and approved by the dean of the college, the MSU Veterinary Teaching Hospital director, and the Chair of the Department of Small Animal Clincal Sciences to be a 1-year, pilot program in May of 2011. Six months of logistical planning, infrastructure to support this practice (such as office space), fee structure, online secure record-keeping system, professional liability insurance, controlled substance licensure, acquisition, and recording system were discussed, revised, and agreed on. Online forms, including owner consent for treatment, individualized cost of care, euthanasia consent, and educational handouts for commonly encountered conditions, were developed. The MSU College of Veterinary Medicine Office of Marketing and Communication aided in the development of informational flyers and brochures about the new service. Similarly, an online Web site for VHC service, including contact information and fee structures, was created. An announcement was sent electronically to the referral community with the date for opening to ensure awareness and garner support.

DEVELOPMENT OF THE INTERDISCIPLINARY TEAM
Primary Care Veterinarian

During this initial 6 months, key stakeholders in the community were also identified and targeted for support, and the interdisciplinary team required to practice strong palliative medicine and hospice care was developed. The primary care/referring veterinarian was identified as a key stakeholder. This author visited many primary care practices throughout the greater central Michigan area to build rapport and learn about their practices. Recognizing that families build strong bonds with, and lean heavily on, their primary veterinarian when the human-animal bond is threatened, the value of these relationships cannot and should not be denied.[17] VHC was to be a referral service that would lead the palliative medicine plan and prepare for a patient's eventual death. Care was taken to ensure that the primary care veterinarian would be part of the team, and that, where possible, referral back for primary care services (such as for euthanasia or need for prescription refills) would be maintained. Additionally, the primary care team was assured that they would receive detailed medical records regarding a patient's changes in plan, similar to all other referral practices. Primary veterinarians, as well as their hospital staffs, were provided with continuing education on palliative medicine and VHC services, and opportunities for dialogue were provided. Flyers about VHC were also dispensed through site visits. These small, interactive, personal meetings with time for open communication about the service provided the cornerstone for referral and engagement.

Other community outreach included consultation with veterinary practitioners of Eastern medicine therapies (ie, holistic practice, reiki, and acupuncture), canine massage therapists, and nutritionists to determine if they would have interest in collaboration for provision of both in-hospital and in-home care. All professionals approached were willing to provide some referral services to VHC patients if needed. Costs for these community practitioners would be established by them independently and paid for directly by clients on referral. A document with contact information for these services was generated for prospective hospice clients.

Specialists

In contrast to human hospice, patients with terminal illness were not excluded from VHC services if their owners continued to seek disease-focused care. Therefore, it was possible for a hospice patient to be simultaneously under the care of veterinary specialists. Within the MSU College of Veterinary Medicine, informational sessions were held at 5 different time points to raise awareness of VHC and allow opportunities for dialogue. These times were chosen to allow for attendance of all staff members, technicians, house officers, faculty, and administrators while maintaining clinical coverage and didactic education and without disruption of hospital management. Specific specialty services (oncology, internal medicine, emergency, and critical care) were additionally targeted for smaller ongoing group sessions because they were anticipated to likely have patients that would meet hospice entrance qualifications. Likewise, private veterinary specialty practices throughout the state were contacted, visited, and offered continuing education and given information on the service for distribution. Other engaged professionals within the MSU Veterinary Teaching Hospital included certified canine rehabilitation technicians and board-certified anesthesiologists.

Mental Health Care

Linda Lawrence, Licensed Master Social Worker, a veterinary social worker concurrently working at MSU Veterinary Teaching Hospital and MSU School of Social Work, was consulted, and she agreed to collaborate to provide hospice families additional layers of mental health support during a pet's duration in hospice and after death. Lawrence established the MSU Companion Animal Loss Support Group in 2006, a group that this author co-collaborated with starting in 2008. Other community mental health care professionals were also engaged and informed about the service.

Disposal, Burial, and Cremation Professionals

Lastly, disposal, burial, and pet crematory professionals throughout the state were contacted. Similar to other stakeholders, these businesses were offered continuing education on VHC services and palliative medicine. Flyers were also dispensed at these locations, because it was recognized that sometimes families plan ahead for currently healthy pets or have multiple animals in the household. The relationships established with this part of the interdisciplinary team would prove extremely valuable as the service grew. Some pet crematory professionals offered to meet this author at a family's home when a euthanasia was scheduled to aid the family in this aspect of care.

State and Regional Veterinary Medical Associations

Prior to accepting the first patient, this author also met with the other veterinary leaders in the state, including the president of the Michigan Veterinary Medical Association, to discuss VHC, to educate and to bring awareness to this new service. Further informational sessions with regional veterinary medical associations across the state were scheduled over the following year. Positive support was engendered toward the start of this new service from state officials.

PATIENT QUALIFICATION FOR VETERINARY HOSPICE CARE

Qualifications for entrance into VHC were established, following the AVMA hospice guidelines.[15] Classically, entrance for human patients into hospice is a life expectancy of less than 6 months.[18] Given that diseases are often discovered later in their course for veterinary patients, temporal consideration for death was not a mandated qualification. Rather, patient-specific qualifications include diagnosis of a terminal illness or a diagnosis of a chronic illness interfering with quality of life. Patients in which a curative treatment of a disease was possible, but was either not pursued or failed, also qualified for hospice care. Similarly, patients diagnosed with progressive, debilitating, life-altering/life-ending disease were also allowed entrance, regardless of how long the trajectory of illness was anticipated to be. Due to the availability of euthanasia in veterinary medicine, families may elect euthanasia due to factors associated with either the patient, the family, or both—even without an inherently life-ending diagnosis. This was considered in determination of appropriateness for VHC services. Additionally, the patients themselves had to be amenable to care, and there needed to be a reasonable expectation that patient comfort could be achieved with increased palliation.

Nonpatient considerations for entrance into hospice include family needs for additional support and willingness to have hospice team members in their home. Families of hospice patients also needed to be willing and able to undertake some caregiving for their own animals, after being provided instruction. Although human hospice is provided at no cost due to the Medicare hospice benefit, VHC would be not be a free service.[13] Therefore, families would have to be willing to pay for services rendered, with fees established and agreed on before being provided.

Patient Referral and Consultation

Patients were acquired through referral from either MSU specialty services, MSU general practice, other specialty referral practices, or community primary care veterinarians. Self-referral was also possible, because families found information on the internet and various media outlets (radio, television, and newspaper). Client-client referral also was possible.

Once contact was made, the initial consultation was scheduled based on a mutually convenient time and took place in a family's home. Similar to human hospice care, VHC was designed to be an in-home service, where families and patients would be most amenable to care.[19] The initial consultation was always with this author. On average, the initial consultation took 2 hours, outside of travel time to and from the location. Prior to this meeting, where possible, the medical record was acquired and reviewed. The initial consultation was adapted from a previously reported stepwise plan[20] and recorded during this visit using a Microsoft Word–based computer system. The first step involved evaluation of family's understanding of the disease, family's and pet's needs, family's beliefs, and preferred mode and place of death. This required a great deal of open-ended questioning and reflective listening to ensure clear communication. Previous experiences with death both in pets and humans was also discussed to ascertain underlying knowledge, fears, and anticipation of future events. As part of evaluating a family's beliefs, care was taken to have the family define what quality of life represents to the patient and the family as well as what constitutes suffering. By helping frame these hard topics of conversation, increased dialogue among not only the hospice care team and the family but also between family members allowed for better understanding and planning for what might lie ahead. As part of understanding a family's values, care was taken to identify current sources of support. These might include one another, other family members or friends, coworkers, spirituality or spiritual leaders, and other pets, for example, These intricate conversations provided the foundation for establishing goals of care for both patient and family. If family members expressed goals of care that were perceived to be unrealistic, open discussion with empathy took place, to try to reframe and refocus the goals. It was common for families to not be able to articulate goals for their patients.

Once goals of care were established, the third step was to provide education about pathophysiology of disease, dying, euthanasia, and palliative care strategies and management. Although many families had received education from their referring veterinarian, the impact of the diagnosis may have prevented them from fully understanding the disease process. After having some time to think, coupled with now being in their own home in a more comfortable atmosphere, many families had questions regarding the anticipated trajectory of illness and what challenges their patient might face. In anticipation of this, information was shared with them both verbally and in writing by the end of the visit to add to their comprehension of disease. Furthermore, additional resources (such as online Web sites or support groups, for example) were shared to provide another layer of support.

After physical examination of the patient and review of information provided by the referring veterinarian (where possible), an individually tailored, relationship-oriented, goal-centered, patient-focused plan of care was created. Plans were carefully and thoughtfully designed to ensure that all interventions would benefit the patient, and would not jeopardize the human-animal relationship. For example, if a patient would benefit from artificial hydration but would hide from the owner, this was deemed non-beneficial to the relationship. The pros and cons for interventions would be determined and other options considered, including the use of an outside person to come in to perform various tasks as well as the associated cost. Current medical therapies were scrutinized to ensure that they were providing increased benefit over risk to the patient and, if not, were discontinued. Care was taken to address potential for pain, nausea, air hunger, hygiene/sanitation, mobility, wound care, sedation, antianxiolytic medications, and others, depending on the needs dictated by the patient. In establishment of the plan, the family's needs were also considered, including but not limited to physical, emotional, and spiritual ability to care for the pet, and human services referral was offered where identified. Each member of the family as well as members of the interdisciplinary team were identified before the end of the visit.

Finally, in developing the care plan, an emergency plan was also created, based on the anticipated needs of the pet, with the family's goals and belief systems in mind. This always included providing the family with after-hours contact information for 24-hour care provided through this author or the MSU Emergency and Critical Care Medicine service. Additionally, identifying the closest 24-hour pharmacy to a family's home was performed and contact information recorded by both this author and the family. Where anticipated, 1 dose to 2 doses of emergency medicines (specifically, antinausea medications and antidiarrheal medications) were often left with the owner, with instructions to contact this author if they believed those medications should be administered. In rare circumstances, 1 dose of anticonvulsant (midazolam or diazepam) was left if it was anticipated to be of benefit for the patient and agreeable to the owner and if the owner signed a consent form that a controlled substance had been received in that case. The owner was educated verbally and left with written documentation about how to properly store this medication and how to dispose of it.

A plan for preferred mode and place of death also was determined. Although this conversation was often difficult and not every plan carried out as hoped, having awareness of mode and place of death improved anticipatory grief and coping in clients. Mode of death was not an exclusionary factor for entrance into VHC. Families could plan for euthanasia or palliated natural death with support and help from the service. Referral for after-death body disposal through the referring veterinarian, other disposal options, cremation, or burial were offered, and resources, where possible, were provided to clients.

In the final part of plan development, all families were offered and provided resources for emotional support though MSU and others in their community where possible. The next point of contact between this author and the family was determined prior to closure of the visit. Typically, this was via telephone contact 24 hours to 48 hours after the initial visit.

Medical Record Keeping

The patient's medical record, generated during the visit, was initially accomplished using a Microsoft Word–based document, later uploaded to the MSU electronic medical record system. This record would then be electronically mailed back to the owner as well as the referring veterinarian. The record documented the entire care plan, including the family's goals and beliefs, the hospice plan, and how and when the next contact with the hospice team would take place. If members of the team (such as an acupuncturist or social worker) were added, then the medical record could be shared electronically as needed. Likewise, referral information from members of the interdisciplinary team would be shared with VHC.

Planning for Emergency

Because the family had access to VHC at all times, changes in the plan were updated and made available to team members by electronic mail or through the electronic medical record. When this author was unavailable, families were directly notified, and an emergency contact person (additional member of interdisciplinary team) was appointed to act as the liaison for the family and the team. The MSU Emergency and Critical Care service was always available to see the patient if the patient had an emergency. This, however, required that the patient and family travel to the hospital for care, which may not have been preferred.

Weekly contact via electronic mail or phone, even if a patient was doing well, was required to ensure that families' and patients' needs were being met. All communication was documented and recorded in the medical record. Follow-up was established for in-home visits as dictated by a patient's illness trajectory or a family's need. Additional visits followed similar structure to the initial visit, with medical record keeping and plan for follow-up. Additional visits shared fee structures similar to those for the initial visit, which were agreed on up front and the responsibility of the family.

RESULTS
Enrollment and Length of Hospice Care

VHC opened to patient enrollment on November 1, 2011, 6 months after inception. In the inaugural year, VHC enrolled 62 patients, characterized by 54 dogs and 8 cats. These numbers far exceeded the expectation of the service and surpassed Colorado State University Pet Hospice (the only other academic hospice practice) 5-year cumulative numbers.[18] This was also unexpected given that the service was not free. The patients ranged in age from 7 years to 19 years, with a mean age of 13 years. As a result of this initial success, VHC was renewed for continuation through MSU.

Over the 3 years that the hospice was open, VHC enrolled a total of 142 patients; 81% of cases were dogs (n = 115), with mixed breeds the most numerous enrolled (27/115; 23.4%), followed by Labrador retrievers (17/115; 14.7%), and golden retrievers (10/115; 8.7%); 49 breeds in total were represented. Of the 27 cats enrolled, only 1, a Singapura, was a purebred cat (1/27; 0.04%), and the remainder were mixed-breed cats. The enrollment age range was 5 years to 21 years, with a mean age of 12.5 years and a median age of 13 years.

During the first 12 months, 62 patients were enrolled. One family was discharged from hospice care due to unwillingness to work with the hospice care team. From the patients enrolled in the first year, the length of hospice care ranged from less than 1 day to 620 days (mean 33 days and median 2 days). Many patients referred within this year were imminently dying or families requesting euthanasia at the time of entrance into the hospice or within the first 24 hours. In the second year of VHC,

52 patients were enrolled. Although the overall number decreased, length of hospice care for patients enrolled in this time frame averaged 62 days (range 1–742 days), with a median of 26 days. This dramatic change represented a shift in referral from late in the disease process to closer to the time of diagnosis. Due to patients living longer in hospice and increased number of patients actively receiving ongoing care, fewer patients could be enrolled in the third year. Only 29 hospice patients were added. Of those patients that died before the end of the third year, the mean length of time in hospice care was 42 days (range 1–257 days) and median 9.5 days. Five patients were still alive at the end of 3 years. Cumulatively, the length of hospice care had a mean 55 days and median 6.5 days; 39 patients enrolled in hospice within 1 day of their death, representing 27.6% of all admissions, and 13 patients were enrolled in hospice less than 24 hours before their death, representing less than 1% of all admissions. Adjusting the values to identify patients exceeding 25 hours in hospice care, 89 patients were identified, representing 63% of the total population. These patients had an average length of time in hospice of 79 days, with a median 24 days.

Referral

Families learned about VHC and were referred for care through various sources. The largest group of referrals came directly from veterinarians, employees, and students affiliated with MSU College of Veterinary Medicine (48 cases, or 33.8% of referred cases). The VHC Web site was responsible for recruiting an additional 20 families to enroll patients (or 14% of cases). Most impressively, a large portion of cases came from word-of-mouth referral, either from previous clients or friends and family member of previous clients, representing 13.3% of cases (19 case referrals). This group exceeded referrals from the primary veterinarian community (14 cases, or 9.8% of referred cases), and other specialty practice referrals (4 cases, or 2.8% of referred cases). The social work community referred 3.5% of cases enrolled in care (or 5 referred cases) and various media sources (including newspaper articles, radio interviews, community events, and flyers) contributed 6% of cases (9 enrolled cases). Eight families cited direct or previous contact with this author as a reason for enrollment, representing 5.6% of cases. Cremation and burial services were responsible for referral of 4 cases to VHC (2.8% of cases referred). The 12 remaining families with hospice patients either did not disclose how they learned about Veterinary Hospice Care, or were simply not queried.

Patient referrals unexpectedly came from greater distances than central Michigan. Although a majority of cases were within a 30-minute radius to MSU, distances of up to 200 miles did not prohibit patient enrollment. As part of the fee structure, mileage fees applied both to and from a patient's home. This fee was discussed and agreed on prior to enrollment. This did not deter patient enrollment but did create new challenges, particularly in regard to the interdisciplinary team and emergency care planning. In these circumstances, additional collaboration with the primary veterinarian and staff were sometimes able to increase the proximity by which a team member could help. Emergency plans for this subset of patients exceeding a 70-mile radius often would necessitate the family being willing to take the patient to a closer emergency veterinary clinic (if one was available). In these cases, a document was issued for the family to provide to the emergency veterinarian identifying that the patient was a hospice patient, with an outline of diagnosis, plan and current treatment, plan for preferred mode and place of death, and this author's contact information. Despite being prepared for this event, no enrolled hospice patient ever required its use.

Requests to have the patient brought to MSU rather than providing in-home care were rarely considered, although for patients that had been hospitalized at MSU and were transitioning to home with the intention of VHC enrollment, an occasional in-hospital visit occurred. These visits were mostly to have an in-person meeting, often in the presence of the referring partner, to determine if hospice care was something that the family wanted to consider. Initial consult with regard to identifying key elements of a family's knowledge and belief systems and the patient care plan were withheld until an in-home visit could take place.

Reasons for Enrollment

Veterinary hospice patients had many reasons for enrollment. Similar to human medicine, the largest reason for enrollment was the diagnosis or the presence of a mass and clinical signs consistent with neoplasia (79/142; 55%).[19] Neurologic disease (22/142; 15.5%), cardiac disease (14/142; 9.8%), and renal disease (11/142; 7.7%) also were common reasons for entrance. Other ailments, including severe osteoarthritis, endocrinopathies, metabolic disease (such as unexplained weight loss, copper storage disease, or hepatic insufficiency), nonhealing decubitus wounds, and others, represented another large group of admitting diagnoses (25/142; 17.6%). Given the average age of patients at the time of enrollment, it was common for patients to have more than 1 illness as the reason for seeking hospice care (10/142; 7%).

Patient Census

In the first year VHC was open, there were anywhere from 0 to 12 patients on the census at 1 time. At the end of the first year, there were 10 active patients remaining on the census. Fourteen months after enrolling the first patient, there were no fewer than 8 active patients on the census. Sixteen months after opening, VHC was averaging 1 to 2 new patients per week. By January 2014, there were no fewer than 12 and as many as 18 active patients receiving care at 1 time. This marked change in the number of active patients was likely a result of earlier referrals in the course of disease—a result of increased awareness in the community and positive feedback from both clients and referral partners. Additionally, dedicated palliative management for these patients likely contributed to them having increased quality life span and more gradual illness trajectories.

Preferred Mode and Place of Death

As discussed previously, hospice represents the time frame between diagnosis of serious or terminal disease and time of death. Therefore, mode of death did not preclude enrollment in hospice. Families were supported and educated in different modes of death, such as palliated natural death (including the use of palliative sedation), and euthanasia. Unpalliated dying in the name of natural death and/or suffering deemed important according to particular spiritual or religious beliefs were not supported by VHC philosophy of hospice and were not part of mode of death for any VHC patients. When questioned about preferred mode and place of death, families overwhelmingly preferred in-home euthanasia over most other options. Feelings expressed about this option included that it could be peaceful, private for the family, and fear-free and stress-free for the patient. Other considerations for this were that other family pets could be nearby. No other family pet was forced to be present at a patient's euthanasia; however, if one chose to be near, this was not discouraged and certainly allowed.

One hundred and thirteen patients were euthanized in their homes in a planned manner through VHC, representing 83% of patients who died in hospice by the end of the third year (n = 136). One family requested their primary veterinarian euthanize their patient in their home. Five percent of families preferred not to have their patient at home and elected to take their patient to their primary veterinarian for euthanasia (7/136). Six patients (4.4%) were euthanized either on an emergency or planned basis by the MSU Emergency and Critical Care service. One family elected for euthanasia of their patient in a neutral, outdoor setting, accomplished through VHC. Hospice often conjures ideations of palliated natural death; however only 9 families achieved their patient's death by this manner, representing a mere 6% of the hospice population.

Outreach

One of the main goals for establishing VHC was providing outreach to the community. Representing alternatives in end-of-life care in veterinary medicine, VHC was featured in 4 community pet-related events. Additionally, VHC was also part of a local human hospice summit, to raise awareness of veterinary hospice with current state leaders in the field of human hospice and palliative care. This program resulted in a partnership with a local human hospice organization, which allowed for sharing of ideas and information. Continuing education sessions in hospice and palliative medicine, the VHC program, end-of-life care, and compassion fatigue were presented at 7 regional veterinary medical associations across the state over a 2-year time frame. In addition to countless in-person visits to primary veterinarians, in-hospital continuing education was presented at 4 veterinary hospitals at their request on hospice and palliative medicine. Four newspaper articles, 1 television interview, and 3 radio interviews featured stories on VHC.

Throughout the time that VHC was open, this author also continued to collaborate with the Companion Animal Loss Support Group, which held twice-a-month meetings at MSU. This support group was offered at no cost to members of the community who were grieving the loss of their animal companions. Families with patients in VHC were offered support through this group, facilitated primarily by Lawrence. Together with VHC, the support group held an annual memorial service for all members of the community to honor their lost companions.

Educational Change

VHC contributed to education in end-of-life care topics to the community, to veterinary students, and to veterinary technician students. As a leader in the field, this author was invited and requested to feature VHC at the Third International Symposium on Veterinary Hospice Care, sponsored by the Nikki Pet Hospice Foundation, the first organization in animal hospice, in July 2012. Similarly, VHC was also featured at the second annual International Association for Animal Hospice and Palliative Care conference the same year. In 2014, VHC was featured at the Michigan Veterinary Conference, and, in addition to discussing the program, this author provided continuing education to attendees on how to establish a hospice care program as well as nutrition in the end-of-life patient and compassion fatigue.

More importantly, the development of VHC at MSU brought increased awareness and visibility of end-of-life issues to veterinary students. Unlike the Colorado State University Pet Hospice model,[21] VHC did not have student participation. Due to the variable and unpredictable hours and travel required as well as liability, administration did not believe that it was in the best interests of students to participate in the direct care of hospice patients. However, 4 hours of lecture were added to the veterinary students' core curriculum to cover end-of-life and related topics, including small animal and large animal content. Previously, end of life was not perceived important in the veterinary curriculum and rarely did veterinary school graduates feel prepared to deal with end of life.[9–11] This vast 5-fold increase was believed to better prepare students in these areas before practice. Additionally, 8 hours of elective material in end-of-life and related topics were also created and offered to the veterinary students, as was a 1.5-hour end-of-life–related discussion session for each 3-week rotation of primary care, mandatory for all students in their senior year.

Five state-wide veterinary technician programs in Michigan (including the program at MSU) also sought to increase end-of-life education after the success of VHC, inviting this author to lecture from 1 hour to 3 hours. For many students in these programs, this was the first and only formal discussion in end-of-life care they received. This author was also contacted personally by 5 other veterinary colleges in the United States and 2 international schools within the first year of opening VHC with inquiries about how to start a program at their respective schools. Despite this, there has been little forward movement in developing end-of-life care services at other academic institutions. To the author's knowledge, no program outside of the Colorado State University program currently exists.[21]

The public response to veterinary hospice was overwhelmingly positive. The need for this care was clearly identified throughout the state, and, during the time that VHC was open, 4 other in-state veterinarians opened hospice care practices. These practices, although all different, were collaborative with ideas for patient care and referral services.

Closure of Veterinary Hospice Care

Despite its success, VHC closed for business in November 2014. Personal reasons made an out-of-state move necessary for this author, and, as the founder and sole practitioner, this unavoidably meant the closure of the hospice service. Families with patients under the care of VHC were made aware in advance that the hospice would be closing, and discussion and preparations were made for referral to other hospice practitioners. With closure of the hospice service, end-of-life care curricular changes were sadly abolished or delegated to others.

SUMMARY

VHC was the second animal hospice established at an academic institution. The program was built on providing a much-needed service to families in the community coping with serious and terminal illness of their beloved animals, while supporting the veterinary community at large with the burden of compassion fatigue and moral distress that inevitably comes from doing this work. Reception for this program was overwhelmingly positive. Changes in core curricula were made for both veterinary students and veterinary technician students as result. Despite its closure for reasons unrelated to its impact or caseload, VHC remains a successful model for academic hospice practice.

REFERENCES

1. McNicholas J, Gilbey A, Rennie A, et al. Pet ownership and human health: a brief review of evidence and issues. Br Med J 2005;33:1252–4.
2. Voith VL. The impact of companion animal problems on society and the role of veterinarians. Vet Clin North Am Small Anim Pract 2009;39(2):327–45.
3. Brown JP, Silverman JD. The current and future market for veterinarians and veterinary medical services in the United States. J Am Vet Med Assoc 1999;215(2): 161–83.
4. Pierce J. Are pets really family? Available at: https://www.psychologytoday.com/us/blog/all-dogs-go-heaven/201510/are-pets-really-family. Accessed May 1, 2016.

5. Pet food industry report. 95% say pets are part of the family. Available at: https://www.petfoodindustry.com/articles/5695-report—say-pets-are-part-of-the-family. Accessed June 1, 2016.

6. Volsche S. Understanding cross-species parenting: a case for pets as children. In: Kogan, Blazina, editors. Clinician's guide to treating companion animal issues: addressing human-animal interaction. London: Elsevier; 2019. p. 130–9.

7. Goldberg KJ. Veterinary hospice and palliative care: a comprehensive review of the literature. Vet Rec 2016;178:369–74.

8. Billings ME, Curtis R, Engleberg RA. Medicine residents' self-perceived competence in end of life care. Acad Med 2009;84(11):1533–9.

9. Rowan AN. The human animal bond in academic veterinary medicine. J Vet Med Educ 2008;35(4):477–82.

10. Tinga CE, Adams CL, Bonnett BN, et al. Survey of veterinary technical and professional skills in students and recent graduates of a veterinary college. J Am Vet Med Assoc 2001;219(7):924–31.

11. Butler C, William S, Koll S. Perceptions of fourth year veterinary students regarding emotional support of clients in veterinary practice in the veterinary college curriculum. J Am Vet Med Assoc 2002;221(3):360–3.

12. National Hospice and Palliative Care Organization. Definition of hospice. Available at: https://www.nhpco.org/about/hospice-care. Accessed November 1, 2018.

13. The Official US Government Site for Medicare. Medicare benefit policy manual. Chapter 9 coverage of hospice services under hospital insurance 2015. p. 1–54. Rev. 209. Available at: www.medicare.gov/coverage/hospice-respite-care. Accessed November 1, 2018.

14. American Medical News. American Medical Association. 2009. Available at: www.amednews.com. Accessed April 5, 2011.

15. Committee on the Human-Animal Bond. Human-animal bond issues. J Am Vet Med Assoc 1998;212(11):1675.

16. CHAB reaffirmed April 2010 guidelines for veterinary hospice care. AVMA. 2007. Available at: www.avma.org/issues/policy/default.asp. Accessed May 1, 2012.

17. Wensley SP. Animal welfare and the human-animal bond: considerations for veterinary faculty, students and practitioners. J Vet Med Educ 2008;35(4):532–9.

18. The Official US Government Site for Medicare. Life expectancy in hospice. Available at: https://www.medicare.gov/what-medicare-covers/what-part-a-covers/how-hospice-works Accessed November 1, 2018.

19. National Hospice and Palliative Care Organization. Facts and figures: hospice care in America. National Hospice and Palliative Care Organization; 2009. Available at: https://www.nhpco.org/sites/default/files/public/newsline/2010/Nov_10_NL.pdf. Accessed April 1, 2011.

20. Shearer TS. Pet hospice and palliative care protocols. Vet Clin Small Anim Pract 2011;41(3):507–18.

21. Bishop GA, Long CC, Carlsten KS, et al. The colorado state university pet hospice program: end of life care for pets and their families. J Vet Med Educ 2008;35(4):525–31.

Pain and Palliative Care Service, Massachusetts Society for the Prevention of Cruelty to Animals-Angell Animal Medical Center

Lisa Moses, VMD[a,b,c],*

KEYWORDS

- Palliative care • Veterinary pain medicine • Palliative program
- Veterinary palliative care • Palliative program development

KEY POINTS

- The development of a veterinary palliative care service required structured planning including development of new knowledge and skills, defining the service configuration, cultivating of a referral community, and most importantly, defining practice values.
- A suitable model and advanced training for the service was mostly derived from experiences at human palliative care services in academic medicine settings.
- Exploring and understanding one's own values surrounding palliative and end-of-life care is important in the development of a palliative care service, to help mitigate moral distress.

THE HOSPITAL SETTING

Angell's Pain and Palliative Care Service is a small division of an independent, nonprofit, teaching institution that is the flagship hospital of the Massachusetts Society for the Prevention of Cruelty to Animals (MSPCA). The hospital was founded more than 100 years ago, 50 years after the establishment of the MSPCA in 1868. Angell is where veterinary post-graduate training originated, with the establishment of the internship program and residencies in 1940. Angell has a large primary care practice in the Boston location along with the better-known referral and specialty services. All told, Angell sees about 75,000 patients of all companion animal species per year, with

No conflicts of interest to disclose.
[a] Pain and Palliative Care, Angell Animal Medical Center, 350 South Huntington Avenue, Boston, MA 02130, USA; [b] Center for Bioethics, Harvard Medical School, Animal Ethics Study Group, Boston, MA, USA; [c] Yale Interdisciplinary Center for Bioethics, New Haven, CT, USA
* Angell Animal Medical Center, 350 South Huntington Avenue, Boston, MA, 02130.
E-mail address: lisa_moses@hms.harvard.edu

more than 30% of them being seen first by the emergency service. The mix of primary care patients and clients who seek out specialty services provides a diverse population of cases referred to the Pain and Palliative Care Service. The long history of the institution in advancing veterinary medicine within the context of a mission-driven and philanthropically supported animal welfare organization played an important role in the development of the service.

HOW AND WHY THE SERVICE DEVELOPED

The Pain and Palliative Care service was developed in 2006 as a pain medicine service. I had spent the prior dozen years as a senior member of Angell's large Emergency and Critical Care Service, as a clinician and overseeing interns and residents. Before that I was pursing residency and board certification in small animal internal medicine. Although I loved emergency and critical care clinical work, I was aware of the tension between my natural (internal medicine type) tendencies to delve deeply into the history and context of a case and the necessary expediency of emergency work and the narrow focus of critical care. A long-standing interest in medical ethics surrounding dilemmas in referral veterinary medicine also became more prominent in the last few years of my emergency and critical care work. Clinical work in chronic pain and palliative care medicine were a good fit for my interests and medical style.

My interest in pain medicine and anesthesiology was known from my self-appointed role as the pain management champion/nag for our intensive care unit and during teaching rounds. Angell's chief of staff approached me with an idea to start a pain service. She saw this idea as a way to fill a void in patient care and hospital services mandated by the hospital's mission while providing me with a new way to challenge myself professionally. I had already been watching the development of the nascent field of veterinary pain management and realized that there were not many examples of such services in a referral hospital, other than as part of a few university anesthesia departments.

The structure of the pain service was developed when I spent a sabbatical pursing extra training in pain medicine and after doing more research on models of pain management services in human health care. As an exploratory step, I did some basic training in rehabilitation and a few other forms of physical medicine, along with pursuing acupuncture certification from the Medical Acupuncture for Veterinarians program. The bulk of my training was in interventional pain management, chronic pain didactic training, and the functioning of a hospital-based pediatric pain medicine department at Boston Children's Hospital. Angell is fortunate to be less than a mile from Harvard Medical School and its expansive campus of teaching hospitals, of which Boston Children's Hospital is one. Boston Children's Pain Service was the first of its kind and provided me with a solid model on which to design Angell's service. This pediatric department consists of an in-patient consultation service and an interdisciplinary outpatient chronic pain clinic. The in-patient service consults on any case where a consult is requested, but also on every patient who fits a set of criteria, such as a particular diagnosis or painful surgical procedure. This is the same structure as which Angell's pain medicine service started. I deliberately chose to focus on pain as a field of medicine rather than structure the service around therapeutic interventions, such as rehabilitation. Because there were other local providers for specific therapeutics it seemed that focusing more on pain diagnosis and cohesive medical management was a bigger need and better suited my background and natural inclinations. I expected and hoped to work with patients with complex medical conditions who were cared for by other specialists, who lacked someone focused on the patient's symptom management. In retrospect, my conceptualization of the service was always better termed "palliative care" or symptom management, but I was not as familiar with palliative care principals at that point.

In preparation for the opening of the service, I met with representatives from all of the hospital departments to assess their need and interest in the service. Those meetings were instructive in shaping how the service was described and marketed, so that specific community needs could be filled. A crucial aspect of this process was meeting with technicians and administrative hospital staff so they understood the point of the service and what was being offered. An unexpected bonus for this effort was that veterinary technicians were the largest source of referrals for the first year of the service. I also enlisted our marketing department to help me reach out to the referring veterinarian community for the same purpose. Marketing materials like a World Wide Web page, brochures, and press releases were created.

While I was doing the planning for what the scope of services would be, how the appointment schedule would be structured, what fees would be charged, what would be needed to create a comfortable examination room, and other such practical details, I was also thinking about my philosophy of care and mission. Much of that was shaped by my past clinical experience, but it was significantly influenced by what I witnessed in pediatric and adult palliative care at various Harvard Medical School teaching hospitals that I was able to visit.

EARLY EXPERIENCES IN THE PAIN MEDICINE SERVICE

When I started seeing patients, it was clear that pet owners felt an unmet need for end-of-life care and support. Even though I was expecting to see patients with complex sources of pain and problems, I was still surprised by how many of my patients were terminally ill or unable to function independently. I was also unprepared for how frequently I saw obvious suffering and how many of them had untreated medical problems contributing to their pain. Many of them were patients whose owners had already been advised by one or more veterinarians to consider euthanasia as the most humane option available. Some immediate, unforeseen challenges became apparent. Appointment times needed to be even longer than anticipated and fees correspondingly larger. Large amounts of time and detective work were needed to track down records, talk to other veterinarians, and fully review histories, diagnostic results, and questionnaires. The typical style of medical records and referral letters used in our hospital did not match what needed to be recorded for these types of visits. How much medical care should I handle myself and how much should I ask the primary care veterinarian or other involved specialists to do? More prosaic problems emerged as well, such as the need for lots of soft furnishings and laundry when your patient population is frequently incontinent.

One of the surprising types of visits were appointments booked because the client did not believe their pet was in pain (despite worried relatives' or veterinarian's contrary opinions). These clients sought my advice to confirm their assessment and prove wrong the other opinion. The visits required a different type of communication than the usual one, including more client education about pain behaviors in nonhuman species. In some of these cases, the pet owners simply could not accept that the animal may be in pain despite obvious signs because of the contradictory behaviors they observed, like a good appetite and attention seeking. Although I was able to explain the evolutionary roots of these behaviors and species-specific differences from humans, it was not until I learned about coping mechanisms and anticipatory grief from palliative care training that I better understood these owners.

TRANSITIONING TO PALLIATIVE CARE

Although I recognized quickly that the service was providing palliative care, not just pain medicine, the name of the service was not changed for many years. This was a purposeful reaction to seeing what seemed like too many cases where the patient was suffering without success in reducing their suffering enough to be acceptable to me. My fear was that if the service name was changed to "palliative care" or I made any mention of hospice care in the marketing materials that the service would be a magnet to pet owners seeking approval for refusing appropriate recommendations of euthanasia or appropriate medical management of pain and suffering. That fear partially stemmed from early experiences with distressing cases when I lacked expertise in advanced symptom management (and so believed I could not help the patient). The other significant factor in this decision was a lack of understanding that approaching all clients without judgment, even if I believed the patient was suffering an untoward amount, would allow me to find some way to help.

Fairly recently the name of the service was officially changed to "Pain and Palliative Care" without much fanfare. The structure and mission of the service did not change. For years preceding the name change I have described the service as providing global improvement in quality of life for patient (and caretakers) with chronic illness, reducing suffering, and lending support in medical decision making, all in keeping with principals of palliative care.

THE STRUCTURE AND FUNCTIONING OF THE PAIN AND PALLIATIVE CARE SERVICE

Currently, the bulk of the service provides outpatient palliative care. The patient load is about 70% dogs, with cats and nontraditional species making up the rest. Occasionally I provide pain medicine services to farm animals at the MSPCA's farm sanctuary for species ranging from chickens to large pigs. Any companion animal species is seen in the clinic, filling a growing need for advanced care of nontraditional species including psittacines, small mammals, and reptiles. With the hiring of several full-time anesthesiologists in the hospital, my former role in providing consultation and locoregional analgesia for perioperative patients has greatly diminished. Likewise, the growing expertise of our emergency and critical care staff in acute pain management has reduced the need for consultations in hospital and allowed me to focus on providing more purely palliative care to chronic patients. I believe that the commitment of the hospital administration in the creation of the service signaled a priority to incorporate palliative care ideals into the medical culture of the institution at large.

The team is still small consisting of myself, a dedicated technician, and a secretary. When available, our hospital social worker attends initial appointments or is brought in to participate near the end of a visit. Ideally, I would like to incorporate a social worker in the management of every case, as is typical in human palliative care, but our social work program cannot provide enough coverage for all of the service's patients at this time.

Appointment are 60 minutes in length and the fees are in line with what other specialists in the hospital charge for their time. Initial appointments and rechecks more than 1 year after the last visit are charged the same fee. Follow-up visits are charged about half the fee because less preparation time is needed to collect and review medical records and coordinate with other practitioners. Pet owners are asked to submit an online, species-specific questionnaire before their appointment (www.angell.org/painsurvey; www.angell.org/catpainsurvey). The questionnaire asks clients several different types of questions including ones designed to elucidate their understanding of the medical problems, ones that help them set goals for the visit, ones that identify problems with functional mobility and independence in their pets, and more existential questions about their pets' "happiness" and how they define quality of life. Reviewing their answers before each appointment has allowed me to shorten the appointment length, identify conflicts between the referring veterinarians and owner's understanding of medical details, and prompt the owner to start thinking about their goals of care.

HANDLING REFERRAL CASES

The caseload is about 60% external referrals/self-referrals and about 40% in-house referrals. I usually do see a spike in external referrals after I give lectures or publish relevant writing. I attribute this to a reduction in the persistent lack of understanding about what palliative care is and how focused pain medicine differs from typical approaches.

Getting to know the local veterinary community has been an on-going strategy to ensure the success of the service. My prior relationships with local veterinarians developed during my tenure on the emergency and critical care service helped get the practice started. I treat the primary care veterinarian or referring specialist clinicians with the same level of communication, including self-referred cases. We generally check in with the referring veterinarian before an initial consultation to make sure I understand their reasons for referral and goals for the visit. After the visit, the entire medical record is shared and a narrative style referral letter is sent the same day, explaining any new problems uncovered during the history taking and physical examination, my assessment, the mutually agreed on goals of care, and a specific plan with immediate actions taken and long-term recommendations. Sometimes the letters include questions I have for them that emerged during the visit. The point of the letter is to share my thought process with other clinicians involved in the case, possibly educate them, but mostly to engage them in team-based care of our patient. If there was some point of conflict reported by the client or something unexpected happened during the visit, I usually call or email the referring clinician immediately, so we can discuss it and there is no miscommunication about sensitive topics. Because many of my clients have solid, trusting relationships with the primary care veterinarian, I frequently engage the veterinarian to be part of determining goals of care, especially when a client feels ambivalent or overwhelmed. Admittedly, this system is labor intensive, but this approach best achieves the goal of supporting the other clinicians to provide good palliative care.

FOLLOW-UP VISITS AND CLIENT COMMUNICATION STRATEGIES

Within the first few years of doing this work, I saw the value of insisting on regular follow-up visits, rather than trying to alter treatment plans via telephone and email communication. I had many examples of dismaying surprises when I eventually re-examined patients after relying on owners' interpretations of their observations during telephone calls. Some of these surprises were simply caused by misinterpretations, but some were related to the common coping phenomenon of "blindness" to difficult realities. There is no substitute for a physical examination, or for watching patients move and navigate a room or engage with their family. All provide invaluable information for the difficult calculus of determining quality of life. For clients having difficulty in seeing changes in their pets, being able to say, "I am noticing that Spot can't get up without help today, but last month he had no trouble" is indispensable. A less obvious reason for in-person visits also arose: face-to-face discussions deepen trust and yield important contextual history that makes me better able to keep adjusting goals of care and treatment plans. The conversations help us move forward, through difficult decisions and scenarios, in a supported way.

My team and I do communicate extensively with clients via email and telephone calls in between scheduled follow-ups. I use these methods for updates on well-defined parameters, such as whether a particular adverse effect has resolved. We are careful to set boundaries, however, and try to avoid allowing owners to believe we are their only available resource. Regarding email communication, I received valuable advice from a psychotherapist client: she suggested not replying to emails immediately to avoid the impression that this took the place of a real conversation. The standard auto-reply to emails in our hospital states that messages will be responded to within 24 hours of a recipient's return to work.

I have developed some personal communication strategies that help me through the many difficult conversations inherent in this work. First, I always start an appointment by sitting down, without a computer in front of me, to talk to clients. I want people to believe they have my full attention when I am listening to them tell their story. I also start by telling people that I have reviewed the medical record, talked to the referring veterinarian, and read their questionnaire, but I want to hear in their words why they are here and what they want help with. It is easy to incorrectly assume that my goals match theirs if I do not ask first. Sometimes I start with a narrative prompt, such as "tell me about your pet," similar to the start of a human palliative care consultation. I have learned many specifics about a family's relationship to their pets, their own past experiences with serious illness and loss, and their fears for this visit by offering them the chance to shape the visit. Those details can help me understand their motivations and values enough to set mutual goals of care.

The overall tone of my communications is empathetic and nonjudgmental, but simple and straightforward about prognosis and my assessment of pain and suffering level. I avoid euphemisms and try to avoid medical jargon if at all possible. Because I am rarely the first veterinary professional to talk with the client about these issues, I know they have come to me for my opinion, which I give. Most of the people who seek my help are already experiencing some level of anticipatory grief and might be easily overwhelmed by choices. I do not offer them a large menu of options and ask them to choose; I prefer to tell them what I think is the best one or two ways to proceed. In rare cases I have serious misgivings about an option they were offered by another professional. Sometimes they are even referred to me because the veterinarian does not think the option chosen by the client is appropriate. If so, I explain without judgment or dismissal of that opinion what those misgivings are and I share that information with the other professional immediately after the examination. I believe that this rarely happens because we begin with establishing values, priorities, and goals of care, before we consider options. Once this is done, it is usually clear which options mesh with those goals and which do not.

FINANCIAL SUSTAINABILITY

The Pain and Palliative care Service, like similar consultation-based services in human health care, has difficulty generating enough revenue to be fully self-sustaining. Also, like human palliative care services, without the financial support of the larger hospital, the service could not endure. But, configured in a different way, veterinary palliative care can be self-sustaining. I have chosen to refer my cases to other hospital specialists when they need diagnostic work-up, losing that substantial revenue potential because keeping my role clearly delineated is important and provides for better patient care. Insisting on regularly scheduled follow-up visits improves patient care and caretaker support, but also provides a revenue stream. If your practice includes provision of specific therapeutic modalities, such as acupuncture, that also provides a predictable revenue stream. Perhaps the most important aspect, however, is making sure that visits are long enough and that your time is charged for appropriately. Clients are seeking help with difficult situations and you will be providing them with a service they cannot usually get elsewhere.

ADVICE FOR STARTING OUT IN PALLIATIVE CARE

The practice of palliative and hospice care is technically complex and emotionally challenging. Be kind to yourself; empathy is the foundation of this work and it should extend to yourself!

Listed next are some practical tactics that were of great help to me in the development of my practice. I hope they are also helpful to others.

- Expand your knowledge base.
  - Form a relationship with local human palliative and hospice care providers and spend time observing and discussing the medicine of their work, their methods for promoting sustainability, and their communication strategies. My experiences with palliative care teams is the foundation of my knowledge and is still how I expand my knowledge.
  - Use resources or attend a meeting for human palliative care continuing education to expand your knowledge. Two great starting places are: The Center to Advance Palliative Care (www.capc.org) and the National Hospice and Palliative Care Organization (www.nhpco.org). Check with your local medical school or teaching hospital to see what they offer.
  - To practice good symptom management, you need to understand the details of your patient's diagnoses and treatments. Educate yourself about common treatments for chronic illnesses, such as heart disease, cancer, and endocrine disorders, so you can better anticipate and manage disease complications and adverse events that impact your patient's quality of life.
- Form a community.
  - Seek like-minded veterinary professionals within your practice and locally. Spend time talking about your vision for this work and what problems you want to solve.
  - Make sure you are working in a practice that understands what palliative care is and what you want to achieve. If they do not you will be facing an even harder time convincing them to support you.
  - Seek the services of local mental health professionals who understand the human-animal bond. You need those people to refer your families to and they can help you learn valuable communication strategies.
  - Even if you do not work in a multidisciplinary hospital as part of an interdisciplinary team, use the team you do have to share the emotional burden of this work. Having someone else in the examination room changes the communication dynamic and gives you someone to corroborate details with if things are especially difficult.
- Make sure you have put into place specific and personalized coping strategies, boundaries, and limits for your palliative care cases.
  - Trust your colleagues to care for your shared cases so you can fully disconnect and your clients have other resources.
  - Be explicit and consistent about communication expectations.
  - Have a list of community resources to give to clients who need help you cannot provide, such as at-home nursing care or help with decision making (remember, decision making involves many nonmedical factors).

○ Figure out what techniques work for you to manage the compassion fatigue that is common when dealing with the cumulative effects of many sad and complex cases. Being exposed on a daily basis to grieving people and suffering animals should impact you. But you can mitigate how and how much.

- Consider additional training in, and/or research medical ethics and health care ethics consultation to help recognize ethical conflict and minimize resultant moral distress in you and your staff.

ETHICAL CONCERNS ABOUT VETERINARY PALLIATIVE AND HOSPICE CARE

As a bioethicist and practitioner, I have spent a lot of time thinking about the ethical implications of palliative and hospice type care for nonhuman patients. Although provision of pain relief and reduction in suffering seems at first glance like a clearly positive intervention, it does raise difficult questions. Most of my concerns surround the ethical defensibility of this kind of care in patients who cannot clearly communicate their wishes, who may be distressed simply by these interventions, and in whom euthanasia is a legal and culturally acceptable option. Of course, that discussion is outside the scope of this article, but a few issues have crept into the design and practice of the service and how I communicate with families. Those include:

- A lack of clear distinction between whether and when we prioritize a patient's needs over the families' needs or wishes. Although this is not often a conflict, it does sometimes erupt, particularly when dealing with requests for nonbeneficial (futile) interventions.
- Conflict over proxy decision making by families stemming from the difference between what a client (or colleague) believes is in the patient's best interest and what the patient might decide for herself. Although most clients do not make a distinction between these two types of proxy decision making, we, as our patient's advocates, often do.
- Lack of widespread availability of at-home care that greatly hampers ability of caregivers to provide adequate care round the clock.
- The reality that veterinary medicine simply does not have the professional infrastructure of home hospice care that exists for people. Because of this lack of availability (and client's lack of understanding about this) we may not be able to adequately manage suffering at home and euthanasia may be a better option earlier than families want it to be.
- No clear humane end point and no "standard of care" outside check on level of intervention at the end of life.

I think we are entering a phase of veterinary medicine where profession-wide conversations about these kinds of issues are ensuing. I hope we work together to define professional ethics for these issues that would provide needed support to all of us.

ACKNOWLEDGMENTS

L. Moses: The development of the Pain and Palliative Care Service at the MSPCA hospital Angell Animal Medical Center (formerly Angell Memorial) was an organic and personal process, inextricably linked with my own professional and intellectual development. Because of that history this article is written as a first-person, narrative account, part how-to and part memoir. Despite the conversational and informal construct of this report, I hope that it provides practical ideas and cautions for veterinary professionals who bring their own passion to advancing palliative care ideals in veterinary medicine. Those well versed in palliative and hospice principals may recognize this article as fitting the category of "legacy work." The hard work of palliative medicine is of great consequence to patients and ultimately so rewarding that I hope many others will share it with me.

Current Topics in Serious Illness and Palliative Medicine
A Curricular Initiative in a US Veterinary Teaching Institution

Katherine J. Goldberg, DVM, LMSW[a,b,c],*

KEYWORDS

- Palliative care • Palliative medicine • Hospice • Goals of care
- End-of-life education • Palliative care training • Veterinary college
- Entrustable professional activity (EPA)

KEY POINTS

- The veterinary profession has much to gain from the history, experience, and knowledge of the human palliative medicine field.
- Core competencies, curricular milestones, and scope of practice for palliative medicine have been identified, with significant overlap between human and veterinary applications.
- A formal palliative care intervention has been implemented in a US veterinary teaching institution.
- Development of rigorous palliative medicine training by veterinary teaching institutions is the keystone for quality advancement of palliative care within the veterinary profession.

A volume such as this one invites the question, What is the current state of palliative care training within the veterinary profession? Although veterinarians historically have provided many of the defining elements of palliative care, establishment of palliative care (and hospice) as a distinct area of veterinary practice is a recent phenomenon.[1] Palliative care is not yet established as a formal discipline within veterinary medicine; however, principles and philosophy of care are identical to those in human medicine, where training programs and corresponding scholarly literature do exist. Many veterinarians in both primary care and specialty practice are already providing palliative

Disclosure Statement: The author has nothing to disclose.
[a] Whole Animal Veterinary Geriatrics and Palliative Care Services, Ithaca, NY, USA; [b] Cornell Health, Counseling and Psychological Services, Ithaca, NY, USA; [c] University of Tennessee Veterinary Social Work Certificate Program, Knoxville, TN, USA
* Counseling and Psychological Services, Cornell Health, Cornell University, 110 Ho Plaza, Ithaca, NY 1453
E-mail address: info@wholeanimalvet.com

care on a regular basis to patients and clients and may choose to further develop this area of practice. Others are cultivating independent practices or services within larger hospital systems dedicated solely to palliative care. As such, professional veterinary organizations, veterinary teaching institutions, and accrediting veterinary organizations stand to benefit from the history and knowledge that the human palliative medicine field offers.

This article aims to first highlight the scope of practice, core competencies, and curricular objectives of hospice and palliative medicine (HPM) as identified by the Accreditation Council for Graduate Medical Education (ACGME) and the American Academy of Hospice and Palliative Medicine (AAHPM). Readers are encouraged to peruse these items with an eye toward educational content areas that are relevant for veterinary medicine and opportunities for cross-pollination between the human and veterinary medical professions. Next, a curricular intervention within a US veterinary teaching institution is described.

DEFINITIONS, SCOPE, AND COMPETENCIES
Definitions

Palliative care, which may be provided to patients of any age, at any time over the course of an illness, is a growing medical specialty that attends to suffering resulting from both serious illness and its treatment. It provides expert pain and symptom relief as well as emotional support and helps navigate the health care system for patients and families. Hospice is a specialized form of palliative care that regards death as a natural process, prioritizes comfort and quality of life over quantity of life as death draws near, and supports the cultural and spiritual aspects of dying. Hospice, simply defined, is palliative care at the end of life. The term, *palliative medicine*, may be used to describe the medical aspects of care provided by licensed medical professionals, whereas *palliative care* typically describes the full complement of interdisciplinary services provided to patients and families. Board certification for human physicians is in HPM; the AAHPM is the professional organization that serves to engage and support physicians practicing HPM.

Scope

The ACGME states the following:

- "The subspecialty of hospice and palliative medicine represents the medical component of the broad therapeutic model known as palliative care. These subspecialists seek to reduce the burden of serious illness by supporting the best quality of life throughout the course of a disease, and by managing factors that contribute to the suffering of the patient and the patient's family."[2]
- "The major clinical skills central to the subspecialty of hospice and palliative medicine are the prevention (when possible), assessment and management of physical, psychological, and spiritual suffering faced by patients with serious illness and their families."[2]

HPM is distinguished from other disciplines by[2]

- A high level of expertise in addressing the many needs of patients with serious illnesses, including skills in symptom-control interventions
- A high level of expertise in both clinical and nonclinical issues related to serious illness, the dying process, and bereavement
- A commitment to an interdisciplinary team approach
- A focus on the patient and family as the unit of care

Competencies

Core competencies, entrustable professional activities (EPAs), and curricular milestones (CMs) in HPM have been comprehensively developed and outlined by the HPM Competencies Project work group (2009) and the HPM CMs/EPAs work group (2015 and 2018), respectively. Detailed distinctions between competencies, EPAs, and CMs in HPM are beyond the scope of this article. Briefly, HPM core competencies are outlined in the 2009 report, version 2.3.[3] HPM EPAs were first outlined by the 2015 work group, each with a detailed description and corresponding list of specific "knowledge, skills and attitudes," which must be demonstrated to fulfill the EPA.[4] CMs are informed by EPAs and core competencies. CMs are "organized as thematically based teachable units"[5] in the 2018 report. Examples of CMs include[5] comprehensive whole-patient assessment, fundamental communication skills for attending to emotion, knowledge of serious and complex illness, and ethics of serious illness. The work group states, "These 22 CMs are a recommended tool to strengthen your program and support a shared curricular structure across the country."[5] The CMs are divided into 4 organizing categories: (1) patient care, (2) communication, (3) HPM processes, and (4) professional development.[5] Within the 2018 report is a detailed list of competencies and actions for each CM. For example,

Category: patient care

CM #2: comprehensive whole-patient assessment[5]
  A. Assess pain and nonpain symptoms
  B. Assess decisional capacity and/or developmental stage (eg, cognitive, behavioral, or emotional)
  C. Identify cultural values as they relate to care
  D. Identify supports and stressors (eg, psychological, psychiatric, spiritual, social, and financial)

CMs share significant overlap with EPAs. EPAs for HPM are shown in **Table 1**. Note that the EPAs are listed in broad category form in **Table 1**, rather than comprehensively. For example, EPA #7: prevent and mediate conflict and distress over complex medical decisions, is listed as "mediate conflict." The detailed description of EPA #7 is as follows: HPM physicians prevent and address clinical conflict, uncertainty, emotionally charged encounters, and value-laden suffering through advanced palliative communication techniques.[4] A list of 18 specific items for EPA #7 categorized

Table 1
Hospice and palliative medicine entrustable professional activities (broad categories)

• Pain management	• Care for the imminently dying
• Nonpain symptoms	• Requests for hastened death
• Emergencies	• Spiritual/existential support
• Prognosis	• Self-care and resilience
• Goals of care	• Transitions across continuum
• Interdisciplinary team	• Hospice medical director
• Mediate conflict	• HPM consultation
• Advanced life-sustaining therapies	• Promote and teach HPM

Data from American Academy of Hospice and Palliative Medicine. Hospice and palliative medicine curricular milestones. Available at: http://aahpm.org/uploads/HPM_Curricular_Milestones.pdf. Accessed February 17, 2019.

into "knowledge, skills and attitudes" follows this description in the original (2015) report. Readers are encouraged to examine the primary source documents for a deeper understanding of HPM structure and concepts within human medicine.

Given veterinarians' frequent encounters with serious illness and death and facilitated death via euthanasia, plus the complex ethical and legal terrain of a veterinarian-client-patient relationship, the veterinary profession is uniquely positioned to benefit from formal palliative care education. Conceptualizing educational initiatives and curricular development from a competency-based EPA and/or thematic framework is consistent with not only HPM education in human medicine but also the Association of American Veterinary Medical Colleges' recent adoption of competency-based education within the veterinary profession.[6] Corresponding EPAs for HPM in veterinary practice are shown in **Table 2**. There is significant overlap with the AAHPM EPAs in **Table 1**. The differences that exist are primarily related to the availability of legal euthanasia for veterinary patients and the veterinarian-client-patient relationship.

These categories as well as additional palliative care topics and objectives for veterinary settings are shared by this author in the spirit of the 2018 HPM CMs/EPA work group, discussed previously, "as a recommended tool to strengthen your program and support a shared curricular structure."

PALLIATIVE MEDICINE TRAINING IN A US VETERINARY COLLEGE
Description

An elective curricular intervention was developed to attend to the needs of seriously ill animals and their human caregivers. To this author's knowledge, it is the only formal palliative care training offered within a US veterinary teaching institution. Curated in accordance with human palliative medicine principles and corresponding competencies and EPAs, the course addresses current the state of the art in serious illness and end-of-life care for companion animals, explores goal-directed communication tools, and tackles several key questions, such as

- How do veterinarians ethically and effectively engage with clients facing the challenges of aging and dying pets?
- How can veterinarians prepare for the issues surrounding prolongation of life versus purposeful ending of it?
- How do veterinarians understand biomedical ethics, aid-in-dying legislation, and the intersection of human and veterinary paradigms of "medicalized" death?

Table 2
Hospice and palliative medicine entrustable professional activities: veterinary medicine (broad categories)

• Pain management	• Transitions across care settings and requests for in-home death
• Nonpain symptoms	• Requests for palliated but not intentionally hastened (ie, natural) death
• Emergencies/crisis plan	• Euthanasia
• Prognosis	• Client support: psychosocial-spiritual and cultural humility
• Goals of care	• Self-care and resilience
• Conflict management	• After-death care and bereavement support
• Life-sustaining therapies, futility, ethical dilemmas	• Interdisciplinary team: veterinary nurses, licensed mental health professionals, other

- How do veterinarians' social locations in terms of race, class, gender, sexuality, age, religion, and (dis)ability affect the way they view problems and solutions?

The course uses lecture material, in-class exercises, online discussion boards, video clips, and full-length documentary film. Reading material is from both human and veterinary medical literature as well as current news media. The following is a representative list of course topics:

- Palliative care principles and practice
- Palliative care assessment and planning
- Preferred place of death
- Hospice in veterinary medicine
- End-of-life ethics and ethical conflict
- Aid-in-dying legislation
- Capital punishment
- Euthanasia technique and pharmacology
- Euthanasia planning and communication
- Objections to euthanasia
- Palliative sedation
- Navigating requests for natural death
- Serious illness communication/goals of care conversations
- Animal-related grief and bereavement
- End-of-life considerations in the emergency room
- Compassion fatigue, moral distress, and burnout
- Veterinarian well-being and serious illness care, self-care planning

After the course, participants are equipped to engage in discussions currently reshaping the landscape of both human and veterinary medicine.

Evaluation

Course participants are surveyed to assess veterinary students' feelings regarding end-of-life issues within the veterinary profession and potential impact of a palliative care educational intervention. All participants are fourth-year veterinary students who took the course immediately prior to graduation and had already completed their clinic rotations. Course content is divided into 6 main categories for the purposes of evaluation:

1. Serious illness conversation/end-of-life communication skills
2. Palliative care principles
3. Euthanasia technique
4. Navigating ritual, aftercare, and/or unique pet death requests
5. Strategies for addressing ethical conflict
6. Addressing own well-being and self-care

Two additional categories were surveyed for the 2018 cohort: euthanasia decision making (in addition to technique) and understanding diverse beliefs regarding death and dying (in addition to navigating ritual and client pet death requests). In all categories, significant improvement in knowledge, skills, and/or ability was reported after the course.

For example, prior to the course, on a scale of 1 (insufficiently prepared) to 5 (sufficiently prepared), 65.2% of 2018 course participants reported 1s and 2s and 21.7% reported 3s (neutral) in response to the statement, "I have an understanding of multiple euthanasia technique options and can utilize them appropriately for my patients." After the course, 87% of participants reported 4s and 5s and 8.7% reported 3s (neutral).

Similar outcomes were reported by the 2017 cohort, in which 82.4% of course participants reported 1s and 2s and 11.8% reported 3s (neutral) in response to the same question prior to the course. After the course, 88.2% of the 2017 cohort reported 4s and 5s and 11.8% reported 3s.

Prior to the course, on a scale of 1 (insufficiently prepared) to 5 (sufficiently prepared), 52.1% of 2018 course participants reported 1s and 2s, and 34.8% reported 3s (neutral) in response to the statement, "I can conduct a Goals of Care conversation in order to help guide treatment of a patient." After the course, 82.6% of participants reported 4s and 5s and 17.4% reported 3s (neutral). Similar outcomes were reported by the 2017 cohort, in which 82.4% of course participants reported 1s and 2s and 17.6% reported 3s (neutral) in response to the same question prior to the course. After the course, 100% of the 2017 cohort reported 4s and 5s.

These examples are included to provide context for the conclusion that formal palliative care training is an effective intervention for veterinary students. Additionally, euthanasia technique data are included to highlight the limited preparedness with which new veterinary graduates enter the profession with regard to euthanasia. Further research is needed to determine the generalizability of these data across veterinary teaching institutions. In the absence of their palliative care course, however, most of these students would be graduating without sufficient knowledge of or comfort with the euthanasia procedure. There is currently a postgraduate opportunity for training and additional certification in companion animal euthanasia.[7] Euthanasia is a fundamental procedure for veterinarians and should not require an elective course or for-profit certification beyond a veterinary degree to achieve competency. Veterinary colleges have an obligation to prepare their graduates for this hallmark responsibility of the profession.

To further assess value of the course related to expectations of new graduates, the 2017 cohort was surveyed at 7 months and 12 months after graduation; 100% of respondents at both time points surveyed agreed that they used knowledge gained in the palliative care course since graduation. At 12 months after graduation, 30.8% of respondents stated that they used knowledge gained in the palliative care course "every day," 23.1% responded "most days," 23.1% responded "weekly," 15.4% responded "monthly," and 7.7% responded "multiple times per week." All 6 of the main content categories listed previously were indicated as used in the 12 months since graduation. In response to the question, "Which of the following course content did you utilize MOST OFTEN in your first year following graduation from veterinary school?" 69.2% responded "serious illness conversation/end-of-life communication"; 23.1% responded "euthanasia technique"; and 7.7% responded "addressing my own wellbeing and self-care." In response to the question, "Which of the following course content did you find MOST USEFUL in your first year following graduation from veterinary school?" 92.3% responded "serious illness conversation/end-of-life communication" and 7.7% responded "euthanasia technique." These results are meaningful in 2 regards: first, they demonstrate the overwhelming importance of serious illness conversation skills for veterinary practice, and, second, it is interesting to note the distinction between "most often" and "most useful. "

Additionally, answers to the most often/most useful questions were different at 12 months than at 7 months after graduation. When surveyed 7 months after graduation, in response to the question, "Which of the following course content have you utilized MOST OFTEN since graduation from veterinary school?" 73.3% responded "serious illness conversation/end-of-life communication, "13.3% responded "strategies for addressing ethical conflict," 6.7% responded "palliative care principles," and 6.7% responded "euthanasia technique." In response to the question, "Which of the following course content have you found MOST USEFUL since graduation from veterinary school?" at the 7-month mark, 46.7% responded "serious illness conversation/end-of-life communication," 20% responded "addressing my own well-being and self-care,"13.3% responded "palliative care principles," 13.3% responded "euthanasia technique," and 6.7% responded "navigating ritual, aftercare and/or unique pet death requests."

Although serious illness conversation skills remain the most frequently used and most useful category of course content, it is interesting to note the variety of other answers at the 7-month mark. This variety may reflect the overwhelming nature of occupying the role of veterinarian ("addressing my own wellbeing and self-care") and/or specific cases that may have been emotionally demanding or uncomfortable ("strategies for addressing ethical conflict" and "navigating ritual, aftercare and/or unique pet death requests") in the first months of practice. It is likely that the importance of euthanasia technique training increased over time as the graduates euthanized larger numbers of patients.

In addition to questions related to specific course content, participants were asked how strongly they agreed or disagreed with various statements; 100% of surveyed participants in all cohorts at all time points agreed or strongly agreed with the following statements:

Serious illness care and end-of-life topics are important knowledge areas for veterinarians.

Serious illness care and end-of-life topics should be addressed in veterinary school.

I have gained knowledge from my palliative care course that I did not learn elsewhere in my veterinary education.

To assess overall impact of the course on preparation for end-of-life issues in the veterinary profession, the question, "How prepared did you/do you feel for addressing end-of-life issues in your veterinary career overall?" was asked. Results are displayed in **Figs. 1–3**.

Significance and Limitations

There are some important considerations and limitations of these particular data (and all data reported in this article, generally). First, overall numbers are low: n = 17 in 2017 and n = 23 in 2018. These numbers reflects 65.4% of registered course participants in 2017 and 88.4% of registered course participants in 2018. Because the course has an open-door policy, these numbers do not reflect participants who audited the course. Data from 2016, the first year the course was offered, are not included because the course changed substantially between 2016 and 2017 and survey questions closely correlated with course content. Broad themes and overall results of surveyed participants from 2016 were consistent with the data reported in this article. Additionally, the data are limited by their retrospective nature. The retrospective nature of the data was necessitated by alterations in course roster between initial registration, when the first precourse survey was administered (data not presented in this article, other than in **Fig. 3**), and final course roster after the add/drop period. This was a more significant issue in 2018 than 2017. Because all survey responses are anonymous, it is not possible to determine which respondents from the initial precourse survey remained registered in the course. Therefore, the postcourse survey repeated the precourse questions, which were then answered

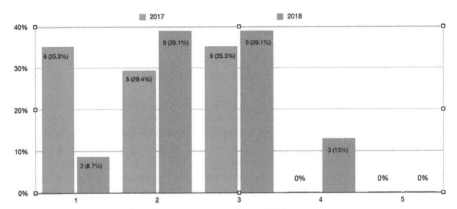

Fig. 1. Post-Course Survey Evaluation, 2017 and 2018 Cohorts.
Prior to taking your palliative care course, how prepared did you feel for addressing end of life issues in your veterinary career overall?

after respondents had completed the course. Admittedly, this is not as methodologically rigorous as is desired. The purpose of this formative data collection and rationale for discussing them, however, are to evaluate trends and assess whether an overall impression of the impact of a formal palliative care intervention may be gained. Initial results show consistent trends, and the overall impression is promising for a positive impact of formal palliative care training for veterinary professionals. A primary goal of this author and additional rationale for sharing these results are to motivate others to develop palliative care curricula in veterinary teaching institutions, guided by ACGME and AAHPM competencies and EPAs as well as the veterinary HPM EPAs listed in **Table 2**.

Fig. 3 is included for several reasons. First, the n = 46, which is 46.9% of the graduating doctor of veterinary medicine (DVM) class, demonstrating a high level of interest in this topic area. The initial roster was 57 students, or 58% of the class. There was significant attrition due to scheduling and other issues, which continued after the add/drop period (recall that the palliative care course is elective), but these initial numbers are significant. Course enrollment has increased steadily each year of the

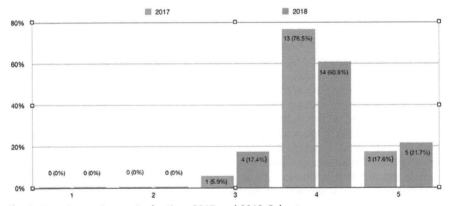

Fig. 2. Post-Course Survey Evaluation, 2017 and 2018 Cohorts.
Following your palliative care course, how prepared do you feel for addressing end of life issues in your veterinary career overall?

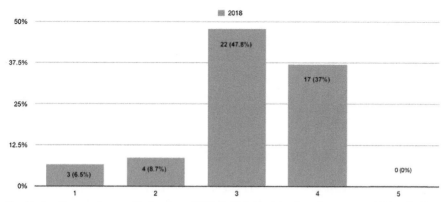

Fig. 3. Pre-Course Survey Evaluation, 2018 Initial Registration (prior to add/drop). Note difference in retrospective assessment of pre-course preparation from those who completed the course, in **Fig. 1**.

How prepared do you feel for addressing end of life issues in your veterinary career overall?

course. This author's belief is that "if you build it, they will come" is an apt philosophy for palliative care education. Experience in human palliative care education, current trends in health care for the aging baby-boomer population, and broad attention to end-of-life issues in the news media and lay literature bear this out.[8–14]

Of additional importance is the distribution of responses in **Fig. 3**. Respondents expressed a higher level of preparation than either of the other cohorts in addressing end-of-life topics, with 37% reporting 4s or 5s prior to the course compared with 13% of respondents who completed the course in 2018 (and 0% of respondents who completed the course in 2017). Due to the anonymity of responses, it is impossible to know which of these initial respondents continued in the course and are included in the final 2018 survey data. It is possible that the reported higher level of preparation pre-course in 2018 reflects an example of illusory superiority, or "not knowing what you don't know," in that prior to taking a palliative care course respondents overestimate their level of knowledge, recognizing deficits only after being exposed to new learning material. Regardless, even if 37% of respondents were sufficiently prepared and competent in end-of-life care delivery prior to the course, 63% reported that they were not. The total number of respondents representing 46.9% of the graduating DVM class of 2018 means that, in the absence of a palliative care course, 29.5% of the class would be graduating ill-prepared for addressing end-of-life issues in the veterinary profession. Given the considerable amount of death, end-of-life stressors, and high frequency of ethical conflict faced by veterinarians,[15–19] this is concerning.

Overall, the survey data reflect significant potential for integration of formal palliative care training into veterinary teaching institutions to have a positive impact on serious illness and end-of-life care delivery of veterinarians as well as veterinarian well-being and ability to cope with the emotional demands of the profession; 91.3% of respondents in 2018 and 88.2% of respondents in 2017 agreed or strongly agreed with the statement, " Having an opportunity to explore my feelings regarding serious illness and end-of-life care is important for my wellbeing as a veterinarian; 84.6% of the 2017 cohort, surveyed 12 months after graduation, agreed or strongly agreed with the statement, "I believe that my palliative care course helped me cope with the emotional demands of the profession in the first year following graduation from veterinary school." Physician well-being related to care of the seriously ill has been examined.[20–25] Self-awareness, self-care, and resilience are all CMs within HPM for physicians. Scholarly attention to the impact of serious illness and end-of-life care on well-being characteristics of veterinarians is warranted.

Free-text survey responses as well as informal feedback from course participants further support the data shared in this article. For example,

I am so much more comfortable talking about goals of care than I was. It was also just amazing to have a forum where we could discuss euthanasia at all because we never discuss it in school.

The palliative care class has been the most helpful thing for me in my internship.

I felt incredibly unprepared to guide people through quality of life/end-of-life discussions and I had very limited exposure to performing euthanasia. This course gave me a lot more options so I can feel more confident...I think that confidence will allow me to devote more energy and attention to the patient/client care in every euthanasia for the rest of my career.

I don't know how I could handle so many difficult conversations with clients in my first 6 months of practice without this class.

The best part of the palliative care course was getting practical advice and best practice recommendations for supporting clients a their pets through difficult end-of-life discussions and palliative care. Nothing else in the curriculum comes close.

Implementation and Considerations

The course described in this article is by no means the only way to implement palliative care training into veterinary education. Each institution has its own curricular format, schedule, strengths, and limitations for integrating this material as well as policy and procedural issues to consider. The aim of this article is to present an example of something that has been implemented, in the hopes of inspiring additional efforts. Preliminary evaluative data are positive but merely lay the groundwork. Most important to this author is that formal palliative medicine training is integrated into the veterinary profession with rigor. This is essential if HPM is to be respected as a legitimate and valued area of contemporary veterinary practice. Although HPM is not currently recognized as a specialized field of veterinary medicine, establishment of training programs and building a base of scientific knowledge re requisite for such efforts in the future.[26]

It is useful to consider that HPM in human medicine was not recognized as a subspecialty by the American Board of Medical Specialties (ABMS) until 2006 and the American Osteopathic Association in 2007. Prior to 2006, the American Board of Hospice and Palliative Medicine (ABHPM) administered board certification to more than 2000 physicians practicing HPM, but ABHPM was not recognized by the ABMS.[27] The first ABMS-recognized board examination was administered in 2008. As of 2014, physicians are required to complete a 12-month ACGME-accredited fellowship in HPM to be eligible to take the examination.[28] Two important lessons emerge for the veterinary profession from this history. First, HPM is a young medical specialty. Medical advances and scholarly research, public policy, legal cases, and years of clinical practice all preceded formal recognition of HPM as an area of specialized care. In this regard, veterinary medicine has a long way to go before American Veterinary Medical Association (AVMA) recognition can reasonably be conferred. HPM has not yet advanced to this level, and this author believes it is wise to focus on more attainable curricular interventions, such as the one introduced in this article. Second, training programs (fellowships) are essential for board certification. This points to the importance of developing clinical training programs in HPM. This is an important step in moving HPM forward within the veterinary profession over the long term. All manner of continuing education may develop online through nonacademic organizations but, without supervised experiential learning and content that is subject to peer review, there are inherent limits to this type of program. Similarly, all classroom-based palliative care initiatives need a clinical component for learners to be able to put content into practice.

FUTURE DIRECTIONS

If the trajectory of HPM in human medicine is any indication, the future is bright for HPM in the veterinary profession. Public perception, media attention, and popular cultural interest around end-of-life issues as well as evolving human-animal relationships and the growth of specialty veterinary care will eventually demand formal palliative care services along with the standard complement of cardiology, neurology, surgery, and other board certified specialties. The question remains, How will veterinary teaching institutions respond to this momentum? Palliative care content may be integrated into areas of veterinary college curricula that are preexisting as well as introduced as stand-alone initiatives in both the preclinical and clinical settings. This is the first step. Once exposed to palliative care in veterinary school, where will veterinarians go to continue their training? A proverbial chicken-or-egg dilemma ensues, with the American Board of Veterinary Specialties stating, "There must be evidence that facilities and programs are available for advanced training of veterinarians that will lead to certification in the veterinary specialty."[26] If there are no advanced training programs, there is little motivation for development of veterinary college curricula and little development of potential trainees. Without trainees and assurance that a program will be successful, how can one be developed? It may be comforting to palliative care pioneers in the veterinary profession to know they are not alone; similar institutional barriers existed in human medicine, but they did not prevail. Baumrucker[29] asserts,

> Graduate education in palliative care presents a Catch-22 for both programs and trainees alike. Palliative care will not become a certified specialty until there are residents and fellows training in graduate education, but residents, fellows, and medical schools would be quite correct in fearing to commit to a program that was not already a certified specialty. Therefore, either palliative care must lift itself up by its bootstraps, or some residents and training programs must show some courage and commitment and open programs despite having a questionable "official" future.[29]

The growth of HPM since 2002 has been nothing short of remarkable. There are now more than 7600 physicians certified in specialty-level HPM and 140 ACGME-accredited fellowship programs as of academic year 2018 to 2019.[28,30] The details of this exponential growth is beyond the scope of this article; however, one strategy this author believes would be wise to emulate in the veterinary profession is the adoption of HPM as a subspecialty. As a subspecialty, HPM is cosponsored by other ABMS specialties (currently there are 10 that support HPM). This creates an inherent and inextricable link between established specialties and HPM, the benefits of which cannot be overstated. Pursuit of a similar relationship within the American Board of Veterinary Specialties in the veterinary profession is worth considering.

Certainly, much progress is still to be made in the basic foundations of veterinary college curricula with regard to serious illness and palliative care; establishment of

HPM as a specialty within the veterinary profession is not the subject of this article nor is it the most urgent initiative for veterinary HPM, in this author's view. No discussion of future directions is complete, however, without mention of this as a possible long-term goal—if not to motivate its pursuit then to caution against doing so hastily.

SUMMARY

Although interest in hospice and palliative care for companion animals is on the rise, formal training in these areas has been extremely limited. Veterinary medicine has much to gain from the history, experience, and knowledge of the human palliative medicine field. Significant overlap exists between human and veterinary applications of HPM competencies, EPAs, and CMs. A formal palliative care intervention has been implemented in a US veterinary teaching institution and is introduced in this article. Preliminary evaluation data reflect significant potential for integration of formal palliative care training into veterinary teaching institutions to have a positive impact on serious illness and end-of-life care delivery of veterinarians. Positive outcomes for veterinarian well-being and ability to cope with the emotional demands of the profession are also suggested. Veterinary students are hungry for this content and have reported positive impacts from palliative care training on their experiences postgraduation. Significant opportunities exist for veterinary teaching institutions to contribute to scientifically rigorous growth of palliative medicine, supporting human-animal relationships in meaningful ways.

REFERENCES

1. Goldberg KJ. Veterinary hospice and palliative care: a comprehensive review of the literature. Vet Rec 2016;178(15):369–74.
2. Acgme. ACGME Program Requirements for Graduate Medical Education in Hospice and Palliative Medicine (Anesthesiology, Family Medicine, Internal Medicine, Pediatrics, Psychiatry, or Radiation Oncology). Available at: https://www.acgme.org/Portals/0/PFAssets/ProgramRequirements/540HospicePalliativeMedicine1YR2018.pdf?ver=2018-02-16-083923-063. Accessed February 17, 2019.
3. Arnold R, Billings J, Block S, et al. Hospice and palliative medicine core competencies version 2.3 2009. Available at: http://aahpm.org/uploads/education/competencies/Competencies%20v.%202.3.pdf. Accessed February 17, 2019.
4. Morrison L, Landzaat L, Barnett M, et al. Hospice and palliative medicine entrustable professional activities. Chicago: American Academy of Hospice and Palliative Medicine; 2015. Available at: http://aahpm.org/uploads/HPM_EPAs_Final_110315.pdf. Accessed February 17, 2019.
5. Gustin J, Landzaat L, Barnett M, et al. Hospice and palliative medicine curricular milestones 2018. Available at: http://aahpm.org/uploads/HPM_Curricular_Milestones.pdf. Accessed February 17, 2019.
6. Molgaard L, Hodgson J, Bok H, et al. Competency-based veterinary education: part 2 - entrustable professional activities. Washington, DC: Association of American Veterinary Medical Colleges; 2018. Available at: https://www.aavmc.org/assets/site_18/files/cbve-publication-1-framework.pdf. Accessed February 17, 2019.
7. Companion Animal Euthanasia Training Academy. 2018. Available at: https://caetainternational.com/. Accessed August 9, 2018.
8. Block SD. Medical education in end-of-life care: the status of reform. J Palliat Med 2002;5(2):243–8.

9. Saft HL, Richman PS, Berman AR, et al. Impact of critical care medicine training programs' palliative care education and bedside tools on ICU use at the end of life. J Grad Med Educ 2014;6(1):44–9.

10. Sullivan AM, Lakoma MD, Block SD. The status of medical education in end-of-life care. J Gen Intern Med 2003;18(9):685–95.

11. Wiener L, Weaver MS, Bell CJ, et al. Threading the cloak: palliative care education for care providers of adolescents and young adults with cancer. Clin Oncol Adolesc Young Adults 2015;5:1–18.

12. Grant M, Elk R, Ferrell B, et al. Current status of palliative care–clinical implementation, education, and research. CA Cancer J Clin 2009;59(5):327–35.

13. Moroni M, Bolognesi D, Muciarelli PA, et al. Investment of palliative medicine in bridging the gap with academia: a call to action. Eur J Cancer 2011;47(4): 491–5.

14. Buss MK, Lessen DS, Sullivan AM, et al. Hematology/oncology fellows' training in palliative care. Cancer 2011;117(18):4304–11.

15. Hart LA, Hart BL. Grief and stress from so many animal deaths. Companion Anim Pract 1987;1:20–1.

16. Batchelor CEM, McKeegan DEF. Survey of the frequency and perceived stressfulness of ethical dilemmas encountered in UK veterinary practice. Vet Rec 2012;170(1):19.

17. Rosoff PM, Ruderman R, Moga J, et al. Response to Open Peer Commentaries on "Resolving ethical dilemmas in a tertiary care veterinary specialty hospital: adaptation of the human clinical consultation committee model". Am J Bioeth 2018; 18(2):W7–10.

18. Moses L. Another experience in resolving veterinary ethical dilemmas: observations from a veterinarian performing ethics consultation. Am J Bioeth 2018; 18(2):67–9.

19. Dickinson GE, Roof PD, Roof KW. A survey of veterinarians in the US: euthanasia and other end-of-life issues. Anthrozoos 2011;24(2):167–74.

20. Meier DE, Back AI, Morrison RS. The inner lifeof physicians and care of the seriously ill. JAMA 2001;286(23):3007–14.

21. Smith L, Hough CL. Using death rounds to improve end-of-life education for internal medicine residents. J Palliat Med 2011;14(1):55–8.

22. Bernacki RE, Hutchings M, Vick J, et al. Development of the Serious Illness Care Program: a randomised controlled trial of a palliative care communication intervention. BMJ Open 2015;5(10):e009032.

23. Rourke MT. Compassion fatigue in pediatric palliative care providers. Pediatr Clin North Am 2007;54(5):631–44, x.

24. Sanchez-Reilly S, Morrison LJ, Carey E, et al. Caring for oneself to care for others: physicians and their self-care. J Support Oncol 2013;11(2):75–81.

25. Rothman MD, Gugliucci MR. End-of-life care curricula in undergraduate medical education: a comparison of allopathic and osteopathic medical schools. Am J Hosp Palliat Care 2008;25(5):354–60.

26. AVMA. ABVS - Standards for the Recognition of Veterinary Specialty Organizations. 2017. Available at: https://www.avma.org/ProfessionalDevelopment/Education/Specialties/Pages/abvs-policies-ii.aspx. Accessed August 11, 2018.

27. NHPCO. Physician board certification in hospice and palliative medicine (HPM) 2006. Available at: https://www.nhpco.org/sites/default/files/public/quality/physician-board-certification-fact-sheet.pdf. Accessed February 17, 2019.

28. AAHPM. HPM Subspecialty certification | AAHPM. Available at: http://aahpm.org/certification/subspecialty-certification. Accessed August 11, 2018.

29. Baumrucker S. The ABMS, the ABHPM, and the future of a specialty. Am J Hosp Palliat Care 2002;19(4):225–7.

30. Accreditation Council for Graduate Medical Education. Hospice and palliative medicine (multidisciplinary) programs 2018. Available at: https://apps.acgme.org/ads/Public/Programs/Search?stateId=&specialtyId=153&specialtyCategoryTypeId=&numCode=&city=. Accessed February 17, 2019.

Section II: Concepts and Essential Viewpoints

Overcoming Obstacles to Palliative Care

Lessons to Learn from Our Physician Counterparts

Lisa Moses, VMD[a,b,c],*

KEYWORDS

- Veterinary palliative care • Obstacles to palliative care
- Development of palliative care • Integrating veterinary palliative care

KEY POINTS

- Pioneering palliative care physicians faced similar obstacles to veterinarians currently working to develop the field.
- Interviews and a literature review identified a wide array of suggestions for veterinary palliative care, ranging from highly practical to conceptual.
- Interviewed pioneers recommended strategic planning to grow the field of palliative care that includes defining the mission and existing problems, classifying obstacles, and building alliances to help integrate palliative care with other veterinary specialties.

INTRODUCTION

Chances are, if you are reading this, you have some investment in the expansion of palliative care in veterinary medicine. You may be well aware of various obstacles blocking that road, such as negative connotations to the phrase "palliative care" or difficulties in generation of revenue for this kind of work. Our physician counterparts have more than 25 years of experience with similar obstacles, although there are important differences in our work.[1] The goal of this article was to identify current systemic, professional, and personal obstacles and use the collective wisdom of palliative care physicians and other professionals to help us solve these problems. This investigation was done using both a literature review and interviews with pioneers and well-known experts in the field of palliative care for human patients. All of the participants

The author has nothing to disclose.
[a] Pain and Palliative Care Service, MSPCA-Angell Animal Medical Center, Boston, MA, USA; [b] Center for Bioethics, Harvard Medical School, Boston, MA, USA; [c] Yale Center for Interdisciplinary Bioethics, New Haven, CT, USA
* Pain and Palliative Care Service, MSPCA-Angell Animal Medical Center, Boston, MA.
E-mail address: lisa_moses@hms.harvard.edu

in this interview research generously gave their time and graciously shared their wisdom for the benefit of our profession.

HISTORICAL CONTEXT

"Palliative care" was a phrase applied first in 1974 by a surgical oncologist in Montreal, hoping to avoid the negative connotations of hospice for French-speaking patients (in France "hospice" had associations different from contemporary meanings).[2] The emergence of palliative medicine in the United States, as a separate and different subspecialty than hospice, did not happen until the 1990s. This rise was catalyzed by the National Institutes of Health analysis, *Approaching Death: Improving Care at the End of Life–A Report of the Institute of Medicine* and a private venture, called *The Project on Death in America* (PDIA).[1,3] The PDIA investigation, originally conceived of and funded by the philanthropist George Soros, brought together professionals from medicine, public policy, law, and social science. The project mapped out a defined strategy to improve care at the end of life for all Americans and granted funding to specific projects that accomplished this aim.[1,2,4] According to PDIA founding member and palliative care pioneer Susan Dale Block, MD, the creation of a strategic plan that assessed what was wrong with end-of-life care and charted a course to change both culture and policy was fundamental to the successful expansion of palliative care (oral communication, 2018). Dr Block credits strategic planning for the growth in the field, but she cautions that it took 25 to 30 years to actually change attitudes (oral communication, 2018). Her advice: be patient! Palliative care is now struggling with such broad acceptance of its importance in good health care that a recent estimate lists the workforce at approximately 11% of what is needed in the United States.[5] There is intense research and written commentary devoted to managing the growing crisis of scarcity in palliative services.[4–7] Veterinary medicine requires cultural shifts and acquisition of knowledge before we face major issues about models of delivery and scarcity. Hopefully our efforts to grow palliative care will progress until demand for services becomes a problem to be solved.

IS THERE A NEED FOR VETERINARY PALLIATIVE CARE?

Before identifying obstacles, we need a cultural and professional consensus, or at least discussion, about what the goals of veterinary palliative care are and what problem(s) we are trying to solve. For example, the reasons for the development of one hospital-based palliative care service were 2 interrelated concerns: inadequate symptom management, and inconsistent communication for persons nearing death. The consensus was that both concerns resulted in the continuation of burdensome, costly, and ineffective treatments at the end of life.[8] During the development of human palliative care there was a broad medical and cultural consensus that end-of-life care for people was in need of reform at all levels.[3,9,10] In the 1990s, the medical profession was coming to the conclusion that physicians were providing expensive and invasive care at the end of life that they would not choose for themselves.[11] The American public was also realizing that a prolonged death in the hospital was not what most people wanted, yet rarely were options for the end of life discussed before death was imminent.[10] An intriguing idea is that palliative care medicine and services arose, at least partially, from the unmet needs of physicians and other clinicians in dealing with difficult family situations, not from poor pain and symptom control (David Doolittle, oral communication, 2018). Indeed, it is still often the case that palliative care services are not requested unless there are psychosocial or physical needs that the current clinical team feels they cannot manage.[12] We, in the veterinary profession, have barely begun to have widespread public discussions about what end-of-life care for animals should ideally be and whether we want to avoid the pitfalls of human health care at the end of life. The veterinary conflict between whether the needs of the client prevail sometimes or always over the needs of the patient adds a layer of complexity to untangling the motivation for growing this field. Consideration of the changing moral and social status of animals and veterinary medical success at prolonging life with chronic disease will help answer the question of what problem are we trying to solve.

STRATEGIC PLANNING: IDENTIFYING AND CLASSIFYING OBSTACLES

Dr Susan Block recommended that we start strategic planning by identifying a small number of like-minded, academic oriented professionals to form a core group (oral communication, 2018). She detailed a procedure for strategic planning that worked for palliative care:

- "Test the waters" to see what level of interest there is in a shared goal of advancing the standard of practice. Nearly everyone interviewed for this article mentioned that we will not be successful until there is a critical mass of veterinarians working on this goal.
- Start with conference calls to establish agenda and priorities.
- Find funding for meeting in person to map strategies.
- Study other successful fields in veterinary medicine to see how they developed and expanded. The pioneers of palliative care studied emergency medicine as it was developing at about the same time and had been very successful in expansion.
- Creating an academic community is fundamental.
- Do research and publish on the initial efforts to pull this community together and establish strategy.

She notes: "Expect that as leaders in the field you will get beaten up a bit." A mental health care professional interviewed said that as pioneers in a new field, it is important to keep on working toward your goal without focusing on how effective you are at changing culture during the genesis. She recommended maintaining faith that other people will take up the cause and contribute. She also advised accepting that you can't evaluate how effective the changes are during "a revolution" (Kate Dare-Winters, oral communication, 2018).

While strategically planning, it will be helpful to classify obstacles into patient factors, owner/client (and maybe cultural) factors, and institutional factors so that they can be addressed systematically (David Doolittle, oral communication, 2018).

Within these categories, expect the barriers to change over time. The hurdles faced by palliative medicine have substantially changed in the past 25 years. The main barriers to palliative care for people were summarized in a 2017 review as follows: lack of resources to refer to, not knowing that resources exist, ignorance regarding what palliative care is, reluctance to refer, reluctance of patient and/or family to be referred, and restrictive specialist palliative care service program eligibility criteria.[13] Veterinary palliative care, being in an earlier stage of development, can use the evolution of these obstacles to predict, and maybe change our future.

SYSTEMIC AND INSTITUTIONAL OBSTACLES

Systemic and institutional obstacles were large barriers to reforming end-of-life care for people. Some of those barriers stubbornly remain, like the US Medicare system requiring the termination of curative treatment in order to cover hospice care. Financial obstacles still remain at the top of the list for many of the professionals interviewed. All hospital-based professionals said that palliative care in the United States struggles to directly generate enough revenue to be self-sustaining and requires institutional support. The reasons for this are mostly based in the structure of third party payments in the United States and because integral members of the interdisciplinary team model cannot directly bill insurers for their services.[14] Dr Michael Spear says that he told his hospital administrators when he was hired that "he wouldn't break even" because programs are not financially sustainable on straight revenue generation (oral communication, 2018). There is a large body of literature devoted to calculating the actual (including indirect) financial benefits of palliative care via cost savings, shorter hospital stays, and referral generation.[15–17]

A less obvious institutional barrier is that hospitals did not necessarily celebrate palliative and hospice departments and there was a perception that these were "secret services" according to Joanne Wolfe (oral communication, 2018). Once it was understood that these services were focused on improving quality of life and not on death, that undercurrent of secrecy was gone and the services usage and reputation improved.

Dr Joanne Wolfe, one of the originators of pediatric palliative care, says that the growth of her field happened more organically than did adult services (oral communication, 2018). She pointed out that managing chronic illness and end-of-life care is quite different in a patient (human or not) who is near the end of the expected life span. End-of-life care for children has "an element of unnaturalness" that was an additional barrier to development compared with adult palliative care (Joanne Wolfe, oral communication, 2018). Dr Wolfe said it took 10 years for pediatric palliative care services to be fully integrated into the hospital workings. She credits word-of-mouth growth and recommends we start by working with clinicians who are receptive, rather than trying to convince those who are resistant.

THE BENEFITS OF ALLIANCE BUILDING

To change cultural and institutional attitudes, we need to convince our profession of the value of palliative care to patients, clients, and to each other. Vicki Jackson, MD, chief of the Palliative Care Division at Massachusetts General Hospital, had pointed advice about the importance of alliance building with colleagues. "Service," both to referring clinicians and patients, is a keystone value in her department. According to Dr Jackson, palliative care should aim to help other clinicians as much as helping patients and families. And, palliative clinicians should demonstrate to families that they hold referrers in high regard. "Palliative care has not done well with a 'holier than thou' attitude or when disparaging referring clinicians" (oral communication, 2018). Michael Spear, MD, counsels that as a consultant, "make it clear that you will never take the place of the primary clinician" (oral communication, 2018). Dr Joanne Wolfe, like many of the other physicians interviewed, stressed the idea of community building and the need for working very collaboratively; she says her field did this well in the early days and it paved the way for their current success (oral communication, 2018).

Mihir Kamdar, MD, director of the Cancer Pain Clinic at Massachusetts General Hospital and a palliative care specialist, is just as emphatic about the imperative to develop interprofessional relations and to show value to other clinicians (oral communication, 2018). He recommends that "being around and available" for casual consultations promotes integration of palliative care principles to skeptics. Also, avoid being oppositional and align with primary clinicians and patients. Celebrating moments with other team members when shared patients do well really helps solidify the alignment. Dr Kamdar recommends finding a champion from outside of palliative care. For example, having an oncologist speak about the value of palliative care at an oncology meeting has a much bigger impact than a palliative care outsider.

Palliative care does need to show value in ways that are visible to convince others. Dr Spear demonstrates the value of having a palliative care service by enhancing educational curriculum, performing quality consultations, facilitating a debriefing program after a patient dies, and by getting nurses and residents involved in educational parts of the program. Dr Kamdar noted that showing primary clinicians how palliative care saves their time (ie, the surgeon can do surgery and less pain management) is obviously valuable to most referrers. But, he cautions, we have to deliver on our promises; we have to prove that we can augment standard medical care. Veterinary medicine is struggling to incorporate the values of alignment and service as the rise in private specialty practice grows. It seems obvious that unless we provide real service to our peers, we will not be able to grow as a field.

THE BENEFITS AND LIMITS OF AN INTERDISCIPLINARY TEAM

For human palliative medicine, the best practice standard is considered the interdisciplinary team model (IDT).[18,19] The function of the IDT is to provide specialized support for each of the primary care domains in palliative care (usually including, at minimum, psychosocial, physical, spiritual, and end of life).[20] Compared with the standard one-on-one model of medical care, the IDT approach usually includes, at least, the medical staff, a social worker, and spiritual caregivers.[18] The IDT improves the experience of patients and families and supports team members.[19] As mentioned previously, it is difficult to generate revenue with this model, but this may be somewhat easier in veterinary medicine because most pet owners pay directly for care. Perhaps an even bigger hurdle is the durability of the traditional veterinarian-client-patient model. For various good reasons, veterinary medicine has not morphed into a fully team-based care delivery system, except in limited ways. In palliative care, a team-based approach might be an effective way to distribute the work and, more importantly, reduce the burden of emotional drain on practitioners. As Susan Block says, even with the team-based approach, the doctor usually is alone in the room with the patient or family member. Despite this, being part of a shared system provides immediate and deep support to the practitioner. Given the difficulties of practitioner sustainability in veterinary medicine, this is a powerful incentive to consider the IDT model.

MODELS OF CARE DELIVERY

In the United States, models of palliative care delivery have been markedly shaped by reimbursement systems.[21] The field originated as a hospital-based consult service, but as is true in veterinary medicine, it has been informally practiced forever.[22] The rapid rise in demand for palliative services, fueled by outcome measures showing improved quality of life and cost savings and by cultural factors like the aging of the population, have driven a search for alternative models. Outpatient services, home-based services, and combined hospice and palliative care services are being intensively studied as models that will improve access to care.[5,6,23,24] An important idea that may have relevance to veterinary palliative care is consideration of creating generalist-level and specialist-level palliative care models. Quill and Abernathy[22] put forth the idea that there are palliative care skills that all clinicians should have and those that require an additional level of knowledge. Of course, we use this model extensively in veterinary medicine and it makes sense to apply it for palliative care.

The investigators propose a list of skills that distinguish the generalist from the specialist. For example, they suggest that primary palliative care includes basic pain and symptom management and basic discussions about prognosis and goals of care. Specialty palliative care should include management of refractory pain and assistance in addressing cases of futility. Although veterinary medicine is developing palliative medicine, perhaps we could start by adopting this structure.

The other aspects of structure to consider are whether palliative care should be embedded or on-demand during the course of a case, how palliative care is integrated into the rest of medicine, and when, during the course of illness, to start providing care. There is an ongoing attempt in human palliative care to answer these questions using empirical data about which models provide better outcomes for quality of life, survival time, and even cost savings.[12,25]

MESSAGING AND THE IMPORTANCE OF CAREFUL LANGUAGE

Dr David Doolittle, a psychologist who trains palliative care fellows in communication and practitioner sustainability, reminds trainees that patients and families often interpret the arrival of the palliative care team at the bedside as the appearance of "the Angel of Death" (oral communication, 2018). Despite all of our care in defining palliative care as being about quality of life rather than death, many of our peers and clients still hold this misconception. And this impression has serious negative implications for our progress, considering how uncomfortable end-of-life discussions are for many. Dr Vicki Jackson believes that other culture changes are difficult to achieve without our peers understanding what palliative care is (oral communication, 2018). She found that joint visits to the patient with referring clinicians really helped combat the misconceptions. Dr Suzana Makowski says that health care professionals have as much misunderstanding about what palliative care is as families do. She hears it equated with "doing nothing," because some physicians consider referral to palliative care as abandonment of care. Dr Makowski suspects that these professionals do not understand what palliative care does, the complexity of it, or that it provides different care than they can offer (oral communication, 2018).

Many investigators have suggested avoiding the use of the phrase palliative care altogether and changing the name of services to avoid the negative connotations. Some providers use the phrase or service name of "symptom management" and talk of "co-management of cases with oncologists" to make it more palatable.[24] Vicki Jackson reports that the Center to Advance Palliative care (www.capc.org) did significant work on messaging language for use in discussions about palliative care. Some of the terms and phrases she includes in her discussions are "serious illness" rather than "terminal" and "....help you live as well as you can, for as long as you can." She repeatedly emphasizes that end-of-life care is a small part of this work; mostly it is about helping people live well in the face of serious illness (oral communication, 2018).

LESSONS IN COMMUNICATION

Along with careful messaging, skillful, empathetic, nonjudgmental communication is the cornerstone of good palliative care. Dr Michael Spear summed up this notion as "Goals of care conversation is what it's all about. If you don't understand what the family wants, and, if they don't understand that the trajectory of illness will be affected by their decisions, you will just keep offering options they don't want" (oral communication, 2018). Dr Suzana Makowski said that sometimes there is an ethical conflict between the care team and family, but mostly it is that care team has not learned how to present prognosis and realistic options. Her trick: "try to always NOT be the messenger." She said that the family usually knows something bad is happening and that is why they sought care. She asks the family what are they afraid of and why. The family usually ends up naming the bad news, then she can say that they are right and asks to "let me tell how I can help." This strategy puts you in the support position rather than in an adversarial role. But, she cautions, recognize that this flips the usual order of a typical hard conversation with a physician and that can be discombobulating to families.

HOW DO WE TRAIN PALLIATIVE CARE VETERINARIANS AND ADVANCE PRACTICE?

Palliative care became a recognized subspecialty in 2008, and most physicians currently working in the field completed a hospice and palliative medicine (HPM) fellowship after residency.[26] This has only recently been the case, as most palliative care physicians who have been practicing for more than 10 years originally attained board certification in other specialties and took a certifying examination for HPM before the establishment of HPM fellowship programs. Because hospice and palliative medicine is a subspecialty, physicians complete a residency in 1 of 10 cosponsoring fields before HPM fellowship and eligibility for board certification.[27] During the past 20 years, there has been debate about whether palliative care should even be a specialty of medicine.[28]

As recently as 2011, there were still fewer than 50 fellowship programs in the United States, although more than 75% of hospitals already had or were planning a palliative care service.[26] As of 2018, there were 140 accredited HPM fellowships.[29] In veterinary medicine, we need to decide whether we want to work toward palliative care (and potentially, hospice) enlarging into a true specialty, whether we want to embed palliative principals into general practice, or both. There have been some attempts to work toward a veterinary hospice and palliative care specialty college, but unlike for physicians, the veterinary effort has largely grown out of general practice and not through academic medicine or specialty colleges. The field of veterinary pain medicine/management has a prior start working through this same situation. The American College of Veterinary Anesthesia added Analgesia (ACVAA) to its name and diplomate titles around the same time that the International Veterinary Academy of Pain Management (IVAPM) was expanding into an educational organization certifying pain practitioners. Both organizations aim to raise the standard of care for pain management; however, there are still widely varying levels of pain management delivered and no consensus on who is a veterinary pain expert. Perhaps using the example of analysis of the problem and strategic planning would help the veterinary profession build agreement about whether we should emulate the example of building a subspecialty from already established board certifications.

One concern about excluding academic centers and specialty colleges from the building of this field is that a new knowledge base needs to be created to advance the practice. Multiple innovators (including Joanne Wolfe, oral communication, 2018) in human palliative care commented that a haphazard and trial-and-error approach to end-of-life care was an important obstacle to be overcome. Without advances in the *medicine* of veterinary palliative care/symptom management and evidence-based outcomes, we run the risk of a lack of credibility besides simply being unhelpful. "In order to show value, we need to be really good" [at palliative care], says Dr Kamdar. He notes that until recently, most practitioners came from other fields, did not do fellowships, and may not have the same knowledge base. He also said that 1 bad case or bad outcome can do a lot of damage to credibility. This problem occurred in palliative care, but more so in hospice medicine (Wolfe, Kamdar, oral communication, 2018). There is still some tension between the fields of human palliative medicine and hospice care separate from the institutional barriers between the fields created by Medicare reimbursement policies. Multiple physicians interviewed characterized this tension as stemming from the relatively different origins of each field; palliative medicine started as a discipline in academic medicine, whereas much of hospice care developed as a practical approach and philosophy without a research and outcomes-based approach. Hospice care was seen as "front line, nonacademic, non–evidence based" and clashed with palliative care early on (Wolfe, oral communication, 2018). Both fields are now working hard on shared goals and they share professional membership organizations. Most recently, there is serious talk about fully integrating palliative care and hospice into a single continuum of practice.[23]

Further evidence of the importance of outcomes-based research in establishing the field came from multiple mentions of seminal research by various physicians interviewed. They asserted that well-done, large-scale research changed attitudes about the value of palliative care in both their peers and the public. Two important articles were most often mentioned: the SUPPORT study (A Controlled Trial to Improve Care for Seriously Ill Hospitalized Patients) in 1995 and Early Palliative Care for Patients with Metastatic Non–Small-Cell Lung Cancer in 2010.[10,30] The SUPPORT Study, despite failing to demonstrate improved outcomes in patients with the intervention trialed, highlighted large gaps in end-of-life communications that provoked intense debate in medical and public culture. Dr Joanne Wolfe, the founder of the first pediatric palliative care service in the United States at Boston's Children's Hospital, credits the SUPPORT study as being the major impetus to examine end-of-life care for children in the United States (oral communication, 2018).

The publication of research in 2010 showing that early palliative care intervention improved survival times and quality of life in addition to reducing costs of care for patients with advanced lung cancer was considered to be a major turning point in the acceptance of palliative care.[30] One of the investigators of that research and subsequent follow-up studies, Dr Vicki Jackson, suggested that we should aim to duplicate that research in veterinary medicine to further our cause.

ADVICE ON PRACTICE PHILOSOPHY AND PRACTITIONER SUSTAINABILITY

Because many of the pioneering physicians interviewed work in leading centers of academic medicine and research, it is not surprising that they value cutting-edge medical care and outcome-based practice. Dr Susan Block characterizes good palliative medicine as being "On Beyond Zebra," referring to the Dr Seuss book about an alphabet that goes past the basic A to Z. Vicki Jackson agrees and pushes the point further. She credits her acceptance by specialists like oncologists and cardiologists to knowing enough about the therapies they prescribe to help them adjust treatment protocols to minimize adverse events. Indeed, in my own veterinary palliative care practice, it was obvious immediately that my training in internal medicine and critical care was central to being able to provide care beyond typical pain management.

In contrast to that approach and possibly more in line with the original impetus for palliative care development (ie, to reform end-of-life care), Dr Suzana Makowski characterizes most palliative care clinicians as "medical minimalists" on a continuum of intervention (oral communication, 2018). She cautions that many patients see more medicine as better, as do some physicians. A good match between where the referring clinician, patient/family, and palliative care staff are on that continuum is important. As an avid pet owner, Dr Makowski expressed concern over her perception that veterinary medicine is trending toward medical maximalism and says she chooses veterinary care based on how much alignment she has with the practitioner.

Michael Spear, MD, who started as a neonatologist/criticalist and has since created and directs a palliative care department at a children's hospital, feels strongly that he could not have done palliative care work when he was a younger and inexperienced clinician (oral communication, 2018). Because the field has only recently transitioned to being a board-certified specialty, there may be big changes in how it is practiced with a larger proportion of younger and less experienced physicians. This idea may relate to the integral role that skilled communication techniques and solid personal coping skills play in sustaining this kind of work. He also recommends that veterinary palliative care education should include training in cultural diversity and interprofessional communication, besides symptom management. Dr Wolfe argued for the importance of fellowships and, like others interviewed, suggested targeting curriculum development and building training courses as important tools for growth.

Dr Susan Block considers peer mentoring very valuable as both support and for new practice ideas. She believes that the development of fellowship programs has been really important to sustainability because it creates structured opportunities for faculty and trainees alike to support each other and to feel part of a shared system. Dr Spear considers structured debriefings an important tool for team stress management because they help make sure people do not feel alone in the work. In addition, his hospital has a tailored wellness curriculum that has been helpful for sustainability. There is a separate version for trainees and for senior physicians. Both include outside trainers in mindfulness, financial counseling, and nutrition, besides other aspects of wellness.

Dr Suzana Makowski voices a decidedly thoughtful answer when asked what advice she has for palliative care veterinarians. She says that "over the years, I've learned a lot of humility" in recognizing the definition of meaningful life is very individual, and that we (and vets) should honor the sadness in ourselves from our work (oral communication, 2018). She wanted us to remember to "listen to your heart, practice with integrity, and listen to your gut. If you have a sense you are about to offer something that doesn't feel right, listen to that gut feeling." Dr Makowski says that we still do not teach medical students that the next step after diagnosis is asking "should we" do this treatment. This is the space where palliative care fits in, according to her practice philosophy.

Dr Mihir Kamdar was a pre-veterinary student when he decided that managing end-of-life care for animals was too hard. Despite that, he chose palliative care because when he arrived for training at the Dana-Farber Cancer Institute, he was "blown away" by how the palliative care team would stay in the room when everyone else felt they did not have anything else to give. He realized as an intern that he was not getting calls about things like what chemotherapy to use, he was getting calls about nausea and pain. In his words, "The Palliative Care team really resonated me. They can immediately improve quality of life. This is really why we have medicine."

Dr Joanne Wolfe provided us with wonderful guidelines for personal sustainability in this difficult work. She said that each person needs his or her own strategy for well-being and you need to be very intentional about ensuring that. Mindset is important to her; she warned do not "beat yourself up about the kids you can't reach" and to "be conscious of the fact that you can't always be available. Make sure you are not the only person who can do everything for a family." She recommended that programs help offer a "menu" of coping strategies for clinicians. Her group does a lot of self-care at work, including a ritualized moment of remembrance when a patient dies and an annual remembrance celebration.

ACKNOWLEDGMENTS

The author gratefully acknowledges the time and effort of the health care professionals interviewed for this article: Susan Block, MD, professor of psychiatry and medicine, Department of Psychosocial Oncology and Palliative Care, Dana-Farber Cancer Institute and Brigham and Women's Hospital, Harvard Medical School, Boston, Massachusetts. David B. Doolittle, Psy.D., clinical psychologist/psychoanalyst, clinical instructor in psychiatry, Harvard Medical School at Massachusetts General Hospital, Boston, Massachusetts. Kate Dare-Winters, LICSW, clinical supervisor/teaching associate, Harvard Medical School, Boston, Massachusetts. Vicki Jackson, MD, MPH, chief, Division of Palliative Care and Geriatric Medicine, Massachusetts General Hospital; co-director HMS Center for Palliative Care, associate professor of medicine, Harvard Medical School, Boston, Massachusetts. Mihir M. Kamdar, MD, associate director, Division of Palliative Care, Director, MGH Cancer Pain Clinic, Division of Palliative Care and Geriatrics, Division of Anesthesia Pain Medicine, Massachusetts General Hospital, Boston, Massachusetts. Suzana K. E. Makowski, MD, chief of palliative care at Exeter Hospital, Exeter, New Hampshire and associate professor of medicine at University of Massachusetts Medical School, Worcester, Massachusetts. Michael L. Spear, MD, MSEdL, director, C.O.R.E. Palliative Care Team, St Christopher's Hospital for Children, professor of pediatrics, Drexel University College of Medicine, Philadelphia, Pennsylvania. Joanne Wolfe, MD, MPH, director, Pediatric Palliative Care at Boston Children's Hospital and Dana-Farber Cancer Institute; division chief, Pediatric Palliative Care Service, Department of Psychosocial Oncology and Palliative Care, Dana-Farber Cancer Institute, associate professor of pediatrics, Harvard Medical School, Boston, Massachusetts.

REFERENCES

1. Clark D, LaMarche G. Transforming the culture of dying: the work of the project on death in America. London: Oxford University Press; 2013. https://doi.org/10.1093/acprof:oso/9780199311613.001.0001.
2. Loscalzo MJ. Palliative care: an historical perspective. Hematology Am Soc Hematol Educ Program 2008;465. https://doi.org/10.1182/asheducation-2008.1.465.
3. Approaching death: improving care at the end of life—a report of the Institute of Medicine. Health Serv Res 1998;33(1):1–3.
4. Ruder DB. From specialty to shortage. Harvard Magazine 2015. Available at: https://harvardmagazine.com/2015/03/from-specialty-to-shortage. Accessed August 3, 2018.
5. Block SD, Billings JA. A need for scalable outpatient palliative care interventions. Lancet 2014;383(9930):1699–700.
6. Bekelman DB, Rabin BA, Nowels CT, et al. Barriers and facilitators to scaling up outpatient palliative care. J Palliat Med 2016;19(4):456–9.
7. Knaul FM, Farmer PE, Krakauer EL, et al. Alleviating the access abyss in palliative care and pain relief—an imperative of universal health coverage: the Lancet Commission report. Lancet 2018;391(10128):1391–454.
8. Norton SA, Powers BA, Schmitt MH, et al. Navigating tensions: integrating palliative care consultation services into an academic medical center setting. J Pain Symptom Manage 2011;42(5):680–90.
9. Wolf SM, Berlinger N, Jennings B. Forty years of work on end-of-life care—from patients' rights to systemic reform. N Engl J Med 2015;372(7):678–82.
10. Connors AF, Dawson NV, Desbiens NA, et al. A controlled trial to improve care for seriously ill hospitalized patients: the study to understand prognoses and

preferences for outcomes and risks of treatments (support). JAMA 1995;274(20): 1591–8.

11. Solomon MZ, O'Donnell L, Jennings B, et al. Decisions near the end of life: professional views on life-sustaining treatments. Am J Public Health 1993;83(1): 14–23.

12. Maltoni M, Scarpi E, Dall'Agata M, et al. Systematic versus on-demand early palliative care: results from a multicentre, randomised clinical trial. Eur J Cancer 2016; 65:61–8.

13. Hawley P. Barriers to access to palliative care. Palliat Care 2017;10. https://doi. org/10.1177/1178224216688887.

14. The challenge of financing sustainable community-based palliative care programs. Available at: https://www.healthaffairs.org/do/10.1377/hblog20141229. 043553/full/. Accessed August 19, 2018.

15. Rabow M, Kvale E, Barbour L, et al. Moving upstream: a review of the evidence of the impact of outpatient palliative care. J Palliat Med 2013;16(12):1540–9.

16. Smith S, Brick A, O'Hara S, et al. Evidence on the cost and cost-effectiveness of palliative care: a literature review. Palliat Med 2014;28(2):130–50.

17. Palliative care impact calculator | CAPC. Available at: https://www.capc.org/ impact-calculator/. Accessed August 24, 2018.

18. Interdisciplinary Team. National Hospice and Palliative Care Organization. Available at: https://www.nhpco.org/interdisciplinary-team. Accessed August 6, 2018.

19. Ciemins EL, Brant J, Kersten D, et al. Why the interdisciplinary team approach works: insights from complexity science. J Palliat Med 2016;19(7):767–70.

20. Anderson EW, Frazer MS, Schellinger SE. Expanding the palliative care domains to meet the needs of a community-based supportive care model. Am J Hosp Palliat Care 2018;35(2):258–65.

21. Morrison RS. Models of palliative care delivery in the United States. Curr Opin Support Palliat Care 2013;7(2):201–6.

22. Quill TE, Abernethy AP. Generalist plus specialist palliative care—creating a more sustainable model. N Engl J Med 2013;368(13):1173–5.

23. Brenner PR. Palliative care and hospice: one approach. Am J Hosp Palliat Med 2000;17(4):241–4.

24. Meier DE, Beresford L. Outpatient clinics are a new frontier for palliative care. J Palliat Med 2008;11(6):823–8.

25. Jackson VA, Jacobsen J, Greer JA, et al. The cultivation of prognostic awareness through the provision of early palliative care in the ambulatory setting: a communication guide. J Palliat Med 2013;16(8):894–900.

26. Palliative medicine career paths. NEJM CareerCenter. Available at: https://www. nejmcareercenter.org/article/palliative-medicine-career-paths/. Accessed August 4, 2018.

27. ABMS subspecialty certification in hospice and palliative medicine, AAHPM. Available at: http://aahpm.org/certification/subspecialty-certification. Accessed August 4, 2018.

28. Vinay P. Should palliative care be a specialty? Can Fam Physician 2008;54(6): 841–3.

29. Accreditation Council for Graduate Medical Education. Advanced program search: hospice and palliative medicine. Available at: https://apps.acgme.org/ ads/Public/Programs/Search?stateId=&specialtyId=153&specialtyCategoryTyp eId=&numCode=&city=. Accessed August 4, 2018.

30. Temel JS, Gallagher ER, Jackson VA, et al. Early palliative care for patients with metastatic non-small-cell lung cancer. N Engl J Med 2010;363(8):733–42.

Goals of Care

Development and Use of the Serious Veterinary Illness Conversation Guide

Katherine J. Goldberg, DVM, LMSW[a,b,c,*]

KEYWORDS

- Palliative care • Goals of care • Serious illness • Serious veterinary illness
- End-of-life communication • Serious illness conversation • Aid in dying • Euthanasia

KEY POINTS

- Goals of care conversations are an essential component of palliative medicine for both human and veterinary patients.
- Goals of care conversations provide formal structure, evidence-based guidance, and dependable support for those involved in serious illness and end-of-life care.
- Serious illness care in veterinary medicine is uniquely positioned to benefit from structured goals of care conversations.
- A goals of care checklist, the Serious Veterinary Illness Conversation Guide, has been modified from human medicine for use in veterinary patients.
- Widespread implementation of high-quality goals of care conversations is a keystone step for quality advancement of palliative care within the veterinary profession.

SETTING THE STAGE: THE UNIQUE NATURE OF SERIOUS VETERINARY ILLNESS AND ITS TREATMENT

In human medicine, end-of-life debates often focus on trying to "die well," being "allowed" to die, and attaining understanding regarding when life-prolonging treatment is no longer in the best interests of patients. This is largely because of the default to treat, which pervades medical intervention for humans. Contemporary medicine in the United States will prolong life at all costs: emotional, financial, and physical, in the name of "doing everything." In the words of oncology nurse Theresa Brown, "Medicine today achieves great things, but too often when patients have no hope of surviving we use technology and drugs simply to keep people alive."[1] Conversations around

Disclosure Statement: The author has nothing to disclose.
a Whole Animal Veterinary Geriatrics and Palliative Care Services, Ithaca, NY, USA; b Cornell Health, Counseling and Psychological Services, Ithaca, NY, USA; c University of Tennessee Veterinary Social Work Certificate Program, Knoxville, TN, USA
* Counseling and Psychological Services, Cornell Health, Cornell University, 110 Ho Plaza, Ithaca, NY 1453.
E-mail address: info@wholeanimalvet.com

Vet Clin Small Anim 49 (2019) 399–415
https://doi.org/10.1016/j.cvsm.2019.01.006
0195-5616/19/© 2019 Elsevier Inc. All rights reserved.

end-of-life care for people consequently tend to focus on upholding the rights of patients to withhold or withdraw life-sustaining treatment, and the many complexities of those rights, including ethical conflicts when patient or family wishes do not match recommendations of the medical team.

In veterinary medicine, where the dominant end-of-life paradigm is euthanasia, the focus is arguably opposite from human medicine. Veterinary end-of-life considerations typically surround questions of life-*ending* versus life-prolonging treatment as well as the "right to live versus right to die," that is, some say that animals have a right to live rather than be euthanized. Meanwhile, the default recommendation for seriously ill or otherwise suffering animals is euthanasia, and disagreement with this tends to be labeled as "resistance." This paradox within end-of-life decision making for human and veterinary patients creates rich ethical terrain for the pet-owning public and veterinary profession alike.

Veterinarians are often in the tricky position of weighing client preferences relative to patient best interests. The "veterinary trilemma," the relationship between the animal, its owner, and the veterinarian, elevates the complexity of these issues,[2] and veterinarians rank resulting ethical conflicts as highly stressful.[3] It is reasonable to wonder when, if ever, euthanasia is a cruelty versus a kindness, and who decides? Within the veterinary profession, there is great interest in preventing suffering in companion animals by euthanizing *before* things get bad (preemptive euthanasia). As a result, those who choose euthanasia later in the disease course, or not at all, are often judged harshly for "letting animals suffer."

An interesting exception to this resistance to prolong companion animal life seems to exist in veterinary intensive care units (ICU), which increasingly resemble their human counterparts. Along with successful outcomes and life-saving interventions, there exists a surprising amount of suffering in the veterinary ICU. Pain is just one unpleasant experience among many for critically ill animals.[4] However, this reality tends to escape judgment because it exists under the purview of veterinary professionals, with an intent to save life. Conversations regarding withhold/withdraw of life-sustaining treatment have yet to be substantively considered in the professional discourse of veterinary critical care, but the boundary between "heroism" and futility in the veterinary ICU has recently been explored.[2,5] Comparatively, discourse around the ethics of advanced care related to futility and nonbeneficial treatment is prevalent in human medicine.[6–12] It is curious that despite increasing availability and social acceptability of advanced care for animals, bringing with it controversies and ethical conflict similar to human medicine, there has been little attention given to the *limits* of this care by the veterinary profession. Largely absent from the conversation not only consideration of animal welfare issues and medical outcomes associated with advanced care but also what veterinarians are obligated to offer, and what they are not, for patients. In addition, formally structured opportunities for discourse around these issues, such as hospital ethics committees, are largely absent from veterinary settings. Moses[13] points to a "deep lack of ethical literacy" in the veterinary profession as an obstacle to widespread acceptance of ethics consultation services. This is an important area for future research.

Similarities between human and veterinary medicine include medical teams sometimes continuing to offer interventions even if they do not think them to be in the patient's best interests, possibly because they think they are obligated to do so. "Resistance" to euthanasia on the part of a veterinary client in the face of veterinarian assessment that it is a reasonable option for her pet is in some ways analogous to "resistance" to discontinuation of life support in the face of physician assessment that it is the most reasonable course of action for a family member. Pressure from both veterinary clients and human patients (and families) to "keep going" with medical interventions is felt by veterinarians and physicians. The dominant paradigms and default actions of human and veterinary medicine may be distinct, but parallel ethical conflicts arise in both settings. In this author's view, all humans are impacted by the ways in which advanced care, the limits of such care, and death are navigated across species and circumstances.

Goals of Care (GOC) conversations, the subject of this article, are the means to exploring these increasingly complex issues. They provide formal structure, evidence-based guidance, and dependable support for those involved in serious illness and end-of-life discussions. Involvement in palliative medicine or end-of-life care without GOC conversations is akin to wandering a trailless wilderness without a map.

What is a Goals of Care Conversation?

GOC conversations focus on what is most important to patients and their families as they face serious illness. They do not presume that the only priority is living longer, but rather recognize that medical treatment plans may, and *ought to* be, altered depending on individual goals and preferences. They foster and prioritize "the ask," the simple yet revolutionary act of asking patients and families what is important to them as their lives are impacted by their illness and its treatment. Although this may sound too simple to warrant scientific inquiry, those who have had a seriously or terminally ill (human) family member know that the impact of these conversations, or lack thereof, is significant. Although GOC conversations have not yet received scholarly attention in the veterinary literature or widespread curricular integration within veterinary teaching institutions, they are established as an essential element of high-quality care in the context of serious illness for people.[14] The structure of, barriers to, and impact of these conversations have all been examined.[14–21] The 2014 article by Bernacki and Block[14] in *Journal of the American Medical Association* "Review and Synthesis of Best Practices" regarding communication of serious illness care goals asserts,

> Communication about goals of care is a low-risk, high-value intervention for patients with serious and life-threatening illness; these discussions should begin early in the course of life-limiting illnesses… Early discussions about end-of-life care issues are associated with improved patient outcomes, including better quality of life, reduced use of nonbeneficial medical care near death, and care more consistent with patients' goals. This approach is also associated with improved family outcomes and reduced costs.[14]

The case for and means of integrating this low-risk, high-value, cost-saving intervention into the veterinary profession are the focus of this article. A complete review of GOC interventions and serious illness communication within human medicine is beyond its scope, but the reader is encouraged to explore the primary source literature cited. Learning from the human medical profession regarding serious illness communication is essential if we are to provide high-quality veterinary care in a goal-concordant way.

Furthermore, rigorous development of palliative medicine within the veterinary profession cannot occur without adequate attention to GOC considerations. Although there have certainly been important contributions to the literature around end-of-life communication,[22,23] the GOC interventions discussed here go beyond the traditional focus on empathic euthanasia decision making and delivery of bad news. It is important to note that frameworks for delivering bad news, which have been evaluated in the literature: SPIKES, PEWTR, ABCDE,[24–26] are only part of a comprehensive GOC conversation; they address *prognosis*, which is one-eighth of the serious illness conversation framework that is outlined here.[15,19,27]

The Serious (Veterinary) Illness Conversation Guide

A user-friendly, scalable tool for serious illness conversation, the Serious Illness Conversation Guide (SICG), was developed by Ariadne Labs: A Joint Center for Health Systems Innovation, and the Dana-Farber Cancer Institute under the leadership of Drs Susan Block, Rachelle Bernacki, Atul Gawande, and others. The SICG is currently in use and has been the focus of a cluster randomized controlled trial that continues to

Serious Veterinary Illness Conversation Guide

CLINICIAN STEPS

☐ **Set up**
- Thinking in advance
- Is this okay?
- Hope for best, prepare for worst
- Benefit for patient/family
- No decisions necessary today

☐ **Guide** (right column)

☐ **Act**
- Affirm commitment
- Make recommendations about next steps
  - Acknowledge medical realities
  - Summarize key goals/priorities
  - Describe treatment options that reflect both
- Document conversation

Katherine Goldberg, DVM
Whole Animal Veterinary Geriatrics &
Hospice Services

© 2015 Ariadne Labs: A Joint Center for
Health Systems Innovation
(www.ariadnelabs.org) and Dana-Farber
Cancer Institute

CONVERSATION GUIDE

Understanding

What is your understanding now of where _____ is with his/her illness?
What questions do you have about information your family veterinarian has already shared with you?

Information Preferences

How much information about _____'s illness would you like from me? How much additional information do you feel you need to help make decisions?

FOR EXAMPLE:
Some families like to have lots of information about what to expect, others do not. Some people are very comforted by lots of diagnostic information and some people find this stressful.

Prognosis

Share prognosis as a range, tailored to information preferences. Understand that euthanasia as end point for most patients has tremendous impact on "prognosis". What is acceptable for one family may not be for another.

Goals

If _____'s situation worsens, what are your most important goals?

Fears / Worries

What are your biggest fears and worries about _____'s health?

Function

What abilities or activities are so critical to _____'s life that you can't imagine him/her living without them?

Trade-offs

If _____ becomes sicker, how much are you willing to go through for the possibility of gaining more time together?

Aid in Dying

What are your beliefs surrounding euthanasia?

Fig. 1. The SVICG. (*Courtesy of* Katherine Goldberg, DVM, LMSW.)[27]

evaluate several research questions.[14,15,28–32] It has also been modified for veterinary use.[27] Curated from its human counterpart following the 2015 Communication in Serious Illness Course in Boston, Massachusetts, the Serious Veterinary Illness Conversation Guide (SVICG) provides veterinarians and their teams with a guide to help conduct comprehensive GOC conversations. It provides a basic framework that may be used in a variety of settings for veterinary patients. Given substantial and compelling evidence for the use of checklists in medicine,[20,33–37] use of a structured communication format for serious illness care is an empirically supported strategy.

They [checklists] ensure completion of necessary tasks during complex, stressful situations in which memory alone may not be sufficient, or when stress and discomfort felt by those participating in the scenarios may cloud clear thought processes, interfere with effective communication, and prevent accomplishment of desired outcomes.[20]

Certainly, serious illness and end-of-life conversations are "complex, stressful situations." Physicians also report discomfort with them, identifying more barriers to having the discussions than patients do.[38] For all these reasons, the checklist structure functions to optimize the likelihood of a quality conversation even when emotions are high. In addition, although the questions explored in the SICG/SVICG are standard topics of GOC conversations, the structure of the checklist provides a systematic approach to developing an individualized treatment plan for each patient.[20] Considering that most veterinarians are less familiar with formal GOC conversations than physicians, using a systematic approach is likely to be beneficial for the introduction of this intervention into veterinary medicine (**Fig. 1**).

Conversation Guide Focus Areas

Understanding
The importance of assessing clients' understanding of where their animal is with his or her disease cannot be overstated. Particularly in a referral setting, where multiple clinicians have seen the patient, much of what has been communicated to the client is often lost. In addition, emotions are frequently high, and clients may be confused or entirely mistaken about what is wrong with their pet. Starting with an open-ended solicitation of the client's understanding of what's going on is invaluable and should not be skipped.

Information preferences
Similarly, gaining an understanding of how much information a client *wants* to receive will proactively establish rapport and help to avoid conflict around communication styles and preferences between clients and veterinarians. The "some people" is a useful tool here: *"Some people like to have a lot of medical information, and some people don't"*; it helps normalize the client's perspective, whatever it may be. The veterinarian is also demonstrating that she or he will support the client, no matter what their information preferences are.

Prognosis
This section tends to dominate "delivering bad news" education, but in fact it is only a fraction of the complete GOC conversation. Still, it is extremely important, and research suggests that targeted approaches are necessary for improvement. For example, one study gathering baseline information about surgeons' experiences and attitudes when delivering bad news was performed at a (human) medical teaching institution.[25]

Ninety-three percent of respondents perceived delivering bad news to be a very important skill, and 7% perceived delivering bad news to be a somewhat important skill; however, only 43% of respondents thought they had the training to effectively deliver such news.[25] In addition, 85% thought they needed additional training to be effective when delivering bad news.[25] Of the 85% of participants who thought they needed additional training, 59% were residents and 26% were attendings.[25] This and other data show that there is an unmet need in educating physicians to empathically and effectively deliver bad news. Corresponding research in the veterinary profession has been limited. One recent study uses the COMFORT model as a framework to organize the communication of "breaking bad news" in veterinary medicine.[39]

As indicated by the SVICG, an important feature of prognosis and delivery of bad news for veterinary patients is the availability of euthanasia. "Prognosis" and survival times, even within the scholarly veterinary literature, are adulterated by euthanasia as the endpoint for most patients. Criteria for euthanasia of client-owned animals are inherently subjective and nonuniform. The importance of this reality relative to GOC conversations is to recognize, and help clients recognize, the profound subjectivity of prognosis. Research methods and limitations within the veterinary profession are beyond the scope of this article; however, randomized clinical trials (RCT) in veterinary research have recently been discussed.[40] Strikingly, mode of death was not mentioned as a factor in interpreting veterinary RCT data. Weighing the relative value of evidence-versus experience-based assessments of prognosis may prove to be an important task for veterinarians and the pet-owning public. The question, *"How much time does he have?"* in the context of euthanasia as an option at any time, often in the absence of a definitive diagnosis, may not be a particularly useful question. The unspoken, yet brutally honest question, *"How much time are you going to give him?,"* is what gets to the heart of "survival times" in veterinary medicine. This reality can be profoundly uncomfortable to recognize, and navigating GOC in this unique context is precisely what makes serious illness communication an essential skill for veterinarians. The burden of responsibility around deciding when to end a pet's life cannot be overstated. Prognosis may be viewed as a 2-part process: first, what do we know about the disease trajectory, and second, what are the client's limits, in terms of seeing the trajectory through?

Goals

Multiple studies in human medicine have shown that people have priorities other than just living longer. Although corresponding research does not exist in veterinary medicine regarding client goals and priorities for their pets, it is reasonable to expect that outcomes could be similar. The goals section of the conversation guide asks what clients want as their pet's disease progresses. What are their goals as time runs short? Goals may be related to the disease and its treatment, for example, maintaining normal behavior patterns and mentation, keeping a pet at home rather than traveling for treatment, avoiding oral medications, or related to shared activities and other "nonmedical" plans, for example, going on a trip to a meaningful place, visiting with now-grown children or others, continuing to go hiking/swimming/another valued activity, being alive for the upcoming birth of a baby, and so on. Open-ended solicitation of client goals is invaluable in its ability to inform treatment planning. It is then the veterinarian's job to assess the feasibility of client goals relative to patient welfare and communicate if alternative planning is indicated.

Fears/worries

Similarly, asking what clients' biggest fears or worries are about their pet's health can be a game-changer. Often, clients are worried about things that veterinarians might not consider, for example, *"I'm worried that her hair won't grow back (after the ultra-sound) before she dies,"* or *"I'm worried that my friends think I'm doing the wrong thing,"* or *"My biggest fear is that I will find him dead in the house,"* or *"I'm worried that he will be scared during the euthanasia."* Medical concerns are also pervasive for clients, that is, fear of pain/not recognizing pain, losing control of bladder/bowels, declining mentation, and so on. Assessing what clients are afraid of/worried about establishes rapport and enables the veterinary care team to address individualized concerns. Client anxiety and distress around unaddressed fears can be considerable and lead to impaired caregiving, which then negatively impacts patient welfare. Proactive communication is an important tool for mitigating this.

Function

Attunement to patient function is essential and often missed in standard "quality-of-life" assessments. For example, despite its title, the popular "HHHHHM Quality of Life Scale" originally developed in 2004 by Villalobos, revised and published in 2007 and 2011, functions as a euthanasia decision tree rather than a quality-of-life assessment tool. Furthermore, it paints with a broad brush functions that are surely experienced differently by individual patients. What is the impact of poor mobility in a Yorkie versus a Newfoundland, for example? Finally, a numerical score determines "acceptable life quality to continue with pet hospice."[41] As is evident from this article, and throughout this issue, such a conclusion is deceptively simplistic, and depending on the level of medical supervision, potentially harmful to patients. In contrast, ascertaining which abilities or activities are so critical to a pet's life that the client cannot imagine him or her living without them enables veterinarians to understand the client's functional "deal-breakers" so to speak, in a nonjudgmental context. Client tolerance and intolerance for immobility, incontinence, and other aspects of illness cannot be assumed. Similarly, for some animals, playing with toys or going on long hikes is essential for their very happiness; others are content to lounge, so long as basic needs are attended to. Patient preferences and individual personalities are relevant, even in nonhuman animals. Humans, caregiver and veterinarian, are responsible for interpreting the animal's behaviors so that individualized treatment planning is optimized. It is here where overlap often occurs between a GOC conversation and palliative-oriented history taking.

Critical to palliative care evaluation, specifically the history or "subjective" part of a Subjective, Objective, Assessment, Plan note, is assessment of activities of daily living (ADLs); for humans this includes things like bathing, dressing, eating, and getting in and out of a car. Extrapolated to animals, ADLs relate to the things that patients need to do to be themselves and move through their day: get in and out of a litter box, go for a walk, ambulate (and/or jump) to a food bowl, eat, groom, play, and interact with people and other animals. Depending on the patient's "job," a list of ADLs may be more involved, service and working animals, for example. A seriously ill working farm dog may require more cognitive stimulation than the average companion dog once their illness prevents them from being able to work. Completion of a GOC conversation using the SVICG will draw on this information in the "Function" section if ADLs have already been assessed, or the ADL assessment may be informed by the SVICG if this has been done first.

Tradeoffs

Tradeoffs are particularly hard to assess by proxy. In human medicine, this is when the patient would be asked, *"How much are you willing to go through for the possibility of gaining more time?"* The question is one of balancing suffering now for possible time later, a complex consideration even for mentally competent humans. Health Care Proxies (HCPs), who speak for patients once they are no longer able to speak for themselves, are charged with best estimating *what the patient would want* and advocating for that preference. In many ways, companion animal owners are HCPs throughout the life of the animal; the veterinary patient never gets to have a choice, although clients may believe they are acting on the patient's behalf. *"I'm asking myself, what would this cat want? I don't want this to be about me."* This point bears further development in future work, because the issue of boundaries between client needs and patient needs is very poorly explored in the veterinary profession (Lisa Moses, personal communication, 2018). It is unfortunately the case that patient suffering occurs, despite client wishes to the contrary, when veterinarians and clients do not examine the rationale behind decision making as closely as is likely warranted.

HCP assessment of tradeoffs becomes particularly challenging when decisions are made that subject the patient to harm with potential (or inevitable) suffering: invasive interventions, surgical recovery time, isolation during hospitalization, and so forth. For veterinary patients and caregivers, consideration of tradeoffs is a complex yet necessary part of the SVICG that assesses information not otherwise obtained via broad questions about goals and priorities. In part, this is because client preferences and limits are also being solicited. How much are *you* (the client) willing to go through for the possibility of more time? Factors to consider here include things like driving long distances to seek specialty care, taking time off from work to care for pets at home, ability/willingness to administer medications, financial budget, environmental modifications of the home, alterations in family schedule, and so on. These factors put the legal status of animal patients (and realities of pet ownership) front and center; although clients may prefer that their own needs not be considered above the animal's, this can hardly be reasonable or possible all the time.

Aid in dying

This final question of the SVICG is what most clearly sets it apart from its human counterpart. The term "Aid In Dying" is intentionally used by the author rather than "Euthanasia" to most appropriately and accurately frame the conversation in the context of GOC. Euthanasia for animals is, in fact, just assisted dying. It is a procedure, the benefits and burdens of which must be considered just as they are for any other medical intervention (inserting a chest tube, obtaining a blood sample, performing pericardiocentesis). In the context of serious illness conversation, which involves patients who are going to die and likely imminently no matter what communication takes place, the question is not about binary modes of death (euthanasia vs not) or language ("natural death," "active euthanasia," "physician aid in dying," "medical aid in dying," "death with dignity") per se, but rather the *intentionality* of the act. What are client beliefs around purposefully choosing to end their pet's life (euthanasia), and what qualifications surround these beliefs? There may be a *preference* for unaided death, for example, but euthanasia is acceptable under certain circumstances. It is then the veterinarian's job to facilitate a conversation about these circumstances and guide treatment planning accordingly. A complete discussion of euthanasia within the veterinary profession, associated ethical conflicts, considerations for clients, and implications for veterinarian well-being is beyond the scope of this article. However, it is important to recognize the depth and complexity of these issues in the context of GOC conversations. The availability of legal euthanasia for companion animal patients alters the landscape of serious illness care, decision making, and treatment planning within the veterinary profession in every possible way. The impact of euthanasia within the veterinary profession cannot be overstated.

Use of the Serious Veterinary Illness Conversation Guide

Ideally, GOC conversations would be implemented for all geriatric, chronically or seriously ill patients, and all clients who are struggling with decisions, but realistically this is unlikely to happen. Case selection, then, is an important consideration and is briefly outlined here. A complete review of triggers and criteria for GOC interventions in human medicine is beyond the scope of this article, but several different approaches have been evaluated in various study populations.[14,30,32,42–46] There are currently no corresponding data in the veterinary literature. The "surprise question" (SQ) has been evaluated extensively in human medicine. It is most appropriately used as a screening tool for palliative interventions (such as GOC conversations) rather than a predictor of death, and studies demonstrate significant utility in several patient populations.[47–55] The SQ simply asks physicians, *"Would you be surprised if this patient died in the next 12 months?"* Physician response of "no" is a trigger for palliative care intervention. Use of the SQ as a screening tool assumes that patients in their last year of life may have unmet palliative care needs; therefore, identifying patients in the last year of life is critical for palliative care provision. Evaluation and validation of the SQ within veterinary medicine, likely with an adjusted timeframe, could prove to be a useful area for future study.

In veterinary medicine, overall outcome data are limited across treatment settings, academic versus private practice ICU, primary care clinic, and so forth. Therefore, it is currently difficult to stratify patients into high/low risk of death (which could be one criterion for a GOC conversation). Although individual institutions may know their own survival-to-discharge rate,[56] these data are not widely known across institutions within the veterinary profession, which further complicates estimates of survival, disease severity, and likelihood of discharge and/or return to function. As a result, it is not easy to determine selection criteria for implementation of serious illness conversation. It is here where GOC interventions and prognostication within veterinary settings (primarily ICU) overlap. Although attention to prognostic stratification in veterinary medicine has been limited, a severity of illness stratification system has been evaluated in a veterinary teaching hospital.[57] Prognosis for neonatal foals in an ICU has also been assessed, with the goal of predicting patient outcomes.[58]

Taking all of this information into consideration, it is this author's recommendation to implement GOC conversations early and often. Certainly, research to evaluate whether GOC outcomes from human medicine hold true in veterinary contexts is warranted. However, given repeated evidence from human studies of significant benefit and no documented harm,[14,16,20,29,32,43,59] there is much to gain from conducting structured GOC conversations with veterinary clients. Few interventions have demonstrated such high value and low risk in either human or veterinary medicine. As Dr Atul Gawande said in his 2015 keynote address at the American Academy of Hospice and Palliative Medicine annual assembly, *"If you (palliative care providers) were a drug, the FDA would approve you!"*

Goals of Care, Veterinary Clients, Pet Death, and Caregiver Burden

Goal-concordant care is vital in veterinary medicine, specifically as relates to end-of-life choices, because it has been shown that reactions, both healthy and potentially harmful, to pet death are more likely to be associated with factors related to the client than the pet.[60] For example, client attitudes toward euthanasia, societal attitudes toward pet death, and level of support received from the attending veterinarian have been shown to be more important modifiers of client grief reactions than the age of pet at the time of death. In addition, these factors more broadly impact client experiences of their pet's death and impressions of their veterinarian's role in that death. Other factors found to increase the intensity of both uncomplicated and complicated grief reactions following pet loss include attachment to pet, level of social support, and preferences regarding means of death/euthanasia.[61] These factors are all explored in GOC conversations, which then function as a modifier of grief reactions following pet loss. Support after the death of a pet is important, but it is not the only opportunity for veterinary professionals to help clients as they face the final phase of their pets' lives.

Of significant importance, and discussed in Mary Beth Spitznagel's article, "Caregiver Burden and Veterinary Client Wellbeing," in this issue, is the issue of caregiver burden related to seriously ill pets. This phenomenon was initially explored by Spitznagel and colleagues[62] and further discussed in an accompanying editorial[63] by this author. GOC conversations are related to caregiver burden insofar as they solicit client goals, preferences, and limits as treatment planning occurs on behalf of a seriously ill pet. Given the intimate involvement of veterinary clients in the care of their ill pets, arguably more than in human medicine, due to fewer established resources, client understanding of, and willingness to participate in, caregiving is critical. Shared decision making is currently promoted as the dominant model and best practice for communication in serious illness for people[46] with goal-concordant care as its aim. It is this author's belief that goal-concordant care is a protective factor against caregiver burden for seriously ill pets and may even mitigate it. Further research is necessary to support this hypothesis. Studies in human medicine have evaluated the bereaved caregiver experience, and it has been suggested that poor quality end-of-life communication may result in bereaved caregivers feeling more anxious, depressed, traumatized, or regretful.[46,64,65]

Serious Illness Conflicts in Veterinary Medicine

By now it is apparent that serious illness care for companion animals is complicated territory. Each experience is unique; however, there are some situations that arise predictably. Some common conflicts for which use of the SVICG may be an effective intervention are now outlined.

Disagreement in family

Family disagreement is a common issue in end-of-life care for people as well as for animals.[66–68] In veterinary practice, differing opinions on everything from whether the pet is eating, happy, or in pain, to fundamental beliefs regarding euthanasia or how much money to spend on a pet's care, often coexist within one family unit. Strategies for dealing with this include recommending that family members assess quality of life as well as answer GOC questions such as those in the SVICG, independently. The process of then coming together to discuss these preferences is often quite useful and aids in communication around difficult decisions. Major family conflicts typically have a long history that will not be resolved before decisions need to be made on behalf of a pet. When this is the case, exemplary symptom management for the animal is critical while the human issues are being worked out.

Traumatic prior experience with animal death/loss

Many clients have unfortunately had negative experiences with animal death and loss. The impact of this on their ability to make decisions on behalf of a current pet cannot be overestimated. Open-ended inquiry regarding past experiences with pets should be part of basic history taking in serious illness contexts, but is certainly essential for GOC conversations. Past experiences with animal death usually come up in the

"Aid in Dying" section of the SVICG, when clients will often share what happened "last time" and how/if they would like things to be different with the current pet. Most people are very willing to share their experiences, and often much useful information can be gained by listening. Relationships with mental health professionals are also important; veterinarians are not trained to recognize or address posttraumatic stress symptoms or concerning features of other disorders. If a veterinarian suspects that a client cannot cope with a previous loss based on comments from the client related to disruptions in ADLs, sleep disturbance, difficulty eating, increased use of alcohol or other substances, physical symptoms, missing work, or thoughts of self-harm, referral to a mental health professional is appropriate. Additional information regarding mental health professionals in veterinary end-of-life care is found in Sandra Brackenridge's article, "The Social Worker: An Essential Hospice and Palliative Team Member," in this issue.

Traumatic prior experience with human death/loss or medical care

Traumatic stress is now thought to occur following several medical experiences, including pediatric injury and illness, chronic disease, and ICU stays.[69–76] This means that a subset of veterinary clients will have experienced trauma from medical intervention, either directly or indirectly. The impact of this on veterinary decision making has not been evaluated. However, clients routinely mention their past negative experiences with human health care over the course of veterinary visits. For example, discussion regarding chemotherapy in a dog turns to the client's mother, currently battling side effects from her own cancer treatment. The statement, "I would never subject my cat to treatment X," is often based on bad experiences with treatment X in people, not pets. These issues typically come up in the "Tradeoffs" and "Function" sections of the SVICG. Veterinarians should be prepared for this information; navigating it can be tricky, but it is important for achieving goal-concordant care for the current patient.

Spiritual conflict

The role of religion in veterinary care has received minimal attention in the scholarly literature. Nevertheless, clients' spiritual or religious beliefs may impact treatment decisions for their pets. This should not come as a surprise, considering that religion is considered standard demographic information in human hospitals, even when the stated religion is "none." Davis and colleagues found that "the religious and spiritual schemata that people use to conceptualize human life and death are applied to companion animals relatively commonly, even among nonreligious people.[77]" In their study, 56% of participants believed in an afterlife for their pet and generally found this belief comforting. Belief in an afterlife for animals has also been related to stronger attachment to a pet and a greater grief response to its death.[77] The Davis and colleagues study did not find that euthanasia raised any religious issues for clients, nor did religious belief impact aftercare choices; however, this is in stark contrast with this author's practical experience, whereby these issues arise commonly and can be quite distressing. One client severed ties with the church that had been central to her life for many decades after the priest said that her ailing dog did not have a soul. Another struggled with pain management recommendations because "suffering is important for enlightenment." Asking, "Is there a spiritual or faith tradition that helps inform decision making for your pet," can help facilitate communication around these issues. Spiritual/religious concerns may come up in any section of the SVICG, but most commonly when discussing "goals/values," "fears/worries," and "Aid in Dying." Patient-tested language from the initial clinical trial with the conversation guide (in human patients) includes *"What gives you strength as you face your illness?"* It is here where people typically mention faith, God, or religion, if these things are important to them. This question is important for veterinary clients as well.

Mental and other illness affecting decision making capacity

This is something of increasing significance that veterinarians have no formal training in. The legal nuances between "competency" and "capacity" are beyond the scope of this brief discussion; concern regarding clients' ability to reasonably make medical decisions on behalf of their pets is the broader issue. Given the legal status of animals, and veterinarians' professional identification as "animal helping" rather than "human helping" professionals, it is not surprising that this issue has received little attention to date. In human medicine, however, it is an area of ongoing engagement.[78–84] The 4 domains in assessment of decision-making capacity are (1) communicating a choice, (2) understanding, (3) appreciation, and (4) rationalization/reasoning. These domains may be affected by anything from memory, attention span, and intelligence, to depression, anxiety, phobias, dementia, and psychosis.[81] Certainly, these factors will be present in the pet-owning public and have the potential to impact veterinary care provision. Again, the reader is referred to Mary Beth Spitznagel's article "Caregiver Burden and Veterinary Client Wellbeing," in this issue for further discussion of the role of mental health professionals.

Goals of Care Conversation Deficits and Application to Veterinary Medicine

Finally, it is important to note that although research in human medicine consistently demonstrates positive outcomes from early GOC discussions,[14,16,20] deficits in the conversations themselves have been identified. Primarily, these have been related to content and timing.[15] Deficits relevant to veterinary practice include conversations occurring too late in the disease course, occurring when patients are in crisis, or occurring when clinicians who know the patient are not available. In addition, physicians tend to focus on choices regarding procedures and treatments rather than on goals and values.[15] Research also shows that "clinicians are underprepared and undertrained" to conduct high-quality conversations and "tend to avoid them."[15,85,86] The structured, checklist format of the SVICG is designed to address these challenges, and research in human medicine has certainly shown promising results related to addressing deficits in, and barriers to, effective GOC conversations. Even still, awareness of these deficits is essential if the veterinary profession is to effectively integrate serious illness communication into the care of its most vulnerable patients.

SUMMARY

Serious illness communication and GOC conversations are at the heart of palliative medicine, insofar as they hold goal-concordant care as their primary objective. These conversations, in combination with exemplary palliation of physical symptoms, have the power to transform serious illness care for veterinary patients and their caregivers. Despite repeated evidence that GOC conversations offer significant benefit and minimal harm to human patients, barriers to widespread and high-quality implementation persist. The veterinary profession can benefit from the experiences of palliative care implementation in human medicine and learn from its challenges. One strategy to overcoming barriers has been utilization of a structured checklist format for serious illness conversations. The SVICG promotes individualized, goal-concordant care planning even when conflict and emotional demands are high. It is this author's sincerest hope that mindful implementation of high-quality GOC conversations will elevate the level of medical care that seriously ill veterinary patients receive and provide much-needed clarity and support for their caregivers.

REFERENCES

1. Brown T. Prolonging death at the end of life. The New York Times 2009.
2. Eddie Clutton R. Recognising the boundary between heroism and futility in veterinary intensive care. Vet Anaesth Analg 2017;44:199–202.
3. Batchelor CEM, McKeegan DEF. Survey of the frequency and perceived stressfulness of ethical dilemmas encountered in UK veterinary practice. Vet Rec 2012;170(1):19.
4. Mellema MS, McIntyre RL. Patient suffering in the intensive care unit. In: Silverstein DC, Hopper K, editors. Small animal critical care medicine. 2nd edition. Philadelphia: Elsevier Inc.; 2015. p. 64–6.
5. Fordyce PS. Welfare, law and ethics in the veterinary intensive care unit. Vet Anaesth Analg 2017;44:203–11.
6. Schneiderman LJ. Defining medical futility and improving medical care. J Bioeth Inq 2011. https://doi.org/10.1007/s11673-011-9293-3.
7. Brett AS, McCullough LB. Getting past words futility and the professional ethics of life-sustaining treatment. Perspect Biol Med 2017. https://doi.org/10.1353/pbm.2018.0003.
8. Wilkinson D, Savulescu J. Knowing when to stop: futility in the intensive care unit. Curr Opin Anaesthesiol 2011;24(2):160–5.
9. DeLisser HM. Medical futility. In: The penn center guide to bioethics. New York: Springer Publishing Company; 2009. p. 761–74.
10. Morparia K, Dickerman M, Hoehn KS. Futility. Pediatr Crit Care Med 2012;13(5): e311–5.
11. Luce JM, Alpers A. Legal aspects of withholding and withdrawing life support from critically ill patients in the United States and providing palliative care to them. Am J Respir Crit Care Med 2000;162(6):2029–32.
12. Mohammed S, Peter E. Rituals, death and the moral practice of medical futility. Nurs Ethics 2009;16(3):292–302.
13. Moses L. Another experience in resolving veterinary ethical dilemmas: observations from a veterinarian performing ethics consultation. Am J Bioeth 2018; 18(2):67–9.
14. Bernacki RE, Block SD, American College of Physicians High Value Care Task Force. Communication about serious illness care goals: a review and synthesis of best practices. JAMA Intern Med 2014;174(12):1994–2003.
15. Bernacki RE, Hutchings M, Vick J, et al. Development of the serious illness care program: a randomised controlled trial of a palliative care communication intervention. BMJ Open 2015;5(10):e009032.
16. You JJ, Downar J, Fowler RA, et al. Barriers to goals of care discussions with seriously ill hospitalized patients and their families. JAMA Intern Med 2015;175(4): 549.
17. Kaldjian LC, Curtis AE, Shinkunas LA, et al. Goals of care toward the end of life: a structured literature review. Am J Hosp Palliat Care 2009;25(6):501–11.
18. Weissman DE, Morrison RS, Meier DE. Center to advance palliative care palliative care clinical care and customer satisfaction metrics consensus recommendations. J Palliat Med 2010;13(2):179–84.
19. Butcher L. Dana-Farber program seeks to improve conversations with patients with serious illness. Oncol Times 2016;14–5.

20. Bernacki RE, Block SD. Serious illness communications checklist. AMA J Ethics 2013;15(12):1045–9.
21. Csikai EL. Bereaved hospice caregivers' perceptions of the end-of-life care communication process and the involvement of health care professionals. J Palliat Med 2006;9(6):1300–9.
22. Shaw JR, Lagoni L. End-of-life communication in veterinary medicine: delivering bad news and euthanasia decision making. Vet Clin North Am Small Anim Pract 2007;37(1):95–108.
23. Shaw JR. Supportive care for the cancer patient: section C) relationship-centered approach to cancer communication. In: Withrow SJ, Vail DM, Page RL, editors. Withrow and MacEwen's small animal clinical oncology. 5th edition. Philadelphia: Elsevier Inc.; 2013. p. 272–9.
24. Bumb M, Keefe J, Miller L, et al. Breaking bad news: an evidence-based review of communication models for oncology nurses. Clin J Oncol Nurs 2017;21(5): 573–80.
25. Monden KR, Gentry L, Cox TR. Delivering bad news to patients. Proc (Bayl Univ Med Cent) 2016;29(1):101–2.
26. Nogueira Borden LJ, Adams CL, Bonnett BN, et al. Use of the measure of patient-centered communication to analyze euthanasia discussions in companion animal practice. J Am Vet Med Assoc 2010;237(11):1275–87.
27. Goldberg KJ. Serious Veterinary Illness Conversation Guide 2015. Modified from the Serious Illness Conversation Guide, © Ariadne Labs: A Joint Center for Health Systems Innovation (www.ariadnelabs.org) at Brigham and Women's Hospital and the Harvard T.H. Chan School of Public Health, in collaboration with Dana-Farber Cancer Institute. Licensed under the Creative Commons Attribution-NonCommercial-ShareAlike 4.0 International License. Available at: http://creativecommons.org/licenses/by-nc-sa/4.0/. Accessed February 17, 2019.
28. Lakin JR, Koritsanszky LA, Cunningham R, et al. A systematic intervention to improve serious illness communication in primary care. Health Aff 2017;36(7): 1258–64.
29. Paladino J, Lakin J, Miranda S, et al. Can we improve the quality of documented end-of-life conversations using a structured, multicomponent intervention? J Clin Oncol 2016;34(26_suppl):49.
30. Bernacki R, Paladino J, Lamas D, et al. Delivering more, earlier, and better goals-of-care conversations to seriously ill oncology patients. J Clin Oncol 2015; 33(29_suppl):39.
31. Bernacki R, Block S. The serious illness care program. J Clin Oncol 2014; 32(31_suppl):12.
32. Paladino J, Bernacki R, Hutchings M, et al. Effect of conversations about values and goals on anxiety in patients. J Clin Oncol 2015;33(29_suppl):9.
33. McCarthy M. WHO surgical safety checklist cuts post-surgical deaths by 22%, US study finds. BMJ 2017;357:j1935.
34. Thomassen Ø, Storesund A, Søfteland E, et al. The effects of safety checklists in medicine: a systematic review. Acta Anaesthesiol Scand 2014;58(1):5–18.
35. Haynes AB, Weiser TG, Berry WR, et al. A surgical safety checklist to reduce morbidity and mortality in a global population. N Engl J Med 2009;360(5):491–9.
36. Clay-Williams R, Colligan L. Back to basics: checklists in aviation and healthcare. BMJ Qual Saf 2015;24(7):428–31.
37. Haynes AB, Edmondson L, Lipsitz SR, et al. Mortality trends after a voluntary checklist-based surgical safety collaborative. Ann Surg 2017;266(6):923–9.

38. Curtis JR, Patrick DL, Caldwell ES, et al. Why don't patients and physicians talk about end-of-life care? Barriers to communication for patients with acquired immunodeficiency syndrome and their primary care clinicians. Arch Intern Med 2000;160(11):1690–6.

39. Nickels BM, Feeley TH. Breaking bad news in veterinary medicine. Health Commun 2018;33(9):1105–13.

40. Oyama MA, Ellenberg SS, Shaw PA. Clinical trials in veterinary medicine: a new era brings new challenges. J Vet Intern Med 2017;31(4):970–8.

41. Villalobos A. Quality of life scale (HHHHHM scale). Hoboken (NJ): Blackwell Publishing; 2007.

42. Schneiderman LJ. Effects of offering advance directives on medical treatments and costs. Ann Intern Med 1992;117(7):599.

43. Mack JW, Weeks JC, Wright AA, et al. End-of-life discussions, goal attainment, and distress at the end of life: predictors and outcomes of receipt of care consistent with preferences. J Clin Oncol 2010;28:1203–8.

44. Wright AA, Zhang B, Ray A, et al. Associations between end-of-life discussions, patient mental health, medical care near death, and caregiver bereavement adjustment. JAMA 2008;300(14):1665.

45. Hofmann JC. Patient preferences for communication with physicians about end-of-life decisions. Ann Intern Med 1997;127(1):1.

46. Sanders JJ, Curtis JR, Tulsky JA. Achieving goal-concordant care: a conceptual model and approach to measuring serious illness communication and its impact. J Palliat Med 2018;21(S2):S17–27.

47. Elliott M, Nicholson C. A qualitative study exploring use of the surprise question in the care of older people: perceptions of general practitioners and challenges for practice. BMJ Support Palliat Care 2017;7(1):32–8.

48. Costantini M, Higginson IJ, Merlo DF, et al. About the "surprise question. CMAJ 2017;189(23):E807.

49. Downar J, Goldman R, Pinto R, et al. The "surprise question" for predicting death in seriously ill patients: a systematic review and meta-analysis. CMAJ 2017; 189(13):E484–93.

50. Hadique S, Culp S, Sangani RG, et al. Derivation and validation of a prognostic model to predict 6-month mortality in an intensive care unit population. Ann Am Thorac Soc 2017;14(10):1556–61.

51. Vickerstaff V, White N, Kupeli N, et al. 60 Can the 'surprise question' be used to correctly identify people nearing the end of life?: a review. BMJ Support Palliat Care 2017;7(3):A371.

52. Hudson KE, Wolf SP, Samsa GP, et al. The surprise question and identification of palliative care needs among hospitalized patients with advanced hematologic or solid malignancies. J Palliat Med 2018;21(6):789–95.

53. Moss AH, Ganjoo J, Sharma S, et al. Utility of the "Surprise" question to identify dialysis patients with high mortality. Clin J Am Soc Nephrol 2008;3(5):1379–84.

54. Javier AD, Figueroa R, Siew ED, et al. Reliability and utility of the surprise question in CKD stages 4 to 5. Am J Kidney Dis 2017;70(1):93–101.

55. Moroni M, Zocchi D, Bolognesi D, et al. The 'surprise' question in advanced cancer patients: a prospective study among general practitioners. Palliat Med 2014; 28(7):959–64.

56. Penn Vet | E&CC | Intensive Care Unit. Available at: http://www.vet.upenn.edu/veterinary-hospitals/ryan-veterinary-hospital/services/e-cc-intensive-care-unit. Accessed September 6, 2018.

57. Hayes G, Mathews K, Doig G, et al. The acute patient physiologic and laboratory evaluation (APPLE) Score: a severity of illness stratification system for hospitalized dogs. J Vet Intern Med 2010;24(5):1034–47.
58. Furr M, Tinker MK, Edens L. Prognosis for neonatal foals in an intensive care unit. J Vet Intern Med 1997;11(3):183–8.
59. You JJ, Fowler RA, Heyland DK. Canadian Researchers at the End of Life Network (CARENET). Just ask: discussing goals of care with patients in hospital with serious illness. CMAJ 2014;186(6):425–32.
60. Adams CL, Bonnett BN, Meek AH. Predictors of owner response to companion animal death in 177 clients from 14 practices in Ontario. J Am Vet Med Assoc 2000;217(9):1303–9.
61. McCutcheon KA. Predictors of complicated and uncomplicated grief after the death of a companion animal [dissertation]. Toronto, ON: York University; 2004.
62. Spitznagel MB, Jacobson D, Cox M, et al. Caregiver burden in owners of a sick companion animal: a cross-sectional observational study. Vet Rec 2017;181(12):321.
63. Goldberg KJ. Exploring caregiver burden within a veterinary setting. Vet Rec 2017;181(12):318–9.
64. Krug K, Miksch A, Peters-Klimm F, et al. Correlation between patient quality of life in palliative care and burden of their family caregivers: a prospective observational cohort study. BMC Palliat Care 2016;15:4.
65. Miyajima K, Fujisawa D, Yoshimura K, et al. Association between quality of end-of-life care and possible complicated grief among bereaved family members. J Palliat Med 2014;17(9):1025–31.
66. Lichtenthal WG, Kissane DW. The management of family conflict in palliative care. Prog Palliat Care 2008;16(1):39–45.
67. Back AL, Arnold RM. Dealing with conflict in caring for the seriously ill. JAMA 2005;293(11):1374.
68. Parks SM, Winter L, Santana AJ, et al. Family factors in end-of-life decision-making: family conflict and proxy relationship. J Palliat Med 2011;14(2):179–84. https://doi.org/10.1089/jpm.2010.0353.
69. Jones C, Bäckman C, Capuzzo M, et al. Intensive care diaries reduce new onset post traumatic stress disorder following critical illness: a randomised, controlled trial. Crit Care 2010;14(5):R168.
70. Jones C, Skirrow P, Griffiths RD, et al. Post-traumatic stress disorder-related symptoms in relatives of patients following intensive care. Intensive Care Med 2004;30(3):456–60.
71. Azoulay E, Pochard F, Kentish-Barnes N, et al. Risk of post-traumatic stress symptoms in family members of intensive care unit patients. Am J Respir Crit Care Med 2005;171(9):987–94.
72. Jones C. Post-traumatic stress disorder in ICU survivors. J Intensive Care Soc 2010;11(2):12–4.
73. National Child Traumatic Stress Network. Medical events and traumatic stress in children and families. Philadelphia: National Child Traumatic Stress Network; 2011.
74. Quossine S, Benbenishty J. PTSD and memory of symptoms during ICU stay. Intensive Care Med 2012;38:S305.
75. Turner J, Kelly B. Culture and medicine: emotional dimensions of chronic disease. West J Med 2000;172:124–8.
76. Hall MF, Hall SE. When treatment becomes trauma: defining, preventing, and transforming medical trauma. Paper based on a program presented at the American Counseling Association Conference. Cincinnati (OH), March 24, 2013.

77. Davis H, Irwin P, Richardson M, et al. When a pet dies: religious issues, euthanasia and strategies for coping with bereavement. Anthrozoös 2003;16(1):57–74.
78. Leo RJ. Competency and the capacity to make treatment decisions: a primer for primary care physicians. Prim Care Companion J Clin Psychiatry 1999;1(5): 131–41.
79. Hindmarch T, Hotopf M, Owen GS. Depression and decision-making capacity for treatment or research: a systematic review. BMC Med Ethics 2013;14(54):1–10.
80. Raymont V, Bingley W, Buchanan A, et al. Prevalence of mental incapacity in medical inpatients and associated risk factors: cross-sectional study. Lancet 2004;364(9443):1421–7.
81. Dastidar JG, Odden A. How do I determine if my patient has decision-making capacity? The Hospitalist 2011. Available at: https://www.the-hospitalist.org/hospitalist/article/124731/how-do-i-determine-if-my-patient-has-decision-making-capacity.
82. Sturman ED. The capacity to consent to treatment and research: a review of standardized assessment tools. Clin Psychol Rev 2005;25:954–74.
83. Appelbaum PS. Assessment of patients' competence to consent to treatment. N Engl J Med 2007;357(18):1834–40.
84. Appelbaum PS, Grisso T. Assessing patients' capacities to consent to treatment. N Engl J Med 1988;319(25):1635–8.
85. Block SD. Medical education in end-of-life care: the status of reform. J Palliat Med 2002;5(2):243–8.
86. Buss MK, Lessen DS, Sullivan AM, et al. Hematology/oncology fellows' training in palliative care. Cancer 2011;117(18):4304–11.

The Animal as Patient
Ethology and End-of-Life Care

Jessica Pierce, PhD

KEYWORDS

• Ethology • Emotion • Quality of life • Pain • Agency • Autonomy

KEY POINTS

- Veterinary hospice and palliative medicine would benefit from interdisciplinary engagement with the field of ethology, in particular, the growing body of research into animal cognition and emotion.
- Pain in animals is interrelated in complex ways with affect, personality, and mood. Attention to animal emotions could improve abilities to interpret and treat pain effectively in animal patients.
- Greater attention to the affective experiences of animals could immensely improve the value and accuracy of quality-of-life assessments. Ethograms and qualitative behavioral assessments might also be added to the palliative care toolbox.
- Respecting each animal patient as a unique individual involves paying attention to the decisional and volitional capacities of animals.

A common refrain in biomedical ethics is "the patient is a person." This admonition is not meant literally, of course, but is symbolic: the patient is not "the liver resection in room 3" or "the 77-year-old female with hip fracture" but is an individual person with unique needs, values, and fears and with her own life story. Against this tendency to flatten out and depersonalize the patient, bioethics asserts a range of moral responsibilities that affirm respect for the patient as a person. The patient has a right to make her own choices, even if these choices are deemed by the medical team not to be ideal; she must be told the truth about her illness, be given the choice to decide which treatment to pursue and when to refuse, have her privacy protected, be treated with fairness, and be allowed to make her own choices about what is important in life. In other words, every attempt should be made to see the patient as a whole person and to remember that health and illness are about far more than just the physical state of an organism.

Veterinary hospice and palliative medicine might heed this same reminder: the patient is a person. In this case, too, person is meant symbolically: the animal patient is a unique

The author has nothing to disclose.
Center for Bioethics and Humanities, University of Colorado Anschutz Medical School, Aurora, CO, USA
E-mail address: jessicapierce.net@gmail.com

individual, with unique needs and wants. As in human medicine, there is a danger that the animal patient can become 1-dimensional during the drama of diagnosis, illness, and caregiving. Because veterinary medicine involves the added layer of a pet owner who represents the patient and who often demands the clinician's attention, it is even easier for the animal patient himself or herself to fade into background.

As veterinary palliative care develops over the next decade, I would like to see a focus on the individual patient diligently kept in view. Thus far, the nascent field has devoted much of its attention to the grieving family and the burned-out and compassion-fatigued veterinary team. I have been to professional conferences where the content was heavily weighted toward handling families in denial, memorializing dead animals, performing euthanasia, and teaching veterinarians and nurses the skills of self-care, with few to no lectures on how to identify behavioral signs of distress or better understand the emotional lives of animal patients. The literature on pet loss and bereavement is many times larger and more robust than the literature on assessing quality of life (QOL) in animal patients, and there are more articles on compassion fatigue than there are on how to accurately identify suffering in animals nearing the end of life.

Surely, veterinarians are wanted who are not burned out and distressed; families are wanted who feel heard and whose grief is handled skillfully. But I would like to see a parallel increase in attention to what animal patients are feeling; how animals themselves experience illness, aging, and dying; and how to best gain access to the subjective experiences of animal patients. To this end, I would like to see veterinary medicine begin to engage more actively with the field of ethology[a], especially the growing body of research into animal emotion and cognition.

In this article, I briefly sketch 3 specific areas in which engagement with the ethology literature and more careful attention to the subjective experiences of animals could improve end-of-life care: (1) interpretation and management of pain, (2) assessments of QOL, and (3) attention to the autonomy of animal patients.

HOW ETHOLOGY COULD HELP IMPROVE DETECTION AND TREATMENT OF PAIN FOR ANIMAL PATIENTS

Pain is arguably the most important clinical and ethical issue in end-of-life care. Research suggests that many companion animals—perhaps numbering in the millions—are not being treated for pain or are being treated inadequately.[1] A significant portion of missed diagnoses, misdiagnoses, undertreatment, and overtreatment likely can be tied to incorrect behavioral assessments, particularly on the part of pet owners but also perhaps on the part of veterinarians.

Research in ethology can nuance understanding of animal pain in a variety of ways, the following 5 of which are briefly sketched: (1) the connection between personality and pain; (2) the compounding of physical pain by the emotional pain of loneliness; (3) the contribution of stress to animal pain; (4) the need for a broader, affective definition of pain; and (5) the problematic role of pet owner in translating animal pain behaviors.

Personality and Pain

Pain is a quintessentially personal experience. The most common medical definition of pain is "what the person says it is." A large body of research has explored how the

---

[a] Ethology is the study of (human and nonhuman) animal behavior, particularly as observed in a natural setting. It focuses on the adaptive significance of behaviors and their genetic, physiologic, and psychological bases.

experience and expression of pain can be influenced by gender, age, past experiences, and cognitive priming. Even individual personality can influence how people experience and express pain. For example, people who rate high on extraversion are more likely to express their experience of pain yet may, at the same time, experience pain less intensely than introverted individuals. People who score high on neuroticism have higher emotional stress responses to pain than those who score low.[2] A similar dynamic seems to be at work in nonhuman animals, with individual personality shaping the experience and expression of pain. (Personality can be understood as individual differences in behavior that remain stable over time.) This has important implications for assessment and effective treatment of animal pain.

Although research into pain and personality in nonhuman animals is still in its early stages, initial results are intriguing. In a 2014 study, Ijichi and colleagues[3] found preliminary evidence that behavioral indicators of pain in horses may not accurately indicate level of tissue damage and that horses' behavioral response to pain varied in relation to personality. Lush and Ijichi[4] conducted a similar study in dogs in 2018, using the Monash Canine Personality Questionnaire–Revised[5] to measure personality and the short form of the Glasgow Composite Measure Pain Scale to measure pain.[6] They found "noticeable individual variation in both behavioral and physiologic responses to pain triggered by the same procedure."[4(p66)]

The investigators also found that behavioral indicators did not correlate with physiologic responses and concluded that "behavior may not indicate when an animal was experiencing poor welfare and that individuals respond differently to the same procedure." Extravert animals scored higher for behavioral expression of pain; more introverted subjects were less likely to exhibit pain-related behaviors. Although the actual pain response may have been the same, the behavioral expression was different. Pain experienced by an introverted animal patient is thus be more likely to be underestimated and also undertreated. (In humans, introverts are also less likely to adopt active coping responses. Might the same be true in other animals?)

It has long been assumed that observable signs of pain, such as those measured in pain scales like the Colorado State University chronic and acute scales for dogs and cats, are reliable indicators not only of the presence of pain but also of the severity of pain experienced. Such behavior-based scales are used to identify whether analgesic drugs are helping and at what dosage. The welfare implications of incorrect assessments of pain are obvious: if underestimated, pain may not be treated effectively; if overestimated, too high an analgesic dosing may be used, leading to adverse effects and possibly also prematurely resorting to euthanasia.[7]

The emerging science of animal personality is vitally important to end-of-life care not only in accurately assessing pain but also in monitoring how patients respond to treatments, how QOL may be impacted by disease or lost mobility, and so on. The better pet owners and veterinarians understand each individual animal, the more effectively they will be able to tailor care to individual needs. Several good personality assessment tools for dogs and cats are available online.[b] These tools could be used by

---

[b] Brian Hare's Dognition Assessment tool (https://www.dognition.com/) and Amanda Jones' Dog Personality Questionnaire (https://gosling.psy.utexas.edu/wp-content/uploads/2014/10/DPQ-forms-and-scoring-keys.pdf) are 2 good validated tools for assessing dog personality. Research into cat personality lags behind dog personality research, and validated tools are still awaited, but Litchfield and colleagues' "The 'Feline Five': An Exploration of Personality in Pet Cats (*Felis catus*)," provides important groundwork, and validated tools will undoubtedly be available soon. Several unvalidated cat personality are available (for example, https://www.catster.com/lifestyle/cat-personality-types); these can still be useful because they encourage cat owners observe their animal more closely.

owners to help build a base of knowledge about canine or feline behavior in general and might nurture a style of close observation and attunement.

Loneliness as Comorbidity

Within the human literature, it is well established that the same neural mechanisms that respond to physical pain also respond to emotional or social pain. The pain of being socially excluded and isolated, for example, is felt in physical ways. A large body of literature in human medicine explores social isolation as a significant risk factor for morbidity and mortality. In "The Psychobiology of Social Pain," McMillan[8] makes a parallel case for social pain and social isolation in animals, suggesting that loneliness and other emotional forms of suffering deserve far more attention from caregivers. "Current research," he says, "leaves little room for doubt that experiences of emotional pain in general, and social pain in particular, can be associated with distress and suffering equal to experiences of physical pain."[8(p166)] Furthermore, there is a marked tendency for humans to underestimate and inadequately empathize with social pain, in particular social pain felt by nonhuman animals.

Loneliness is just one type of social pain experienced by companion animals—but is probably one of the most common forms of suffering in dogs, cats, and other animals kept as pets. Loneliness may be an unexpected comorbidity for animals with chronic disease and perhaps also for animals who are dying. Loneliness could increase sensitivity to pain and perhaps heighten distress associated with other conditions. Illness can exacerbate loneliness and vice versa; on the flip side, social connectedness can enhance mental and physical health. Social support has a significant stress buffering effect.

Social behavior and inflammatory processes are powerful coregulators: sickness leads to characteristic changes in social behavior or what Eisenberg and colleagues[9] call "sickness behaviors." Inflammation increases neural sensitivity to negative social experiences and, in turn, exposure to social stressors increases proinflammatory activity. Individuals who are lonely show increased inflammatory activity. Although Eisenberg and colleagues[9] are writing about human behavior, much of the research on which they build their case was conducted using animal models, and it can be assumed that loneliness and social isolation in other social mammals may similarly increase inflammatory response and thus increase sensitivity to pain.

McMillan,[8] Dodman,[10] Pierce,[11] and others have warned of an epidemic of loneliness in companion dogs in the United States, United Kingdom, and other places where dogs are kept intensively captive. Millions of dogs are left home alone for long periods or are denied adequate social interaction. The problem of loneliness is likely epidemic among cats, too, although little research has explored the social needs of cats, due to the persistent (and undoubtedly inaccurate) stereotyping of cats as aloof and independent. (There are hundreds of research studies about cats being beneficial to humans who feel lonely; I am not aware of a single peer-reviewed article exploring loneliness in cats.) Loneliness is likely a significant welfare problem for the vast array of other species kept as pets as well.

Given than loneliness, social isolation, and separation anxiety affect millions of pet dogs and likely also many cats and other pet animals, greater attention within palliative and hospice medicine to the social well-being of animal patients could be of tremendous benefit. Part of any palliative care counseling should include discussion with owners about taking care of the emotional and social needs of their animal. Owners are generally unaware of the negative effects of leaving dogs alone for long periods and need to be educated about appropriate timeframes for leaving a dog. Although empirical research in this area is lacking, there is loose consensus among behaviorists and trainers that leaving a dog alone for 4 hours is probably fine, but periods longer than this may compromise canine well-being.[a] Many dogs are regularly left alone for much longer periods, some for as many as 12 hours to 14 hours a day.[12] Older and ill animals may have even less tolerance for being alone and likely need additional social support. Compromised mobility, pain, and hearing or vision loss can increase social isolation, and owners may need to take extra steps to keep animals with physical limitations adequately engaged.

Stress, Pain, and Illness

Loneliness and other kinds of social and emotional pain trigger a stress response in the body, and disease and stress are intimately related. Chronic stress can induce and exacerbate disease. For example, research has found that dogs with nonadrenal diseases had significantly higher stress levels than healthy controls,[13] and stressful behavioral conditions in dogs are predictive of skin disorders and shortened life span.[14] Based on these research findings Nicholson and Meredith[15] argue that stress management should be part of clinical care provided to all chronically ill dogs. Cats with high levels of stress are almost 5 times more prone to developing upper respiratory tract infection than cats with lower levels of stress,[16] and stress is linked to development or exacerbation of various other feline diseases.[17]

In addition to counseling about social isolation and loneliness, hospice and palliative medicine veterinarians might consider a general stress audit for their patients, involving a careful discussion with caregivers about a wide range of potential stressors that might be affecting an animal patient (for example, time alone, exposure to noise and activity, and sources of fear, such as slippery floors or steep stairs).

Novel behavioral reactions to stressors also can be used as cues that an animal may be in pain. For example, an older dog who suddenly develops noise phobias should be evaluated for potentially painful conditions. Building on the well-established relationship in the human literature between pain and the development of fear-related avoidance responses, with hypersensitivity to sound a possible indicator of pain, Lopes Fagundes and colleagues[18] looked for a similar relationship in canine patients. They found that older dogs who suddenly develop noise sensitivities are also those who have a chronic health issue that is likely painful. Late-onset noise sensitivities also have been linked to comorbidities with other behavioral problems in dogs. For instance, chronic pain can lead to decreased social play and can heighten aggression toward other dogs. This reinforces what veterinarians often advise pet owners: behavioral changes in animals that occur later in life should always prompt a thorough physical examination, to look for possible signs of pain or discomfort.

Broadening the Definition of Pain

The definition of pain in veterinary medicine needs to extend beyond the International Association for the Study of Pain (IASP) classic definition of pain as "an unpleasant sensory and emotional experience associated with actual or potential tissue damage, or described in terms of such damage," to a definition that invokes a broader range of social and emotional sources of distress. In 2016, prominent pain researchers Williams and Craig[19] proposed an update to the IASP definition: pain is "a distressing experience associated with actual or potential tissue damage with sensory, emotional, cognitive, and social components."[19] This new definition highlights the interactions among health, behavior, mood, affect, and personality. Future research into the complex associations between health problems and affect in elderly and ill dogs, cats, and other companion animals will be of keen interest to clinicians providing care for animal patients nearing the ends of their lives.

Educating Pet Caregivers About Pain Behaviors

Veterinary hospice and palliative medicine relies heavily on owner assessments of how an animal is doing. These assessments are generally inadequate, and it is likely that a great deal of suffering simply falls through the cracks, raising questions about the ethical appropriateness of promoting home-based hospice care for companion animals. Various studies have shown that pet owners are not reliable historians, are not good at assessing how their animal is feeling, and, furthermore, may have only a rudimentary understanding, if any, of the natural history, biology, and behavior of the animals they keep as pets.

Studies repeatedly show owners missing important behavioral cues. Although pet owners usually can recognize sudden changes in behavior, they are not skilled at recognizing subtle behaviors related to pain or the presence of disease or at identifying gradual changes in behavior over time.[20] For example, in a large survey of dog owners by Mariti and colleagues,[21] only half of respondents were able to correctly identify what stress is (a short-term or long-term alteration of homeostasis that can lead to illness). Although many owners were able to recognize overt behavioral indicators of stress, such as trembling, whining, and panting, few could identify more subtle stress behaviors, such as an averted gaze, nose licking, or yawning. Packer and colleagues[22] found that 58% of owners of dogs showing clinical signs of brachycephalic obstructive airway condition did not believe their dog had any breathing problem. Brown and colleagues[23] found that owners had difficulty remembering the time their dog was in pain, and pain scales conducted by owners did not correlate with vertical force produced by arthritic dogs, suggesting that dog owners may not be good at detecting when their pet is in pain.

These and other similar studies highlight the critical need for caregiver education. Ideally, the education of pet owners into the basics of ethology would begin before an animal is even brought into the home and would continue throughout the animal's lifetime. (A recent UK study found that fully a quarter of all people acquiring a pet knew nothing about the type of animal they chose to buy and had done no prior research.[24]) It goes well beyond the ethical obligations of veterinarians to provide this education for pet owners, but as long as there are such enormous gaps in pet owners' understanding of animal behavior, veterinarians need to do what they can to plug the holes.

HOW ETHOLOGY COULD IMPROVE QUALITY-OF-LIFE ASSESSMENTS FOR ANIMAL PATIENTS

Arguably, the QOL assessment could be and should be one of the most important elements of caring for ill or aged animals nearing the end of life. At its best, a QOL assessment would provide a relatively objective measure of how an animal patient is feeling and how illness, age-related changes, and treatment protocols are affecting the life-experience and well-being of the animal patient, from the patient's own point of view. The purpose of such an assessment would be to fine-tune pain protocols, look for improvements to an animal's physical environment, reduce sources of stress and fear where possible, and identify and fill gaps in meeting an animal's emotional and social needs.

Unfortunately, QOL assessment tools have not yet come into their own in hospice and palliative medicine. Many tools, such as the ubiquitous Pawspice QOL scale, are available online to pet owners, and veterinarians often recommend the use of such tools for clients. Yet, although these simplified tools can sometimes help owners see gaps in care, more often they function as decision trees for euthanasia and not rigorous ones at that. The Pawspice QOL and other pet owner scales are rarely statistically validated and often lack the nuance required to carefully assess subjective states of an animal. They instruct people to look for certain behaviors, such as incontinence, but give no guidance about how such behaviors might reflect an animal's internal state nor do they given any hint at just how complex reading an animal's behavior can be. They do not account for the individuality of animal patients and pay no attention to the complex interplay of affect, illness, and behavior.

Clinicians recommending the use of tools, such as the Pawspice QOL scale, need to understand their function and limitations and be attuned to the limitations of pet owners in assessing an animal's behavior, including lack of observational skills and behavioral training and the potential for human emotional contamination of behavioral observations. Given that the purpose of the QOL assessment is to measure the subjective state of an animal, more attention to how to observe, record, and interpret canine or feline behavior surely would be beneficial. Instead, QOL tools tend to focus on what the caregiver believes is important—which may not track well onto what the animal wants or is experiencing.

A handful of good validated and reliable QOL instruments has been developed, mainly to measure clinical outcomes in research settings (eg, comparing outcomes for 2 different treatment protocols for cancer). Although statistically validated and often highly detailed, these clinical instruments may be too complex and involved for most pet caregivers and have limited usefulness in the home setting. The development of a variety of validated and reliable instruments for use in the home setting, and focused by species, diagnosis, and other refining features, would improve end-of-life care.

One final note about QOL. The term is vague, and this creates some ethical hazards. Even clinical veterinary studies evaluating the success of various treatments often refer to QOL without carefully defining the term.[25] Moreover, the parameters used to assess QOL are primarily clinical, ignoring behavioral parameters that might be involved in a broader assessment of an animal's welfare, including the impacts of a treatment on an animal's emotional and social well-being. Interdisciplinary dialogue between ethologists and veterinarians could help improve animal welfare assessments within a veterinary context, both in the clinical setting and within the home environment.

Qualitative Behavioral Assessments and Ethograms

No matter how good the QOL assessment tools, they only capture part of what is important to an animal. In addition to a larger and better set of QOL assessment options, hospice and palliative medicine could make use of a broader behavioral assessment toolbox. Pain scales are one important adjunct to QOL assessments (despite their limitations, as discussed previously). Two additional tools that might further augment end-of-life care (and care throughout the life span of an animal) are ethograms and qualitative behavioral assessments (QBAs).

Briefly, an ethogram is an inventory or catalog of species-specific and, for this article's purposes, individual-specific behaviors. The ethogram is one of the basic tools used by ethologists to observe and record an animal's behavior. Bekoff and Pierce[26] argue that simple ethograms could be used by pet owners to enhance their knowledge and understanding of their individual animal and thereby improve the quality of the human-canine or human-feline (or human-other) bond. The ethogram approach focuses on the full range of behaviors, not just those behaviors that have been identified (by caregiver or veterinarian) as problematic, negative, or illness related. Creating ethograms can help pet owners establish a baseline of normal behavior and can encourage them to revel in and get to know the individual quirks of their animal.

The use of ethograms by pet owners with ill or aged animals could augment care in important ways, by encouraging close observation, curiosity about behavioral patterns, and attention to change. Unlike QOL assessments, which focus heavily on negative experiences and involve highly subjective judgments by pet owners ("Did your animal have a good day or bad day?"), ethograms are descriptive and focus simply on what an animal is doing.

The QBA is an approach to whole-animal behavioral profiling, pioneered by Wemelsfelder.[27] A QBA is designed to give the observer a window into an animal's own perception of his or her world and into the animal's affective state. It is an enhanced QOL assessment tool: it is more comprehensive and focused on the entire range of an animal's behavioral repertoire, not just pain or sickness behaviors. The QBA is a "validated methodology for the study of animal expressivity (body language) and subjective experience" and "focuses on observation of the whole animal and characterizes and quantifies the animal's dynamic demeanour as an expressive body language."[28] Work has been done to develop QBA tools to assess the welfare and coping ability of dogs in shelters, with the goals of providing the dogs an opportunity to express a wide repertoire of behaviors and helping shelter staff make comprehensive assessments of dogs' welfare state. Thus far, QBAs have not been developed or applied to end-of-life care, but I believe this would be a fruitful avenue for further work.

Quality-of-Life and Euthanasia Decisions

Researchers know little about how and why people choose euthanasia for chronically ill animals and what determines the decision point. But it is likely that judgments about an animal's QOL are often driving the decision to request euthanasia, whether or not these QOL judgments are guided by some kind of formalized assessment or are simply a gestalt judgment made by pet owners at some point in an animal's life. The life-and-death nature of these judgments suggests the profound importance of getting behavioral assessments as right as possible.

Researchers in New Zealand combed through a medical records database to investigate how chronic disease conditions and clinical signs of illness influenced decision making about euthanasia for aging companion animals.[29] They found that more than 90% of cat and dog patients were euthanized (with a high frequency of these deaths occurring, for whatever reason, in December). Cost was a driving factor in approximately one-fifth of the euthanasias; in the remaining cases, most animals "were recorded as having >1 clinical sign associated with a decreased quality-of-life,"[29] with inappetence[c] and nonspecific decline the 2 most common factors. This study highlights the fact that pet owners are using behavioral cues (QOL indicators), such as inappetence, to drive the decision to euthanize. It is essential to find ways to make behavioral assessments as informed and accurate as possible. The study also elucidates an additional key point: many older animals are living with chronic

---

[c] Inappetence is often cited by pet owners as contributing to euthanasia decisions, and veterinarians actively treat inappetence as a problem (for example, by prescribing drugs to stimulate appetite). Yet there is virtually no empirical research on the role of inappetence in serious illness in companion animals, particularly not in end-of-life care. Most animals are euthanized preemptively when illness and decline set in, so there is never an opportunity to observe what cessation of eating and drinking before death would look like for them or to gather data on inappetence at the end of life. It is not known, then, whether and when inappetence might be unpleasant for an animal and whether it should be labeled as suffering. In sharp contrast, most humans cease eating and drinking before death, and this is taken to be a natural and inevitable (and, incidentally, relatively comfortable) part of the dying process.

disease conditions and may suffer, if care is not taken to observe, interpret, and respond to behavioral cues of stress, pain, or discomfort.

Another reason the QOL assessment may be playing an outsized role in euthanasia decisions is that some animals are euthanized by a veterinarian (or, in a few states, perhaps a veterinary nurse) who has never seen the patient before the euthanasia appointment. In these cases, the pet owner is relying on her own assessments of how the animal patient is feeling and when it is time, although hopefully with at least some input from the animal's regular veterinarian. In the United States, approximately 10% to 15% of pets are euthanized by a mobile euthanasia service seeing the animal for the first time. As mobile euthanasia services proliferate, this scenario is likely to become more common. What kind of QOL assessments have been made, if any, is unknown.

Finally, the actual, practical outcomes of QOL assessment use or nonuse need to be understood as part of a larger question of whether QOL scales do more harm than good. On their face, a QOL assessment tool seems hard to argue with. Who would not want a caregiver to pay more attention to how their animal is feeling? Yet it is far from clear that seat-of-the-pants assessments improve animal well-being or contribute to good end-of-life care. As far as I am aware, no research has yet looked at what happens to animal patients when veterinarians and family caregivers initiate use of a QOL tool. Does quality of care improve? Does QOL improve? In what ways (eg, Are dogs whose owners use a QOL tool more likely to be treated appropriately for pain?)? Does the use of QOL scales initiate earlier euthanasia? How many of these euthanasias might be premature, from the animal's point of view? Can tools developed for use in palliative care situations to increase an animal's comfort be distinguished from those developed as euthanasia decision trees?

Quality of Life and Caregivers

Optimizing end-of-life care and QOL for animals is an extraordinarily complex endeavor and, as discussed previously, relies on an extremely nuanced appreciation of how pain and behavior intersect. As if gaining access to how an animal is feeling were not hard enough, there are layers of additional complexity arising from a patient's relationship to his or her human caregiver(s). The knowledge, attitudes, and attentiveness of pet owners influence how well they read their animal and how responsive they are. Their own emotional state can influence what they see in their pet. For instance, hospice and palliative care veterinarians often report that owners seem blind to their animal's suffering, because the owners themselves are so caught up in anticipatory grieving or denial.

How closely bonded a human is with his or her animal can influence both how well the human is able to read and interpret behaviors and what level of care an ill or dying animal receives. For example, the type of relationship a dog and owner have can influence the behavior of a dog during a clinical examination with a veterinarian[30]—information that is useful for clinicians and caregivers alike, when trying to understand normal behavior patterns for a given animal. Csoltova and colleagues[31] showed that veterinary encounters produce an acute stress response in dogs, with dogs showing significant increases in lip-licking, heart rate, and maximal ocular surface temperatures. An owner's touching and talking to her dog during the examination had an attenuating effect on the dog's stress level.

Another key area for further work is on the interconnections between what Spitznagel and colleagues[32] call "caregiver burden" and the quality of an animal's care. When caregivers are so stressed that they suffer from reduced psychosocial functioning, their ability to provide good care—including, presumably, their ability to make and report objective and accurate behavioral observations of their animal—may be compromised.

Although attention to a patient is always the priority, effective care cannot occur in isolation from an animal's family.

RESPECT FOR PATIENT AUTONOMY

The concept of patient within biomedical ethics discussion typically evokes a range of associations linked to the unique moral responsibilities owed by physicians, researchers, and health care systems to people who are placed in this role. Perhaps the most likely association that springs to mind is respect for patient autonomy.

There is a strong tendency to be paternalistic toward animal patients and to assume that they cannot speak for themselves or decide on or engage in their own care. Yet even a cursory reading of the literature on animal cognition and emotion establishes that animals share with humans the decisional and volitional capacities that underlie autonomy and agency. In relation to animal patients, I would like to see the field of veterinary hospice and palliative medicine engage the ethically important components of care related to respecting patients as autonomous agents who can and should participate in decision making and for whom the concepts of consent and dissent are meaningful.

A careful discussion of these issues goes well beyond the scope of this article. Interested readers might begin with Beauchamp and Wobber's[33] article; Fenton's[34] article; Bekoff and Pierce's[35]; and Peña-Guzmán's[36].

An example of how the ethological literature on animal agency and autonomy might stimulate discussion in veterinary medicine is to raise the question of when, if ever, allow animals should be allowed to refuse treatments. To take a concrete case related to end-of-life care, how can the behavior of a dog or cat who decides, at some point, to stop eating and drinking be understood? An animal refusing food or losing interest in food is a common problem in palliative and hospice care. On the one hand, many animals who are ill or in pain experience decreased appetite. Inappetence is a medical condition to which veterinarians should respond. Yet how can medical inappetence and an animal's decision to stop eating and drinking as an autonomous act, a refusal of continued life, be distinguished?

Voluntary refusal of food and fluid seems to fall into a compendium of what Peña-Guzmán[36] calls "self-initiated behaviors that ultimately produce self-harm or death." How can all the threads in a patient's refusal to eat or drink be untangled, so that the response to individual animals affirms their choices, if they are indeed making a choice, to produce death, while ensuring that uncomfortable symptoms, such as nausea and pain, are responded to? Refusal to eat is often met with 1 of 2 responses: (1) medication to stimulate appetite and, perhaps more likely, (2) what the poet Billy Collins calls "the needle of oblivion." But what about a third option? When, if ever, might an animal's autonomous choice to end his or her own life by not eating be respected? A refusal to eat points to a larger issue of dissent. Animals have the cognitive ability to dissent from various kinds of interactions with humans, and this is a morally salient capacity.

Within the realm of companion animal end-of-life care, finding ways to provide medical care that is attentive to consent, assent, and dissent should be continued. Too often a throw-away point is simply made: "animals cannot speak so we have to decide for them." This paternalism often goes unchecked and is always unwarranted. There is an opportunity to do much better to accommodate the volitional and decisional capacities of animals.

SUMMARY

Treating the animal patient as a person involves refining the capacity to see the patient as clearly as possible. Veterinary end-of-life care can usefully engage with the science of animal emotion and cognition to help bring the patient into 3-D. The word, *patient*, derives etymologically from the Latin word *patiens*, which means "one who suffers." It is by attending as carefully as possible to the subjective experiences of each individual animal, to who each animal is, and to what he or she is feeling that addressing suffering and providing effective support during the final months, weeks, days, and moments of each animal's life will be best situated

REFERENCES

1. Simon BT, Scallan EM, Carroll G, et al. The lack of analgesic use (oligoanalgesia) in small animal practice. J Small Anim Pract 2017. https://doi.org/10.1111/jsap.12717.
2. Soriano J, Monsalve V, Gómez-Carretero P, et al. Vulnerable personality profile in patients with chronic pain: relationship with coping, quality of life and adaptation to disease. Int J Psychol Res 2012;5:42–51.
3. Ijichi C, Collins L, Elwood R. Pain expression is linked to personality in horses. Appl Anim Behav Sci 2014;152:38–43.
4. Lush J, Ijichi C. A preliminary investigation into personality and pain in dogs. J Vet Behav 2018;24:62–8.
5. Ley JM, Bennettt PC, Coleman GJ. A refinement and validation of the Monash Canine Personality Questionnaire (MCPQ). Appl Anim Behav Sci 2009;116:220–7.
6. Reid J, Nolan A, Hughes JML, et al. Development of the short form Glasgow Composite Measure Pain Scale (CMPS-SF) and derivation of an analgesic intervention score. Anim Welf 2007;16:97–104.
7. Ashley H, Waterman-Pearson AE, Whay HR. Behavioural assessment of pain in horses and donkeys: applications to clinical practice and future studies. Equine Vet J 2005;37:565–75.
8. McMillan FD. The psychobiology of social pain: evidence for a neurocognitive overlap with physical pain and welfare implications for social animals with special attention to the domestic dog (*Canis familiaris*). Physiol Behav 2016;167:154–71.
9. Eisenberg N, Moieni M, Inagaki T, et al. In sickness and in health: the co-regulation of inflammation and social behavior. Neuropsychopharmacology 2017;42:242–53.
10. Dodman N. Pets on the couch. neurotic dogs, compulsive cats, anxious birds, and the new science of animal psychiatry. New York: Atria Books; 2017.
11. Pierce J. Run, spot, run: the ethics of keeping pets. Chicago: University of Chicago Press; 2016.
12. Pierce J. How long can you leave a dog home alone? Psychology Today. Available at: https://www.psychologytoday.com/us/blog/all-dogs-go-heaven/201802/how-long-can-you-leave-dog-home-alone. Accessed February 15, 2019.
13. Kaplan AJ, Peterson ME, Kemppainen RJ. Effects of disease on the results of diagnostic tests for use in detecting hyperadrenocorticism in dogs. J Am Vet Med Assoc 1995;4:445–51.
14. Dreschel NA. The effects of fear and anxiety on health and lifespan in pet dogs. Appl Anim Behav Sci 2010;125:157–62.
15. Nicholson S, Meredith J. Should stress management be part of the clinical care provided to chronically ill dogs? J Vet Behav Clin Appl Res 2015;10:489–95.

16. Tanaka A, Wagner DC, Kass PH. Associations among weight loss, stress, and upper respiratory tract infection in shelter cats. J Am Vet Med Assoc 2012;240: 570–6.

17. Amat M, Camps T, Manteca X. Stress in owned cats: behavioural changes and welfare implications. J Feline Med Surg 2016;18:577–86.

18. Lopes Fagundes AL, Hewison L, McPeake KJ, et al. Noise sensitivities in dogs: an exploration of signs in dogs with and without musculoskeletal pain using qualitative content analysis. Front Vet Sci 2018;5:17.

19. Williams DE, Craig KD. Updating the definition of pain. Pain 2016;157(11): 2420–3.

20. Reaney S, Zulch H, Mills D, et al. Emotional affect and the occurrence of owner reported health problems in the domestic dog. Appl Anim Behav Sci 2017;196: 76–83.

21. Mariti C, Gazzano A, Lansdown Moore J, et al. Perception of dogs' stress by their owners. J Vet Behav Clin Appl Res 2012;7:213–9.

22. Packer RMA, Hendricks A, Burn CC. Do dog owners perceive the clinical signs related to conformational inherited disorders as 'normal' for the breed? A potential constraint to improving canine welfare. Anim Welf 2012;21:81–93.

23. Brown DC, Boston RC, Farrar JT. Comparison of force plate gait analysis and owner assessment of pain using the canine brief inventory scale in dogs with osteoarthritis. J Vet Intern Med 2013;27:22–30.

24. People's Dispensary for Sick Animals. PAWS report 2017. Available at: https://www.pdsa.org.uk/media/4371/paw-2018-full-web-ready.pdf. Accessed February 15, 2019.

25. Christiansen SB, Forkman B. Assessment of animal welfare in a veterinary context – a call for ethologists. Appl Anim Behav Sci 2007;106:203–20.

26. Bekoff M, Pierce J. Unleashing your dog: a field guide to freedom. Novato (CA): New World Library; 2019.

27. Wemelsfelder F. How animals communicate quality of life: the qualitative assessment of behaviour. Anim Welfare 2007;16:25–31.

28. Arena L, Wemelsfelder F, Messori S, et al. Application of free choice profiling to assess the emotional state of dogs housed in shelter environments. Appl Anim Behav Sci 2017;195:72–9. Available at: http://openaccess.sruc.ac.uk/handle/11262/11266.

29. Gates MC, Hinds HJ, Dale A. Preliminary description of aging cats and dogs presented to a New Zealand first-opinion veterinary clinic at end-of-life. N Z Vet J 2017;65:313–7.

30. Lind AK, Hydbring-Sandberg E, Forkman B, et al. Assessing stress in dogs during a visit to the veterinary clinic: correlations between dog behavior in standardized tests and assessments by veterinary staff and owners. J Vet Behav Clin Appl Res 2017;17:24–31.

31. Csoltova E, Martineau M, Boissy A, et al. Behavioral and physiological reactions in dogs to a veterinary examination: owner-dog interactions improve canine well-being. Physiol Behav 2017;177:270–81.

32. Spitznagel MB, Jacobson DM, Cox MD, et al. Caregiver burden in owners of a sick companion animal: a cross-sectional observational study. Vet Rec 2017. https://doi.org/10.1136/vr.104295.

33. Beauchamp TL, Wobber V. Autonomy in chimpanzees. Theor Med Bioeth 2014; 352:117–32.

34. Fenton A. Can a chimp say "no"? Revisioning chimpanzee dissent in harmful research. Camb Q Healthc Ethics 2014;23:130–9.

35. Bekoff M, Pierce J. The animals' agenda: freedom, compassion, and coexistence in the age of humanity. Boston: Beacon Press; 2017.
36. Peña-Guzmán DM. Can nonhuman animals commit suicide? Animal Sentience 2017;20(1). Available at: https://animalstudiesrepository.org/cgi/viewcontent. cgi?article=1201&context=animsent.

Caregiver Burden and Veterinary Client Well-Being

Mary Beth Spitznagel, PhD[a],*, Mark D. Carlson, DVM[b]

KEYWORDS

- Pet caregiver burden • Veterinary client • Serious illness • Palliative care

KEY POINTS

- Caregiver burden is present in about one-half of veterinary clients in the context of serious illness, and is greater in this group than matched healthy controls.
- Greater caregiver burden correlates with poorer client psychosocial functioning, including greater stress, symptoms of anxiety and depression, and lower quality of life.
- Factors associated with caregiver burden include a difficult patient care plan, the frequency of clinical signs in the patient, and client reactivity and sense of mastery.
- Best practices for decreasing caregiver burden have yet to be established, but research-based suggestions for veterinarians working with clients who face these issues are provided.

INTRODUCTION

The management of a companion animal's serious disease in a palliative care setting can be complex and time consuming for the client, possibly leading to emotional distress or caregiver burden. Even when the gift of time, energy, love, and care is willingly given, it can cause strain. Caregiver burden is the term used to describe the response of distress to difficulties encountered while providing care for an individual with an illness.[1] This reaction is typically multidimensional, with repercussions ranging across physical, financial, social, and mental health domains.[2] A person in this situation often "gives until it hurts."

Particularly in a palliative care setting, working with veterinary clients is not just a matter of customer service. Emotions run high and the client may not feel equipped to deal with everything they are facing. Although it is not within the veterinarian's scope of practice to treat mental health issues in clients, it is important to understand the perspective of the client experiencing caregiver distress.

In this article, we describe caregiver burden, including how it differs from other key client experiences in the palliative care setting, particularly client quality of life and grief.

Disclosure Statement: The authors have nothing to disclose.
[a] Department of Psychological Sciences, Kent State University, 144 Kent Hall, Kent, OH 44242, USA; [b] Stow Kent Animal Hospital, 4559 Kent Road, Kent, OH 44240, USA
* Corresponding author.
E-mail address: mspitzna@kent.edu

We briefly review caregiver burden in human relationships, and summarize research to date examining veterinary client caregiver burden in the context of serious illness (also referred to as pet caregiver burden [PCB]). We describe the influence of PCB on the client's psychosocial well-being, discuss risk factors for who develops burden in this context, and begin to address how it might be ameliorated or prevented. Finally, we provide suggestions for veterinarians coping with these issues in a palliative care setting.

DIFFERENTIATING CAREGIVER BURDEN FROM CLIENT QUALITY OF LIFE AND GRIEF

Before beginning a discussion of PCB, it is important to distinguish this concept from other veterinary client experiences in the context of serious illness, including grief and the client's quality of life. These 3 issues are each important and should not be confused with one another (**Table 1**).

Caregiver Burden

As noted, caregiver burden is a response to the many problems and challenges faced by a person providing care for a loved one who is ill.[1] Burden is viewed as a combination of both objective aspects of providing care, including time and physical demands of caregiving, as well as subjective experiences, such as perceptions and emotional responses to caregiving.[3] Consider the many daily needs provided by a caregiver: meal preparation, medication administration, personal care, managing health care appointments, and so on. Caregivers may forgo their own self-care to provide for a loved one, depleting their own time, energy, physical, emotional, and financial resources. Burden usually lasts throughout the time spent providing care, and increasing over time[4] with worsening illness and rising care demands. As a product of dealing with difficulties associated with caregiving, the burden should abate when caregiving activities discontinue, for example, after the loved one dies.

Caregiver and Veterinary Client Quality of Life

Whereas burden describes strain experienced by the caregiver owing specifically to the caregiving role, quality of life is a broad multidimensional concept that involves an assessment of the overall "goodness" of the person's life across multiple domains, such as physical and psychological wellness, and social relationships.[5] A close link is observed between caregiver burden and quality of life,[6] that is, someone who is feeling burdened in caregiving is likely to experience lower quality of life; however, these phenomena are conceptually distinct. Burden focuses specifically on strain owing to caregiving, whereas quality of life is an assessment of satisfaction with different facets of life. Quality of life has recently been evaluated in veterinary clients caring for dogs and cats with diseases, including diabetes and dermatologic presentations.[7–10] Measures considering how a companion animal's illness impacts the owner have also been developed in the context of oncology[11] and seizure disorder,[12] although the term quality of life is not explicitly used in these cases, and these instruments have not been validated against established measures of human quality of life. As veterinarians continue to conceptualize client experiences, it is important to understand the difference between quality of life and caregiver burden, because research suggests that findings in one domain may not directly translate to the other.[13]

Grief

In contrast with both caregiver burden (ie, strain from caregiving) and veterinary client quality of life (ie, goodness of life), grief is a reaction to loss. After the death of a loved one, emotional reactions such as sadness, anger, guilt, anxiety, and despair are

Table 1
Key client experiences in palliative care settings

	Caregiver Burden	Quality of Life	Grief
What is it?	Strain owing to caregiving; subjective (emotional) response plus objective (physical) demands of caregiving	Sense of life's "goodness;" client's subjective evaluation of positive and negative aspects of own life	Bereavement reaction; feelings of sadness and despair owing to a loss (or anticipated loss in anticipatory grief)
What is the course?	Increases in intensity with greater duration of caregiving; abates when caregiving stops (eg, death)	Changes according to context, for example, may be lower in the context of caregiver burden	Typically decreases in intensity over time; may be acute reaction or prolonged (complicated grief)
How is it measured?	Self-reported experiences of stress, anger, uncertainty, embarrassment, financial strain, lack of time, etc owing to caregiving	Self-reported satisfaction with various life domains, such as physical health, mood, work, social relationships, and financial status	Self-reported difficulty accepting death, avoidance, reduced daily functioning, feeling distant, depressed, fatigued, and hopeless
When is it measured?	During period of caretaking for a loved one's illness	Any time, of particular interest during periods of difficulty (eg, caretaking, grief)	After a death, unless examining anticipatory grief

common; physical effects such as reduced sleep and feeling ill can also occur.[14] Grief comes in waves, especially when thoughts turn to memories of the deceased,[15] but tends to decrease in intensity within approximately 6 months.[14] Grief has been evaluated in the context of veterinary medicine and pet loss. Early work[16] showed severe grief was present in 30% of owners who had lost a dog or cat within the past 2 weeks. Later research[17] demonstrated that subclinical grief and sadness lasting 6 months or more occurred in about 30% of pet owners; the more distant time point may account for the lower severity of grief compared with the prior work. Importantly, for some clients, grief may begin before the companion animal's death, in the form of anticipatory grief, a grief process that occurs before, and in preparation for, actual loss.[18] When anticipatory grief occurs, grief and burden may cooccur. Otherwise, the 2 generally differ in timeframe, with burden occurring while the patient is alive and grief after the patient's death, and certainly differ in fundamental emotional experience.

Grief and veterinary client quality of life are important issues for the palliative care veterinarian to be aware of, but these phenomena are more commonly recognized in veterinary medicine compared with caregiver burden. A better understanding of the full range of client experiences in this setting, including caregiver burden, might facilitate empathic communication and relationship-centered interactions with a distressed client, which could in turn leading to greater gratification for both the client and the veterinarian.[19,20]

LESSONS FROM HUMAN MEDICINE

Although to date little research has attended to the issue of caregiver burden in veterinary medicine, it is well-studied in human medicine. We thus briefly turn to the human caregiving literature to provide a foundation to better understand PCB.

Correlates and Consequences of Burden

The human caregiving literature demonstrates physiologic consequences of burden, such as higher daytime levels of cortisol,[21,22] as well as negative emotional outcomes including anxiety and depression.[23,24] Depression is especially common, with up to 70% of caregivers exhibiting clinically meaningful symptoms of depression, and 50% meeting diagnostic criteria for a major depressive disorder.[25] Although depression and caregiver burden often cooccur, they are independent constructs, with some investigators suggesting that prolonged burden may lead to depression.[3,26] Poorer caregiver functioning (eg, experiencing significant burden and depression) shows strong links to increased risk of mortality for the caregiver[27] and institutionalization for the care recipient.[28] These problems are not just an emotional reaction to the fact that a loved one is ill, but seem to be related specifically to the role of caregiving. Research shows greater burden is present in the individual providing care compared with noncaregiver relatives.[29]

Predictors of Caregiver Burden

Not all caregivers experience significant distress; considerable individual variability in burden exists. Recent data show that nearly 60% of caregivers report moderate or greater burden, with the remaining approximately 40% not endorsing substantial burden.[30] Many different factors predict caregiver distress, and are often considered contributors to burden, such as the care recipient's symptom severity and behavior problems, number of tasks and amount of time spent caregiving, longer duration of the caregiving role, and lower relationship satisfaction before onset of caregiving.[23,31–33] Ongoing research efforts in human medicine are identifying risk and protective factors for caregiver burden; these data are essential to incorporate when considering interventions.

Interventions for Caregiver Burden

A substantial literature demonstrates that it is possible to ameliorate burden. For example, behavioral interventions can decrease distress and anxiety[34] as well as symptoms of caregiver burden[35] among family caregivers. A review[3] suggests the most effective interventions are of at least 6 months duration,[36] extend beyond education to address various components of burden,[37] and are agile, targeting the caregiver's specific needs.[38] Most recently, an emphasis has been placed on low-cost, technology-based (ie, telephone, Internet) efforts to reduce burden, which have been effective in a manner similar to face-to-face interventions for human caregiving relationships.[39,40] This trend will likely continue, because common caregiver stressors including time pressure and financial strain, necessitate that interventions be easily available and cost effective.

IS CAREGIVER BURDEN PRESENT IN OWNERS OF SICK PETS?

The concept of caregiver burden, as understood in human medicine, is just beginning to gain traction in veterinary medicine. Although companion animals have long been viewed by their owners as members of the family,[41] until recently, few data existed to address whether burden within the context of human–animal interaction occurs in a manner similar to human caregiving relationships. Christiansen and colleagues[42] examined this issue in a qualitative study, interviewing 12 owners of aged or ill dogs. They identified several issues suggesting the presence of caregiver burden, including the need to provide additional care, limitations related to work, social life, and finances, and emotional strain including sadness and frustration in the context of their dog's changes in health and activity. This work suggested a need for further study.

Assessing Presence and Psychosocial Correlates of Burden

Study 1: Social media sample
To quantitatively measure caregiver burden in the context of a companion animal's serious illness, Spitznagel and colleagues[43] asked 238 owners of a dog or cat about experiences related to burden using a standard measure called the Zarit Burden Interview,[1] adapted for use in veterinary medicine. This measure taps into many aspects of burden, for example, feeling like there is insufficient time in the day or financial resources to provide care, or emotional responses like guilt, anger, or fear in the context of caregiving. Established measures of stress, anxiety, depression, and quality of life were also used. Questions were posed in an online format. Participants were recruited via social media, in large part through pet disease support groups. Owners of a dog or cat with a serious illness, such as cancer, diabetes, renal failure, or other disease requiring daily management, were blindly matched with healthy controls according to owner age and gender, and animal species.

The results (**Fig. 1**) showed that owners of a sick dog or cat reported high levels of caregiver burden—on average, about twice as high as those with a healthy dog or cat ($P<.001$). The level of burden reported by those with a sick companion animal was above the cutoff that would be considered clinically meaningful if that burden were being reported in a human caregiving situation. Poorer psychosocial functioning was observed for stress and symptoms of depression and anxiety (ie, higher levels in owners of a sick companion animal), whereas quality of life showed the opposite pattern (ie, higher in healthy controls). Further, as expected, these problems were correlated with caregiver burden ($r_s = 0.41$ through 0.54; $P<.001$).

This first study to formally measure PCB thus showed that burden is present in owners of a seriously ill cat or dog and is closely related to the client's psychosocial

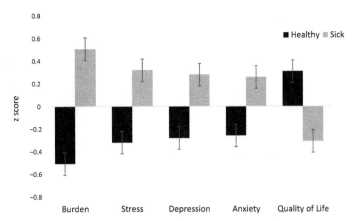

Fig. 1. Greater caregiver burden, stress, anxiety, and depressive symptoms was observed in owners of dogs and cats with a serious illness compared with age and gender (owner) and species-matched healthy dogs and cats (all *P*<.001). Higher quality of life was observed in owners of healthy dogs and cats (*P*<.001). (*Data from* Spitznagel MB, Jacobson DM, Cox MD, et al. Caregiver burden in owners of a sick companion animal: a cross-sectional observational study. Vet Rec 2017;181:321.)

well-being. Importantly, this sample was recruited online through social media, and it is possible that persons experiencing a particularly great amount of distress would turn to social media pet disease groups for support, introducing potential bias. As such, although this study was an important step in understanding PCB, it was necessary to replicate the work in veterinary clients.

Assessing the Presence and Psychosocial Correlates of Burden

Study 2: Veterinary client sample
Methods from the first study were repeated and extended in a sample of veterinary clients recruited through a small animal general veterinary hospital via mass email.[44] The participants, 124 clients (62 with a dog or cat with an illness defined by the client as chronic or terminal, and 62 demographically matched clients with a healthy pet) completed the online measures described elsewhere in this article. A similar pattern of results emerged—greater burden and poorer psychosocial functioning, including greater stress, symptoms of anxiety and depression, and lower quality of life in the context of serious illness (*P*<.01; **Fig. 2**). Again, burden was robustly correlated with all measures of psychosocial functioning in the direction of greater burden being linked to reduced client well-being (r_s = 0.50 through 0.59; *P*<.001).

Importantly, although caregiver burden was higher in the context of serious illness, approximately one-half of the owners with a sick companion animal showed meaningfully increased levels of burden. This finding is consistent with statistics from the human medicine literature,[30] and highlights that, although caregiver burden is present for many, not all caregivers experience high levels of burden.

Assessing the Presence and Psychosocial Correlates of Burden

Summary of current research
Together, these works demonstrate that caregiver burden can be detected in the context of serious illness in the companion animal, and that its presence is linked to negative psychosocial outcomes including stress, symptoms of anxiety and

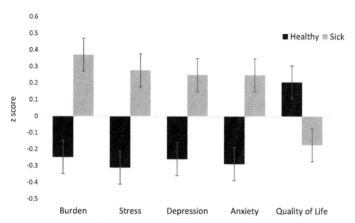

Fig. 2. Greater caregiver burden, stress, anxiety, and depressive symptoms was observed in small animal veterinary clients with dogs and cats with a serious illness compared with age and gender (client) and species-matched healthy dogs and cats (all *P*<.01). Higher quality of life was observed in owners of healthy dogs and cats (*P*<.01). (*Data from* Spitznagel MB, Cox MD, Jacobson DM, et al. Assessment of caregiver burden and associations with psychosocial function, veterinary service use, and factors related to treatment plan adherence among owners of dogs and cats. J Am Vet Med Assoc 2019;254(1):124–32.

depression, and diminished quality of life. As cross-sectional observations, these studies cannot determine if the burden of caregiving is the root of these problems. However, they demonstrate the importance of continued research to determine who develops PCB, and if it can be prevented or reduced when it occurs.

WHY DO SOME EXPERIENCE BURDEN, WHILE OTHERS DO NOT?

In the context of serious illness, some veterinary clients develop PCB while others do not. It is thus important to identify primary contributors to burden. Are there certain risk factors that, if present, increase the likelihood that a client will experience burden?

Predicting Caregiver Burden in Veterinary Clients: A First Look

To examine predictors of PCB, Spitznagel and colleagues[44] looked at elements of the care plan to determine if specific challenges related to caregiving in the context of serious illness are linked to greater burden in the 62 veterinary clients described elsewhere in this article. For example, does difficulty administering medication or otherwise following a care plan increase the likelihood of burden? Key correlates of burden included changes in daily routine and difficulty following new routines. Although these factors were significantly correlated with burden (*P*<.001), the magnitude of the relationship was only moderate ($r_s = 0.43$), suggesting that the development of caregiver burden is more complex than just difficulty managing a care routine.

Predicting Caregiver Burden in Veterinary Clients: Follow-Up

To further investigate potential factors underlying PCB, Spitznagel and colleagues[45] examined a broad model of possible contributors to burden in veterinary clients managing serious illness in a dog or cat. Demographic characteristics such as the client's income were considered alongside the companion animal's clinical signs and behavior problems (both frequency of occurrence and the client's level of distress in response), as well as the client's personal resources, such as coping style, problem-solving skills, sense of control over the situation, emotional support (eg, having some-one to talk to), and tangible support (eg, having someone to help out) in a sample of 95 owners of a seriously ill companion animal, recruited through a small animal general veterinary hospital.

Consistent with findings in the human literature, the frequency of the companion animal's clinical problems were strongly related to burden ($P<.001$), with greater correlations found for presentations including weakness, a change in personality, seeming sad, depressed, or anxious, the animal being in pain or discomfort, frequent urination, and excessive sleeping or lethargy. Although a relationship with lower burden was observed for greater coping skills and better social support, these factors did not predict burden, or the client's reaction to their companion animal's problems ($P = .01$), or the sense of control ($P = .04$) in this context.

Predicting Caregiver Burden in Veterinary Clients: Summary of Current Research

Taken together, findings suggest that caregiver burden arises from factors beyond a difficult care plan or the companion animal's specific clinical signs and behavior problems. These issues are important, but must be considered within the framework of the individual client's reactivity, including how well-equipped the client feels to deal with these problems. Other important risk and protective factors for PCB will likely emerge with continued research, and should ultimately help to target appropriate strategies for prevention or intervention.

FIXING THE PROBLEM: CAN WE RELY ON EMPIRICAL EVIDENCE FROM HUMAN MEDICINE?

To date, no interventions for PCB have been established empirically, but it is natural to ask if methods used to alleviate burden in human caregiving would translate to successful interventions for PCB. To begin addressing this question, it is worth considering not only burden, but also the influence of positive experiences in caregiving.

The Role of Positive Experiences

Although the negative consequences of caregiving are often highlighted, there can be many positive aspects of providing care for a loved one with an illness, such as emotional satisfaction, personal growth, experiencing a sense of competency, spiritual growth, and sense of fulfillment of duty.[46,47] Positive aspects of caregiving are assessed via self-report, with questions assessing whether providing care makes the respondent appreciate life more, feel needed, or feel more useful.[48] Interventions for negative outcomes in caregiving often rely on enhancing positive aspects of caregiving, because having a more positive appraisal of caregiving can be protective against burden, depression, and even health concerns.[47,49] This finding makes it a crucial factor when considering potential treatments for burden.

Comparing Family and Pet Caregiving

In a study to cross-sectionally compare burden and positive aspects of caregiving for human family and pet caregivers,[50] 369 caregivers (117 pet caregivers and 252 family dementia caregivers) were recruited via social media. Owing to the many expected differences in these 2 groups, analyses were repeated in a subset of caregivers (n = 75 per group) with similar demographic profiles, including caregiver age, education, gender, race, income, living situation (all caregivers lived with the care recipient), and duration of caregiving experience (>1 or <1 year). Although burden was clinically elevated in both groups, it was higher overall for dementia caregivers (P<.001 for both samples), whereas greater positive aspects of caregiving were seen in pet caregivers (P<.001 for both samples; **Fig. 3**A, B). The positive aspects of caregiving were negatively associated with burden in both groups (P<.001). The aspects of burden were also explored to determine if groups reported any similar experiences; results showed comparable levels of guilt, fear of what the future holds, and financial strain.

Although an increased burden was present for both caregiver groups, and some similar issues of burden were observed, the overall caregiving experience was not fully equivalent. Companion animal caregivers in this sample reported a lower burden and a more positive appraisal of caregiving than did family caregivers. This finding might be expected for many reasons, most notably the option of euthanasia in companion animal caregiving. Whereas assuming the role of caregiver may not be optional in human caregiving relationships owing to financial limitations or lack of other support,[51] the companion animal owner is making a choice to provide care, because euthanasia is an available alternative. Having chosen this path, the companion animal caregiver could be more positively predisposed to the caregiving experience.[50]

As noted elsewhere in this article, treatments for burden in the human medicine literature often aim to increase positive aspects of caregiving; however, because pet caregivers already report positive caregiving experiences, they may be at a ceiling for such effects.[50] Prior work from human medicine showed that persons reporting a more negative view of caregiving derive greater benefit from this type of intervention, whereas those starting with more positive perceptions of caregiving required a decrease in the load of actual daily care to ameliorate the experience of burden.[49] The differences in caregiving experiences between companion animal and human family caregiving groups thus highlight the importance of tailored models for understanding and intervening with burden associated with PCB.

Can We Rely on Empirical Evidence from Human Medicine? Not Entirely

Although caregiver burden research from the human medicine literature offers a solid foundation for understanding PCB, the work reviewed herein suggests that a thoughtful approach will be needed for intervention. Successful treatments for PCB may not directly translate from methods used in human caregiving relationships. Best practices must be established, but the current state of science is that we are just beginning

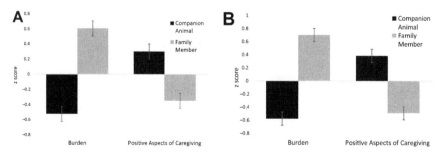

Fig. 3. Caregiver burden and positive aspects of caregiving in caregivers for a seriously ill companion animal compared with a family member with dementia, full sample (A) and matched subsample (B). Companion animal caregivers reported lower (although still clinically meaningful) burden (P<.001) and greater positive aspects of caregiving (P<.001) for both samples. (*Data from* Britton KB, Galioto R, Tremont G et al. Caregiving for a sick pet compared to a family member: Burden and positive experiences in caregivers. Front Vet Sci 2018;5:325.)

to recognize and understand the phenomenon of PCB. More research is needed to determine what might be done to improve it.

COPING NOW WITH CAREGIVER BURDEN IN A PALLIATIVE CARE SETTING

Given that best practices for decreasing PCB have not been developed, what can the veterinarian do in the meantime? First and foremost, it is important to emphasize that it is not the role of the veterinarian to treat mental health issues in the client. The veterinarian's goal should be identifying caregiver burden when it occurs and understanding the perspective of the client in distress. With this caveat in place, we can provide potentially helpful suggestions based on caregiver burden research.

1. Treat every client as an individual. Research suggests that high levels of burden are experienced by about one-half of owners of a seriously ill companion animal.[44] The burden is thus not the only outcome in caregiving—making the choice to provide care to a sick loved one can give people a sense of purpose, a greater appreciation for their own strengths, and an opportunity to practice patience. Do not assume that all clients in a palliative care setting are experiencing burden.
2. Avoid minimizing the feelings of burden. If your client tells you about their distress, be careful with the trust they have placed in you. It may be helpful to share that it is easy to feel overwhelmed by the demands of caregiving and research shows that companion animal caregiving is stressful for many owners. Emphasize that acknowledging the burden of caregiving does not mean that the pet itself is a burden—the term burden refers to personal strain that is experienced owing to the challenges of caregiving. Experiencing stress while caregiving does not make a person weaker, uncaring, or uncommitted to the care of their pet.
3. Share the power of knowledge. Although education alone is unlikely to decrease the burden,[3] it is a necessary first step to the client experiencing mastery of the situation, which is linked to lower burden.[45] Provide the client with trusted resources about the patient's disease. If your client is interested in learning more about caregiver burden, our team has created a science blog dedicated to helping pet owners understand caregiver burden www.petcaregiverburden.com.
4. Collaborative care plan and goals of care conversations. Discuss care plan needs with the client, rather than simply handing out a new routine. Research shows that greater caregiver burden correlates with the degree to which the client's daily routine is altered, and the client's perception that the animal's care plan is difficult to follow.[44] A clear and concrete plan that is developed with consideration of the client's typical routine could help to decrease burden. Client preferences, fears, and limits are all explored in a goals of care conversation (see Katherine Goldberg's article, "Goals of Care: Development and Use of the Serious Veterinary Illness Conversation Guide," elsewhere in this issue).
5. Help the client to problem solve. Research shows that PCB is predicted by both the frequency of and the client's reaction to clinical signs and problem behaviors of the pet.[45] Help the client apply problem-solving skills for difficult situations, such as a cat that is difficult to medicate or a dog that will not eat. Encourage the client to focus on small actions that can be taken to manage the problem directly in front of them.
6. Offer words of encouragement. Research shows that one predictor of PCB is the degree to which the client feels a sense of control.[45] Pointing out successful problem solving when the client demonstrates it may increase sense of self-efficacy[52] in this difficult situation, which in turn could help to decrease the burden.
7. Practice within your competence. As a veterinarian, it is important to understand these issues and use the information to optimize positive client communication,

but it is not appropriate to attempt individual counseling for mental health issues, unless you have an advanced degree in a mental health field and are licensed to do so.

SUMMARY

PCB is important to consider in the palliative care setting, and should be differentiated from other client experiences, such as quality of life and grief. It is present in nearly one-half of veterinary clients in the context of serious illness, and is significantly greater in this group compared with matched healthy controls. Greater PCB correlates with reduced psychosocial well-being in the client, including greater levels of stress, symptoms of anxiety and depression, and a lower quality of life. Factors strongly associated with PCB include a difficult care plan, greater frequency of clinical signs in the patient, a higher level of client reactivity, and lower sense of mastery felt by the client. Although extensive caregiving research has been conducted in human relationships, PCB seems to differ in some ways, and must be thoughtfully approached in future research. Until best practices for reducing PCB can be established, several suggestions based on the current state of the research can be offered for veterinarians dealing with clients facing these issues in a palliative care setting.

REFERENCES

1. Zarit SH, Reever KE, Bach-Peterson J. Relatives of the impaired elderly: correlates of feelings of burden. Gerontologist 1980;20(6):649–55.
2. Paradise M, McCade D, Hickie IB, et al. Caregiver burden in mild cognitive impairment. Aging Ment Health 2014;19:72–8.
3. Tremont G. Family caregiving in dementia. Med Health R I 2011;94(2):36–8.
4. Adelman RD, Tmanova LL, Delgado D, et al. Caregiver burden: a clinical review. JAMA 2014;311(10):1052–60.
5. World Health Organization. Annotated bibliography of the WHO quality of life assessment instrument – WHOQOL. Geneva, (Switzerland): World Health Organization; 1999.
6. Rha SY, Park Y, Song SK, et al. Caregiving burden and the quality of life of family caregivers of cancer patients: the relationship and correlates. Eur J Oncol Nurs 2015;19:376–82.
7. Favrot C, Linek M, Mueller R, et al, International Task Force on Canine Atopic Dermatitis. Development of a questionnaire to assess the impact of atopic dermatitis on health-related quality of life of affected dogs and their owners. Vet Dermatol 2010;21:63–9.
8. Noli C, Borio S, Varina A, et al. Development and validation of a questionnaire to evaluate the quality of life of cats with skin disease and their owners, and its use in 185 cats with skin disease. Vet Dermatol 2016;27:247–58.
9. Noli C, Minafo G, Galzerano G. Quality of life of dogs with skin diseases and their owners. Part 1: development and validation of a questionnaire. Vet Dermatol 2011;22:335–43.
10. Niessen SJ, Pownet S, Guitian J, et al. Evaluation of a quality of life tool for cats with diabetes mellitus. J Vet Intern Med 2010;24:1098–105.
11. Giuffrida MA, Farrar JT, Brown DC, et al. Psychometric properties of the Canine Symptom Assessment Scale, a multidimensional owner-reported questionnaire instrument for assessment of physical symptoms in dogs with solid tumors. J Am Vet Med Assoc 2017;251:1405–14.
12. Nettifee JA, Munana KR, Griffith EH. Evaluation of the impacts of epilepsy in dogs on their caregivers. J Am Anim Hosp Assoc 2017;53:143–9.

13. Spitznagel MB, Solc M, Chapman K, et al. Caregiver burden in the veterinary dermatology client: comparison to healthy controls and relationship to quality of life. Vet Dermatol 2019. https://doi.org/10.1111/vde.12696.

14. Prigerson HG, Horowitz MJ, Jacobs SC. Prolonged grief disorder: psychometric validation of criteria proposed for DSM-V and ICD-11. PLoS Med 2009;6(8): e1000121.

15. American Psychiatric Association. Diagnostic and statistical manual of mental disorders (5th ed.). Arlington, (VA) American Psychiatric Publishing; 2013.

16. Adams C, Bonnett BN, Meek AH. Predictors of owner response to companion animal death in 177 clients from 14 practices in Ontario. J Am Vet Med Assoc 2000; 217(9):1303–9.

17. Adrian JA, Deliramich AN, Frueh BC. Complicated grief and posttraumatic stress disorder in humans' response to the death of pets/animals. Bull Menninger Clin 2009;73(3):176–87.

18. Reynolds L, Botha D. Anticipatory grief: its nature, impact, and reasons for contradictory findings. Counselling, Psychotherapy, and Health 2006;2(2):15–26.

19. McArthur ML, Fitzgerald JR. Companion animal veterinarians' use of clinical communication skills. Aust Vet J 2013;91:374–80.

20. Shaw JR, Adams CL, Bonnett BN, et al. Veterinarian satisfaction with companion animal visits. J Am Vet Med Assoc 2012;240:832–41.

21. Gallagher-Thompson D, Shurgot GR, Rider K, et al. Ethnicity, stress, and cortisol function in Hispanic and non-Hispanic white women: a preliminary study of family dementia caregivers and noncaregivers. Am J Geriatr Psychiatry 2006;14(4): 334–42.

22. Wahbeh H, Kishiyama SS, Zajdel D, et al. Salivary cortisol awakening response in mild Alzheimer disease, caregivers, and noncaregivers. Alzheimer Dis Assoc Disord 2008;22(2):181–3.

23. Schulz R, Martire LM. Family caregiving of persons with dementia: prevalence, health effects, and support strategies. Am J Geriatr Psychiatry 2004;12(3):240–9.

24. Ornstein K, Gaugler JE. The problem with "problem behaviors": a systematic review of the association between individual patient behavioral and psychological symptoms and caregiver depression and burden within the dementia patient–caregiver dyad. Int Psychogeriatr 2012;24(10):1536–52.

25. Family Caregiver Alliance. Caregiver assessment: voices and views from the field. Report from a National Consensus Development Conference (Vol. II). San Francisco, CA, 2006.

26. Epstein-Lubow G, Davis JD, Miller IW, et al. Persisting burden predicts depressive symptoms in dementia caregivers. J Geriatr Psychiatry Neurol 2008;21(3): 198–203.

27. Schulz R, Beach SR. Caregiving as a risk factor for mortality. JAMA 1999;282(23): 2215–9.

28. Cohen CA, Gold DP, Shulman KI, et al. Factors determining the decision to institutionalize dementing individuals: a prospective study. Gerontologist 1993;33(6): 714–20.

29. Fredman L, Cauley JA, Hochberg M, et al. Mortality associated with caregiving, general stress, and caregiving-related stress in elderly women: results of caregiver study of osteoporotic fractures. J Am Geriatr Soc 2010;58:937–43.

30. National Alliance for Caregiving (NAC) and the AARP Public Policy Institute. Caregiving in the U.S. 2015. Available at: http://www.caregiving.org/wp-content/uploads/2015/05/2015_CaregivingintheUS_Final-Report-June-4_WEB.pdf. Accessed August 21, 2018.

31. Pinquart M, Sorensen S. Differences between caregivers and noncaregivers in psychological health and physical health: a meta-analysis. Psychol Aging 2003;18(2):250–67.

32. Davis J, Tremont G. Impact of frontal systems behavioral functioning in dementia on caregiver burden. J Neuropsychiatry Clin Neurosci 2007;19:43–9.

33. Steadman P, Tremont G, Davis J. Premorbid relationship satisfaction affects caregiver burden in dementia caregivers. J Geriatr Psychiatry Neurol 2007;20:115–9.

34. Kwok T, Au A, Wong B, et al. Effectiveness of online cognitive behavioral therapy on family caregivers of people with dementia. Clin Interv Aging 2014;9:631–6.

35. Losada A, Márquez-González M, Romero-Moreno R, et al. Cognitive–behavioral therapy (CBT) versus acceptance and commitment therapy (ACT) for dementia family caregivers with significant depressive symptoms: results of a randomized clinical trial. J Consult Clin Psychol 2015;83(4):760–72.

36. Sorensen S, Pinquart M, Duberstein P. How effective are interventions with caregivers? An updated meta-analysis. Gerontologist 2002;42(3):356–72.

37. Brodaty H, Green A, Koschera A. Meta-analysis of psychosocial interventions for caregivers of people with dementia. J Am Geriatr Soc 2003;51:657–64.

38. Belle SH, Burgio LD, Burns R, et al. Enhancing the quality of life of dementia caregivers from different ethnic or racial groups: a randomized, controlled trial. Ann Intern Med 2006;145(10):727–38.

39. Lee E. Do technology-based support groups reduce care burden among dementia caregivers? A review. J Evid Inf Soc Work 2015;12:474–87.

40. Tremont G, Davis JD, Papandonatos GD, et al. Psychosocial telephone intervention for dementia caregivers: a randomized, controlled trial. Alzheimers Dement 2015;11:541–8.

41. Berryman J. Pet owner attitudes to pets and people: a psychological study. Vet Rec 1985;117(25–26):659–61.

42. Christiansen SB, Kristensen AT, Sandoe P, et al. Looking after chronically ill dogs: impact on the caregiver's life. Anthrozoos 2013;26:519–33.

43. Spitznagel MB, Jacobson DM, Cox MD, et al. Caregiver burden in owners of a sick companion animal: a cross-sectional observational study. Vet Rec 2017; 181:321.

44. Spitznagel MB, Cox MD, Jacobson DM, et al. Assessment of caregiver burden and associations with psychosocial function, veterinary service use, and factors related to treatment plan adherence among owners of dogs and cats. J Am Vet Med Assoc 2019;254(1):124–32.

45. Spitznagel MB, Jacobson DM, Cox MD, et al. Predicting caregiver burden in general veterinary clients: contribution of companion animal clinical signs and problem behaviors. Vet J 2018;236:23–30.

46. Lloyd J, Patterson T, Muers J. The positive aspects of caregiving in dementia: a critical review of the qualitative literature. Dementia 2014;15(6):1534–61.

47. Cohen CA, Colantonio A, Vernich L. Positive aspects of caregiving: rounding out the caregiver experience. Int J Geriatr Psychiatry 2002;17(2):184–8.

48. Tarlow BJ, Wisniewski SR, Belle SH, et al. Positive aspects of caregiving: contributions of the REACH project to the development of new measures for Alzheimer's caregiving. Res Aging 2004;26(4):429–53.

49. Hilgeman MM, Allen RS, Decoster J, et al. Positive aspects of caregiving as a moderator of treatment outcome over 12 months. Psychol Aging 2007;22(2): 361–71.

50. Britton KB, Galioto R, Tremont G, et al. Caregiving for a sick pet compared to a family member: burden and positive experiences in caregivers. Front Vet Sci 2018;5:325.
51. Quinn C, Clare L, Woods RT. Balancing needs: the role of motivations, meanings and relationship dynamics in the experience of informal caregivers of people with dementia. Dementia 2015;14(2):220–37.
52. Tremont G, Davis JD, Spitznagel MB. Understanding and managing caregiver burden in cerebrovascular disease. In: Paul RH, Cohen R, Ott Br, et al, editors. Vascular dementia: cerebrovascular mechanisms and clinical management. Totowa (NJ): Humana; 2005. p. 305–21.

Section III: Advances and Information to Guide Clinicians

Advances in Pain Management: Palliative Care Applications

Jordyn M. Boesch, DVM

KEYWORDS

- Analgesia • Epidural • Interventional • Intrathecal • Locoregional
- Neuromodulation • Pain • Radiofrequency

KEY POINTS

- Opioids are the mainstay of severe pain management in terminally ill humans and are commonly delivered via intravenous or subcutaneous infusion at home.
- Short-term ketamine and lidocaine intravenous infusions are used in humans to treat neuropathic and cancer pain, and the effects of these infusions outlast their duration.
- Biological toxins that act at various points in nociceptive pathways have tremendous potential as therapeutic agents for severe pain.
- Joint and myofascial trigger point injections are commonly performed in human pain practice; these relatively straightforward procedures can be performed in a general practice or home setting and deserve further investigation.
- Many of the modalities used to control severe pain in humans are *interventional*, minimally invasive procedures conducted under the guidance of an imaging modality; some of these are performed in dogs and cats but are not as well established in the veterinary profession, whereas others are completely novel but urgently require development.

INTRODUCTION

The relief of pain, and the suffering it begets, is one of the most important goals of palliative medicine and hospice care. Advances in pain management, both pharmacologic and nonpharmacologic, are increasing the quantity and quality of time that a dog or cat with a chronic or terminal condition has with his or her family. However, severe pain is still difficult to control, especially in the home setting, and often results in euthanasia even when the pet is systemically healthy.

The author has no conflicts of interest to disclose.
Section of Anesthesiology and Pain Medicine, Department of Clinical Sciences, Cornell University Hospital for Animals, Cornell University College of Veterinary Medicine, 930 Campus Road, Box 32, Ithaca, NY 14853, USA
E-mail address: jmb264@cornell.edu

Vet Clin Small Anim 49 (2019) 445–461
https://doi.org/10.1016/j.cvsm.2019.01.011
0195-5616/19/© 2019 Elsevier Inc. All rights reserved.

vetsmall.theclinics.com

Pain control as part of palliative medicine and hospice care is far more advanced in human than in veterinary medicine and uses a wide variety of drugs and procedures, from simple, over-the-counter oral analgesics and physical modalities to novel drugs and advanced interventional techniques. Some of these are already widely used in veterinary medicine; others are relatively nascent or unavailable. This article focuses on means of pain control in chronically or terminally ill humans that are not as well established in veterinary as in human medicine or that are completely novel to veterinary practice, but urgently deserve further attention. Most of these are *interventional pain medicine* procedures, minimally invasive techniques conducted under the guidance of an imaging modality. Many of these procedures hold tremendous potential for the relief of pain that is unresponsive to currently available therapies. This article is not intended to review oral analgesic/pain-modifying drugs in current use, physical therapies, or regenerative medicine, and the reader is directed to other recent publications on these topics.[1–3]

SOURCES OF CHRONIC PAIN

Before beginning a discussion of advances in pain management, it is important to identify chronic pain generators in dogs and cats that can be difficult to control and might respond to the treatments discussed later (**Table 1**).

DRUGS AND EQUIPMENT

An exhaustive review of the drugs and equipment used in pain management is beyond the scope of this article. The specific drugs and equipment at a given practice depend on the type of pain management practiced by the clinician or clinicians. For instance, the Anesthesiology and Pain Medicine Service at the author's institution uses a combination of pharmaceuticals and interventional pain medicine procedures (**Figs. 1** and **2**), extrapolating from human data in many cases. However, they work closely with the Sports Medicine and Rehabilitation Service, which can provide physical pain management modalities, and other services as applicable (eg, Surgery, Neurology, Oncology).

Table 1
Examples of chronic pain generators in small animals

- Musculoskeletal/neurologic
  - IVDD
  - Degenerative LS stenosis
  - OA
  - Hyperalgesia and allodynia following decompressive spinal surgery
  - Chronic tendinopathies
  - Medial shoulder syndrome (instability)
  - Spondylosis deformans
  - Myofascial pain
  - Chiari malformation/syringomyelia
  - Postamputation neuropathic pain
- Dental
  - Periodontal/endodontal disease
  - Stomatitis
  - Feline odontoclastic resorptive lesions
- Neoplasia
- Dermatologic
  - Otitis
- Ophthalmologic
  - Glaucoma
  - Uveitis
  - Keratoconjunctivitis sicca
  - Keratitis/corneal ulcers
- Gastrointestinal/genitourinary
  - Esophagitis
  - Gastroduodenal ulceration
  - Inflammatory bowel disease
  - Pancreatitis
  - Hepatitis/cholangitis
  - Urinary tract infection
  - Urolithiasis

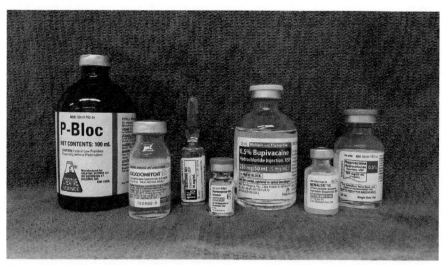

Fig. 1. Drugs used in interventional pain medicine. Lidocaine is used for skin and SC infiltration to decrease pain on insertion of the larger needle used to perform the procedure in sedated patients. Otherwise, longer-acting local anesthetics, such as bupivacaine and ropivacaine (preservative free if used for epidural injection), are used. A variety of other drugs are also used, alone or in combination with local anesthetics, depending on the procedure; refer to text for details.

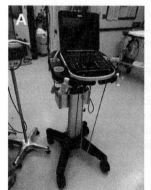
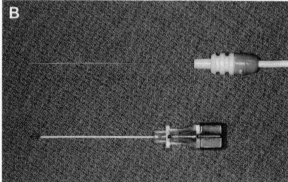

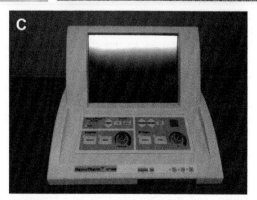

Fig. 2. Examples of equipment used in interventional pain medicine. (*A*) SonoSite Edge ultrasound machine with high-frequency 6- to 15-MHz linear array transducer (FUJIFILM SonoSite, Inc, Bothell, WA). (*B*) RF cannula (5 cm) with 5-mm active tip and a 5-cm RF electrode (model SL-S505–22 and model RFDE-10, respectively; Abbott, Abbott Park, IL). (*C*) RF generator (Neurotherm, NM1000; St. Jude Medical).

SPECIFIC THERAPEUTIC MODALITIES

For each of the therapeutic modalities discussed later, **Table 2** summarizes their advantages and disadvantages in veterinary patients.

Subcutaneous Opioid Infusion and Other Opioid Delivery Routes

When human patients with cancer are no longer able to take oral opioids as end of life approaches, alternative routes become necessary. Opioids, such as morphine, diamorphine, hydromorphone, methadone, fentanyl, and sufentanil, can be administered to humans by a variety of alternatives routes. Continuous subcutaneous infusion (CSCI) is an effective alternative and is commonly used (although the intravenous [IV], rectal, and transdermal routes are comparable in terms of efficacy and safety).[4,5]

Veterinary applications

If a suitable commercial device were available for dogs and cats, CSCI of opioids might prove to be an excellent way of controlling moderate to severe pain from a variety of pain generators (eg, neoplasia, musculoskeletal, or neurologic disease) at home when other treatments (eg, oral medications, physical therapies) are insufficient. This modality would be particularly useful for relief of pain from areas that cannot be easily treated with a locoregional technique (eg, extensive oropharyngeal neoplasia). It would also be useful in patients whose owners do not wish their pets to undergo a more invasive or complex pain management procedure, or in patients who have been diagnosed with a painful terminal illness whose owners wish to take them home to spend a short time with them before euthanasia (eg, a dog with appendicular osteosarcoma and pulmonary metastasis).

After routine clipping and aseptic preparation as for an IV catheter, a subcutaneous (SC) catheter, which exits the skin under a sterile dressing and connects to an external pump worn by the patient, could be placed. The pump could be placed either on an outpatient basis or at home by the primary care or palliative/hospice care veterinarian in a patient with only a few days to live. For longer-term pain management, insertion of a totally implantable device could be placed under light sedation and local anesthetic infiltration in a general practice setting or at home.

Nonopiate Intravenous Infusions

Pain physicians use IV infusions (eg, lidocaine, ketamine, dexmedetomidine, bisphosphonates) to treat neuropathic and cancer pain; the effects of the infusions outlast their duration, often by weeks to months.[6] Lidocaine and ketamine have been studied most extensively in humans, with several randomized, placebo-controlled studies demonstrating superiority to placebo.[6] Lidocaine dose and duration of infusion typically range from 1 to 5 mg/kg or higher, given over a period of time from 30 minutes to several hours. A bolus of ketamine of 0.5 mg/kg or less is usually administered over less than an hour and may be followed by an infusion; however, ketamine may be administered daily for over a week in some cases.

Veterinary applications

Infusions of lidocaine, ketamine, and dexmedetomidine are commonly used in veterinary medicine for relief of acute pain. However, minimal data exist to support their use for relief of chronic pain, and they are used far less commonly for this purpose. Bisphosphonates like pamidronate are used in dogs with bone malignancies to decrease pain by inhibiting osteoclast activity, but efficacy is unclear.[7] This author, as well as the Oncology Service at this author's institution, administers ketamine and lidocaine infusions at doses similar to those used in humans. Patients are typically

Table 2
Therapeutic modalities

	Advantages	Disadvantages
CSCI of opioids	• Useful in patients in which IV access difficult • Could be used at home • Totally implantable device could likely be implanted in private general practice; SC catheter could be placed at home for short-term use	• Placement of totally implantable device would likely require light sedation and local anesthetic infiltration
IV infusions (eg, ketamine, lidocaine)	• Simple • Inexpensive • Could be performed at home by palliative care clinician	• Requires IV catheter (technically difficult in some patients and could be removed by patient)
Toxins	• Dependent on toxin used	• Cost or availability unclear • Intrathecal administration currently necessary for some
Joint and myofascial injections	• Simple • Inexpensive, could be performed at home	• Requires light sedation due to procedural pain
ESI	• May cause fewer systemic side effects compared with oral anti-inflammatory drugs • Can be performed without imaging in general practice by properly trained clinicians	• Should be performed in hospital • Requires heavy sedation or general anesthesia • Complications include nerve damage and epidural hematoma
Peripheral nerve blocks	• Some performed without special equipment • May provide long duration of analgesia depending on drugs used	• Special training and equipment required for many • Many must be performed in hospital • Requires heavy sedation or general anesthesia • Other complications depending on nerve to be blocked
Neurolysis	• Long duration of analgesia	• Equipment may be cost-prohibitive • Eventual nerve regeneration • Only for use on sensory nerves • Complications include postprocedure pain (with TRF) • Requires special training • Must be performed in hospital • Requires heavy sedation or general anesthesia
PRF	• Can be used on any nerve (sensory or motor)	• Equipment may be cost-prohibitive • Requires special training • Must be performed in hospital • Requires heavy sedation or general anesthesia
IDDS and SCS	• Automated, long-term pain relief, allows patient to remain at home and perform normal activities	• Cost • Requires special training and equipment • Must be performed in hospital • Requires general anesthesia

Known or potential advantages and disadvantages to using modalities discussed above in dogs and cats, assuming (1) proven safety and efficacy and (2) equipment for some becomes commercially available. The potential advantages of all of these obviously are (1) analgesia superior to that which can be achieved with current treatments and (2) ability to be performed on an outpatient basis. Risk of infection is possible with all; other possible complications are listed under *Disadvantages*.

admitted as day cases. An IV catheter is placed, and the patient receives the infusion throughout the day while other procedures, such as thoracic radiographs or radiation therapy planning, are performed. Empirically, these infusions appear to be most effective against pain from primary bone tumors (eg, of the skull or mandible, appendicular skeleton, ribs, or vertebral bodies, which likely has both inflammatory and neuropathic components), although patients with extensive soft tissue tumors and other neuropathic pain generators also seem to respond. Blinded, randomized, placebo-controlled clinical trials are sorely needed. These infusions are relatively inexpensive and could be administered easily in a general practice setting.

Toxins

A wide variety of toxins produced by animals or other organisms selectively modulate ion channels and receptors in pain pathways.[8] Research into these substances has generated novel drugs used in humans to treat chronic pain (and continues to uncover exciting prospects for further drug development). For instance, ziconotide (Prialt), a Food and Drug Administration–approved drug administered by intrathecal infusion for severe chronic pain, is the synthetic form of the conotoxin MVIIA, a peptide produced by a marine cone snail that selectively antagonizes the voltage-gated calcium channel, $Ca_V2.2$.[9] Botulinum toxin is also used to treat a wide variety of pain syndromes (see later discussion).[10]

Veterinary applications

In 2 recent studies, intrathecal injection of resiniferatoxin (an agonist of the nonselective cation channel transient receptor potential vanilloid 1 found in the plant *Euphorbia resinifera*) and substance P-saporin (a conjugate of the neurotransmitter, substance P, and the neurotoxin saporin) produced positive outcomes in dogs with naturally occurring pain from bone malignancy.[11,12] Intra-articular (IA) resiniferatoxin has also been shown to relieve osteoarthritis (OA) pain in dogs.[13] Theoretically, toxins could be used to relieve pain from a wide variety of other pain generators too, from other types of neoplasia to chronic musculoskeletal and neurologic diseases (eg, intervertebral disc disease [IVDD], lumbosacral [LS] stenosis, postamputation neuropathic pain).

Joint Injections for Osteoarthritis

IA injection of steroids is commonly performed in humans with OA when they fail more conservative management with treatment, such as nonsteroidal anti-inflammatory drugs (NSAIDs), weight loss, and exercise; good evidence for short-term anti-inflammatory effects and analgesia exists.[14] In horses, there is evidence of a beneficial effect of triamcinolone acetonide in normal joints and joints with experimentally induced OA.[15,16] Intraarticular steroid injection in dogs is performed by some veterinarians. However, this practice appears to be less common than in humans and equine athletes, likely due in part to the paucity of data on analgesic effects and effects on articular cartilage in dogs with naturally-occurring OA.[15] Fear of side effects, such as chondrotoxicity, and problems secondary to systemic absorption, including adrenocortical suppression and iatrogenic hyperadrenocorticism, likely also limit this practice. Early studies in rabbits demonstrated deleterious effects on articular cartilage; however, many of these were of poor quality, and some studies tested doses and frequencies of administration much higher than those used clinically in humans, horses, or dogs.[15] On the other hand, studies in dogs with experimentally induced OA of the stifle demonstrated unambiguously positive effects of triamcinolone hexacetonide on cartilage.[17–19] In these studies, low doses (0.2–0.25 mg/kg) were injected only 2 to 3 times.

Veterinary applications

Empirically, IA steroid injections provide excellent analgesia in dogs with OA of the shoulders, elbows, hips, stifles, and other joints. At this author's institution, this is typically done when dogs with moderate to severe pain have failed conservative treatment (ie, NSAIDs and other oral drugs, physical therapies, weight loss, and controlled exercise). However, until more is known about the systemic effects of IA steroids and their effects on articular cartilage, clinicians should exercise caution. Injection of low doses when patients fail more conservative therapies is recommended.

Myofascial Injections

Myofascial pain is a term that refers to muscle strain, myofascial trigger points, and myofascial pain syndrome, a chronic regional pain syndrome that often involves the muscles of the neck and back (eg, piriformis or iliopsoas pain) in humans.[20] Myofascial trigger points are palpable, irritable, taut bands or knots within a muscle that causes pain that radiates into a specific "reference pain zone"; muscle twitch will sometimes occur on palpation. They are common in myofascial pain syndrome. Trigger points can be active (producing spontaneous pain) or latent (producing pain only on palpation).

A wide variety of treatments are used for myofascial pain in humans, including "dry needling" (inserting and withdrawing a fine-gauge needle), injection of local anesthetic with or without steroid, or botulinum toxin A.[21–23] Specific muscles (eg, piriformis) can be injected as well using fluoroscopic guidance.[24] Ultrasonography can be used to visualize trigger points.[25]

Veterinary applications

Myofascial pain has been recognized in veterinary medicine, but many veterinarians remain unaware of this important pain generator.[26,27] Palpation of these points often elicits vocalization, anxiety, and escape behaviors. This author has identified what appear to be myofascial trigger points in the cervical muscles of dogs with cervical IVDD or dogs recovering from decompressive cervical spinal surgery as well as muscles in the stump of dogs following limb amputation. Empirically, injection of small volumes (<1 mL to as much as 3 mL, depending on the size of the patient and the trigger point) of 2% lidocaine or 0.5% bupivacaine, combined with triamcinolone (0.1 mg/kg), has been highly effective. However, the injection can be painful, and sedation is recommended.

Epidural Injection

Epidural injection is one of the most common interventional pain management procedures performed in humans. Cervical, thoracic, lumbar, or caudal epidural injections in humans are used for treatment of many chronic, nonmalignant pain syndromes. Epidural steroid injection (ESI) for unilateral or bilateral radiculopathy/radiculitis due to IVDD or spinal/foraminal stenosis is most common, but other indications include phantom limb pain, vertebral fractures, diabetic polyneuropathy, postherpetic neuralgia, and cancer pain.[28,29] Commonly used steroids include triamcinolone, methylprednisolone, and dexamethasone; local anesthetics (eg, bupivacaine) and other drugs are often combined with the steroids.[30]

In humans, epidural injection can be performed on an outpatient basis under local anesthesia with or without sedation. Injection is ideally guided by fluoroscopy (or, less commonly, computed tomography [CT] or ultrasonography); when fluoroscopy or CT is used, radiopaque water-soluble contrast medium (eg, Omnipaque [iohexol]) is injected first to produce an epidurogram to confirm proper needle placement in the epidural space and spread of injectate around the nerve root or roots generating the pain.[31] However, a "blind" injection using the loss-of-resistance (LOR) technique can be used when such imaging modalities are unaffordable.[32] In dogs, false negative results can occur with the well-known "hanging drop" test. The LOR technique can serve as either a primary or a backup method of identifying the epidural space. Saline is aspirated into the LOR syringe, which is then attached to the hub of the needle. The clinician applies pressure to the plunger as the needle is pushed through sequential layers of tissue; when the needle enters the epidural space, the plunger surges ahead effortlessly.

Box 1 describes techniques used for cervical, thoracic, and lumbar injections in humans.

Veterinary applications

Some veterinarians perform this procedure routinely in patients with IVDD or LS stenosis. This author performs ESI in dogs with a definitive diagnosis of IVDD or LS stenosis made on CT or MRI, or patients with certain other sources of neuropathic pain that are unresponsive to conservative therapy (**Fig. 3**). However, epidural injection for chronic pain management is not as well established in veterinary medicine, primarily because of the paucity of data on the subject. To this author's knowledge, only one study has examined epidural injection for chronic pain management.[34] In dogs with

---

Box 1
Common epidural injection techniques used in humans

- Midline (median) interlaminar
  - Technique used in veterinary medicine
  - Technique
    - Needle is inserted on midline between 2 laminae/spinous processes
    - The posterior epidural space may be absent in humans above C7-T1; thus, some physicians may insert the needle at an inferior interspace (eg, C7-T1) and either (1) pass an epidural catheter cranially to the appropriate level to deposit injectate or (2) use an injectate volume large enough to spread cranially to the appropriate level.

- Paramedian interlaminar
  - Indications
    - Patients with unilateral pathologic condition (eg, radiculopathy)
    - Patients who have difficulty flexing the vertebral column or have calcified ligaments due to previous surgery
    - Injection at interspaces between T3-T9, where the angle of the spinous processes makes the midline interlaminar technique difficult
  - Technique
    - Needle inserted lateral to midline (ipsilateral to side of pain) at level of inferior border of the superior spinous process, then directed medially and cranially

- Transforaminal
  - Used to deposit smaller injectate volume into anterior epidural space, closer to affected nerve root
  - Technique
    - Needle inserted just inside posterior intervertebral foramen of affected nerve root
  - Not used by some in cervical region due to possibility of major complications[33]

- Caudal
  - Used in humans who have undergone low-back surgery or are anticoagulated
  - Technique
    - Needle inserted on midline at the sacral hiatus (sacrococcygeal space)

Data from Waldman DS. Atlas of interventional pain management. 4th edition. Philadelphia: Elsevier Saunders; 2015.

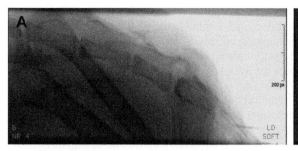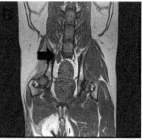

Fig. 3. (A) Fluoroscopic image of an epidurogram in an 11-year-old domestic shorthair cat with a chief complaint of severe neuropathic pain (paroxysms of vocalization and self-mutilation resulting in hemorrhage) following tail amputation for a nonhealing wound. A diagnosis of presumptive postamputation pain (possibly due to neuroma) was made. After iohexol injection, a combination of buprenorphine, bupivacaine, and triamcinolone was injected at the sacrococcygeal space. Complete pain relief was achieved until euthanasia from unrelated illness 6 months later. (B) MRI of the LS region of a 5-year-old mixed breed dog that presented for lameness and self-mutilation of the right distal pelvic limb; paresis, decreased proprioception, and hyperesthesia were noted on examination. Note the thickening of the right L6-7 nerve roots and sciatic nerve (*arrow*). The primary differentials were nerve sheath neoplasm or lymphoma. The patient was unresponsive to multiple oral analgesics. LS epidural injection of buprenorphine, bupivacaine, and triamcinolone resulted in complete resolution of signs of pain for 6 weeks.

confirmed LS stenosis, methylprednisolone acetate was injected at 1 mg/kg every 2 weeks for a total of 3 injections. The study was retrospective, was not blinded, and had no positive or negative control groups. However, 53% of dogs in this study were judged to be "cured" by the owners, whereas almost 80% showed some improvement. Clearly, ESI in dogs deserves further study. It may be a good option in patients with IVDD or LS stenosis whose owners do not want them to have surgery, want to exhaust other options before going to surgery, or cannot afford surgery; it may also be an alternative to surgery in patients who are poor surgical and/or anesthetic candidates (eg, a dog with LS stenosis who also suffers from dilated cardiomyopathy).

Peripheral Nerve Blocks

A staggering array of peripheral nerve, ganglion, and plexus blocks, from the trigeminal nerve block for trigeminal neuralgia to the celiac plexus block for pancreatitis and pancreatic cancer to medial branch blocks for low back pain, are performed in humans for diagnostic, therapeutic, and/or prognostic purposes. For instance, occipital nerve block with local anesthetic and steroid is used to determine if a person's headaches are caused by occipital neuralgia. If significant short-term pain relief is achieved, a neurolytic procedure, such as thermal radiofrequency (TRF) or cryoneurolysis (see later discussion), may be used to provide long-term analgesia.

Peripheral nerve blocks can be performed using palpation of landmarks, electrolocation, or imaging modalities, such as ultrasonography. Not surprisingly, the perineural injection of local anesthetic is virtually ubiquitous; however, several adjuvants have been added to the local anesthetic in an attempt to prolong the duration of the block, a concept known as multimodal perineural analgesia (MMPNA) (see **Fig. 1**).[35,36] Buprenorphine, the alpha-2 agonists clonidine and dexmedetomidine, dexamethasone, and magnesium have most consistently demonstrated prolongation of analgesia.[35] Buprenorphine, like local anesthetics, is a potent voltage-gated Na^+ channel blocker.[37] In a small randomized, double-blind, placebo-controlled study in humans, buprenorphine displayed analgesic and antihyperalgesic effects.[38] Although both clonidine and dexmedetomidine are vasopressors, which could extend block duration by decreasing the rate of systemic absorption of local anesthetic, they have been shown to block the inward cation current, I_h (also known as I_f, or funny current) that flows through hyperpolarization-activated nucleotide-gated channels.[39,40] These channels have been implicated in both inflammatory and neuropathic pain.[41] Bupivacaine plus dexmedetomidine for combined femoral and sciatic nerve block provided analgesia for tibial plateau-leveling osteotomy that lasted as long as 24 hours in dogs.[42] Although dexamethasone has been shown to prolong analgesia after peripheral nerve block, it is unclear if this is due to systemic absorption. However, local administration of steroids can produce beneficial effects that reduce neuropathic pain. For instance, triamcinolone acetate applied to the L5 dorsal root ganglion (DRG) immediately after ligation and transection of the L5 spinal nerve in rats reduced mechanical hypersensitivity, as well as cellular changes in the DRG known to occur following nerve damage.[43] Both magnesium alone and a combination of magnesium plus lidocaine increased excitation threshold in C fibers in explanted rat saphenous nerves.[44]

One substance that veterinarians, particularly equine veterinarians, recognize more often than physicians is Sarapin, an aqueous solution of soluble salts of the volatile bases of *Sarracenia purpurea* (pitcher plant) in an alkaline solution that also contains 0.75% benzyl alcohol as a preservative. Although Sarapin was discontinued by the manufacturer (High Chemical Company Manufacturing Pharmacists), P-Bloc (Creative Science LLC), a similar product, is available at the time of this writing. Sarapin is intended to be injected paravertebrally, perineurally, or intramuscularly for the relief of neuralgic pain, with dosage dependent on site of injection. Experiments conducted in the mid-twentieth century on the saphenous nerves of cats demonstrated that action potentials in C fibers ceased after immersion in Sarapin.[45] However, high-quality clinical trials of Sarapin are lacking.[45,46]

Veterinary applications

This author performs peripheral nerve blocks using electrolocation, ultrasonography, or both. Various combinations of local anesthetic and the aforementioned adjuvants have provided analgesia lasting from several days to as long as a month (**Fig. 4**). Examples of patients who have received such blocks include dogs and cats with oral tumors or chronic stomatitis, appendicular bone tumors, rib tumors, iatrogenic nerve

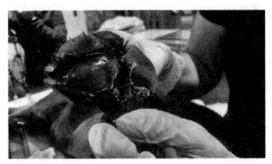

Fig. 4. Foot pad sloughing in a Labrador retriever receiving radiation therapy for mast cell tumor. Using the concept of MMPNA, intermittent sciatic nerve blocks with bupivacaine, dexmedetomidine, triamcinolone, and Sarapin were performed.

injury during surgery, chronic pain after major surgery such as femoral head ostectomy or fracture fixation, mucositis or dermatitis after radiation therapy, postamputation neuropathic pain, and peripheral nerve sheath tumors. For more information on specific peripheral nerve blocks in dogs and cats, the reader is referred to textbooks on the subject.[32,47]

Neurolysis

Neurolysis, or destruction of nervous tissue (as opposed to a block, which does not damage nervous tissue), has been used for decades for long-term relief of intractable pain. Three methods are currently used.

Chemical neurolysis

Chemical neurolysis is the method still used by some veterinarians but has largely been replaced in human pain medicine by other methods. Today its use is primarily limited to celiac plexus neurolysis for pain from terminal neoplasia (although celiac plexus *block* is used for nonmalignant pain such as that from chronic pancreatitis). Nociceptive primary afferent neurons pass through several sympathetic ganglia/plexuses on their way to the dorsal horn of the spinal cord; thus, injection of a neurolytic agent into a given ganglion or plexus can relieve pain from specific anatomic structures. Destruction of the celiac plexus will decrease (but not abolish) pain from the pancreas, the gastrointestinal tract from the esophagus to the transverse colon, the liver, the adrenal glands, and the ureters; reduction in opioid requirements is the goal.[48] Ethanol (50%–100%) and phenol (5%–10%) are most commonly used.[49] Wallerian degeneration of neurons occurs distal to the injection site.[50,51] Complications are uncommon; postprocedural pain, transient diarrhea, and hypotension are most common complications.[52]

Radiofrequency therapy

Radiofrequency (RF) therapy is applied to nerves to produce long-term (months to a year or more) analgesia. The biophysical concepts underlying radiofrequency therapy are complex and are discussed in detail elsewhere for those interested.[53,54] Briefly, an RF cannula coated with insulation, except for a short (usually 5–10 mm) length at the distal end (the "active tip"), is used (see **Fig. 2**). This cannula is positioned so that the active tip is adjacent to the nerve to be treated. An electrode connected to an RF generator is then inserted through the cannula until its tip reaches the active tip of the cannula (see **Fig. 2**). The RF generator produces an alternating current at radio wave frequency (250 kHz to 1 MHz). The current creates an electromagnetic field that induces oscillations in dipole molecules (such as water) in the tissues surrounding the active tip/electrode, generating heat. A thermocouple in the electrode allows the generator to automatically adjust its power output to maintain a preset target temperature.

TRF (also known as continuous or conventional RF, RF ablation, or RF neurolysis) was first described in humans in the 1970s.[55] With TRF, a target temperature of $\sim 80^{\circ}$C is maintained for 1 to 2 minutes, resulting in localized necrosis of axons, myelin breakdown, and hemorrhage.[56] This thermal neurodestruction, known as "lesioning," induces Wallerian degeneration of neurons, which prevents transmission of nociceptive impulses. Because Wallerian degeneration can take up to 2 weeks, onset of analgesia in humans can be immediate or delayed. Because axons, myelin, and endoneurium are disrupted, the lesion is classified as third-degree peripheral nerve injury (PNI). Functional, but incomplete regeneration can occur but can take months to years.[57,58] Thus, TRF can only be used on sensory nerves.

The procedure is typically performed under local anesthesia only, and steroid is often injected perineurally at the lesion site to provide postprocedure analgesia and prevent neuritis.[59] In humans, this procedure is most often used to lesion the medial branches of the dorsal rami of lumbar spinal nerves to relieve low back pain caused by zygapophyseal (facet) joint OA.[60] However, lesioning of many other nerves has been described.[61,62]

Cryoneurolysis

Cryoneurolysis (or cryoablation) uses a special probe to freeze nerves. Pressurized gas (usually N_2O or CO_2) travels down the inner tube of the probe and passes through a tiny aperture into a larger outer tube; the gas expands rapidly into the tip of the probe, and heat is extracted (Joule Thompson effect).[58] This process generates temperatures as low as $-88°C$ to $-79°C$ at the tip, and an ice ball measuring several millimeters is formed.[58] Wallerian degeneration ensues, but because myelin and endoneurium remain intact (second-degree PNI), the nerve will eventually regenerate.[57,58] Cryoneurolysis is an alternative to TRF that some physicians use to avoid the risk of postprocedure neuritis with TRF.[58]

Veterinary applications

An approach to the celiac plexus has not been developed in dogs and cats but, because pancreatitis, inflammatory bowel disease, and abdominal neoplasia are common chronic pain generators, celiac plexus injection with alcohol or phenol is worthy of further investigation. TRF or cryoneurolysis could be used on any sensory nerve or certain sensory-motor nerves that could be treated without producing motor deficit that would significantly impact the patient; examples include the inferior alveolar nerve in patients with mandibular tumors, the auriculotemporal and great auricular nerves in patients with severe, chronic otitis or painful otic tumors, intercostal nerves in patients with rib tumors, or the saphenous nerve in patients with stifle OA.

Pulsed Radiofrequency

The biophysical concepts underlying pulsed radiofrequency (PRF) are the same as described for TRF (above). However, with PRF, the RF generator produces current in short, high-voltage bursts, known as "pulses." The "silent period" between pulses allows for heat dissipation, resulting in an average tissue temperature of $\sim 40°C$, which is below the temperature ($45°C–50°C$) considered lethal for neurons.[63] PRF has many different effects that could account for the analgesia it produces, including ultrastructural changes in neurons and changes in gene expression in the DRG; however, elucidation of the precise mechanism whereby PRF relieves pain has lagged behind its clinical application in humans.[53,64–66] Because PRF does not cause clinical motor deficits, it is used on numerous mixed sensory-motor nerves to treat a multitude of painful conditions.[67,68]

Veterinary applications

PRF could be used on any sensory or mixed sensory-motor nerve conducting nociceptive signals. In the author's practice, it has been used successfully on mixed sensory-motor nerves, such as the sciatic nerve in dogs with appendicular bone tumors.

Implantable Intrathecal Drug Delivery Systems

The first intrathecal drug delivery system (IDDS) for intrathecal morphine administration was implanted in 1981.[69] Today, other full mu opioids, as well as local anesthetics, the alpha-2 agonist clonidine, and ziconotide, are also delivered intrathecally for malignant and nonmalignant pain.[70] Deposition of drug in cerebrospinal fluid in such close proximity to its receptors means that doses far lower than those given systemically can be used, reducing side effects, such as nausea and constipation.

The SynchroMed™ II from Medtronic (Minneapolis, MN, USA, https://www.medtronic.com/us-en/healthcare-professionals/products/neurological/drug-infusion-systems/synchromed-ii.html) is what is known as a programmable rate device. It is typically implanted SC over the anterior abdomen. The pump is comprised of an inner compartment, or reservoir (available in two sizes), containing the drug to be administered and an outer compartment filled with propellant that, once warmed to body temperature, exerts constant pressure on the reservoir. Battery-powered electronics and a motor move the drug from the reservoir into an intrathecal catheter using a peristaltic pump. The dose is programmed into the device by the clinician and can be changed using an external programmer. The reservoir can be filled percutaneously via a reservoir fill port. The catheter access port allows injection of drug directly into the catheter, bypassing the pump.

Veterinary applications

Unfortunately, these pumps would currently be cost-prohibitive for most pet owners, and a veterinary product is not currently available. If such a pump were available, it would likely prove useful in the management of pain from neoplasia, hip and stifle OA, LS stenosis, IVDD, zygapophyseal (facet) joint OA, spondylosis deformans, postamputation neuropathic pain, and many other sources.

Spinal Cord Stimulation

Neurostimulation devices relieve chronic, intractable pain by stimulating neurons with electricity, replacing it with paresthesias (eg, tingling). The Gate Control Theory (GCT) is typically cited to explain how electrical energy interrupts nociceptive transmission.[71] However, GCT does not explain why spinal cord stimulation (SCS) is more effective at treating neuropathic than nociceptive pain or why the analgesic effects persist after SCS is discontinued. Several other mechanisms appear to play a role.[72] This technology is most commonly used for relief of neuropathic pain, such as radiculopathy, complex regional pain syndrome, or diabetic neuropathy.[72]

SCSs consist of electrodes (leads) implanted into the epidural space (percutaneously or via a small laminotomy), anchors to attach the electrodes to lumbar fascia to minimize lead migration, extensions that connect to an implantable pulse generator (IPG, or battery), a programmer, and a charger (if IPG is rechargeable).[73] Several companies manufacture these devices (eg, Abbott, https://www.sjm.com/en/professionals/disease-state-management/chronic-pain/spinal-cord-stimulation).

Veterinary applications

SCS might prove useful in the management of pain from IVDD, LS stenosis, postamputation neuropathic pain, and many other sources.

REFERENCES

1. Millis DL, Ciuperca IA. Evidence for canine rehabilitation and physical therapy. Vet Clin North Am Small Anim Pract 2015;45(1):1–27.
2. Bradbrook CA, Clark L. State of the art analgesia- recent developments in pharmacological approaches to acute pain management in dogs and cats. Part 1. Vet J 2018;238:76–82.
3. Bradbrook C, Clark L. State of the art analgesia-Recent developments pharmacological approaches to acute pain management in dogs and cats: part 2. Vet J 2018;236:62–7.

4. Radbruch L, Trottenberg P, Elsner F, et al. Systematic review of the role of alternative application routes for opioid treatment for moderate to severe cancer pain: an EPCRC opioid guidelines project. Palliat Med 2011;25(5):578–96.

5. Herndon CM, Fike DS. Continuous subcutaneous infusion practices of United States hospices. J Pain Symptom Manage 2001;22(6):1027–34.

6. Kosharskyy B, Almonte W, Shaparin N, et al. Intravenous infusions in chronic pain management. Pain Physician 2013;16(3):231–49.

7. Fan TM, Charney SC, de Lorimier LP, et al. Double-blind placebo-controlled trial of adjuvant pamidronate with palliative radiotherapy and intravenous doxorubicin for canine appendicular osteosarcoma bone pain. J Vet Intern Med 2009;23(1):152–60.

8. Cardoso FC, Hasan M, Zhao T, et al. Toxins in pain. Curr Opin Support Palliat Care 2018;12(2):132–41.

9. Safavi-Hemami H, Brogan SE, Olivera BM. Pain therapeutics from cone snail venoms: from Ziconotide to novel non-opioid pathways. J Proteomics 2019;190:12–20.

10. Shim SR, Cho YJ, Shin IS, et al. Efficacy and safety of botulinum toxin injection for interstitial cystitis/bladder pain syndrome: a systematic review and meta-analysis. Int Urol Nephrol 2016;48(8):1215–27.

11. Brown DC, Agnello K, Ladarola MJ. Intrathecal resiniferatoxin in a dog model: efficacy in bone cancer pain. Pain 2015;156(6):1018–24.

12. Brown DC, Agnello K. Intrathecal substance P-Saporin in the dog efficacy in bone cancer pain. Anesthesiology 2013;119(5):1178–85.

13. Iadarola MJ, Sapio MR, Raithel SJ, et al. Long-term pain relief in canine osteoarthritis by a single intra-articular injection of resiniferatoxin, a potent TRPV1 agonist. Pain 2018;159(10):2105–14.

14. McAlindon TE, Bannuru RR, Sullivan MC, et al. OARSI guidelines for the non-surgical management of knee osteoarthritis. Osteoarthritis Cartilage 2014;22(3):363–88.

15. Vandeweerd JM, Zhao Y, Nisolle JF, et al. Effect of corticosteroids on articular cartilage: have animal studies said everything? Fundam Clin Pharmacol 2015;29(5):427–38.

16. Frisbie DD, Kawcak CE, Trotter GW, et al. Effects of triamcinolone acetonide on an in vivo equine osteochondral fragment exercise model. Equine Vet J 1997;29(5):349–59.

17. Pelletier JP, Martel-Pelletier J. Protective effects of corticosteroids on cartilage lesions and osteophyte formation in the Pond-Nuki dog model of osteoarthritis. Arthritis Rheum 1989;32(2):181–93.

18. Pelletier JP, Martel-Pelletier J. In vivo protective effects of prophylactic treatment with tiaprofenic acid or intraarticular corticosteroids on osteoarthritic lesions in the experimental dog model. J Rheumatol Suppl 1991;27:127–30.

19. Pelletier JP, DiBattista JA, Raynauld JP, et al. The in vivo effects of intraarticular corticosteroid injections on cartilage lesions, stromelysin, interleukin-1, and oncogene protein synthesis in experimental osteoarthritis. Lab Invest 1995;72(5):578–86.

20. Shah JP, Thaker N, Heimur J, et al. Myofascial trigger points then and now: a historical and scientific perspective. PM R 2015;7(7):746–61.

21. Misirlioglu TO, Akgun K, Palamar D, et al. Piriformis syndrome: comparison of the effectiveness of local anesthetic and corticosteroid injections: a double-blinded, randomized controlled study. Pain Physician 2015;18(2):163–71.

22. Liu L, Huang QM, Liu QG, et al. Evidence for dry needling in the management of myofascial trigger points associated with low back pain: a systematic review and meta-analysis. Arch Phys Med Rehabil 2018;99(1):144–52.e2.

23. Khalifeh M, Mehta K, Varguise N, et al. Botulinum toxin type A for the treatment of head and neck chronic myofascial pain syndrome: a systematic review and meta-analysis. J Am Dent Assoc 2016;147(12):959–73.e1.

24. Albayrak A, Ozcafer R, Balioglu MB, et al. Piriformis syndrome: treatment of a rare cause of posterior hip pain with fluoroscopic-guided injection. Hip Int 2015;25(2):172–5.

25. Kumbhare DA, Elzibak AH, Noseworthy MD. Assessment of myofascial trigger points using ultrasound. Am J Phys Med Rehabil 2016;95(1):72–80.

26. Wall R. Introduction to myofascial trigger points in dogs. Top Companion Anim Med 2014;29(2):43–8.

27. Janssens LAA. Trigger points in 48 dogs with myofascial pain syndromes. Vet Surg 1991;20(4):274–8.

28. Kaye AD, Manchikanti L, Abdi S, et al. Efficacy of epidural injections in managing chronic spinal pain: a best evidence synthesis. Pain Physician 2015;18(6):E939–1004.

29. Waldman DS. Atlas of interventional pain management. 4th edition. Philadelphia: Elsevier Saunders; 2015.

30. Cohen SP, Bicket MC, Jamison D, et al. Epidural steroids: a comprehensive, evidence-based review. Reg Anesth Pain Med 2013;38(3):175–200.

31. Shim E, Lee JW, Lee E, et al. Fluoroscopically guided epidural injections of the cervical and lumbar spine. Radiographics 2017;37(2):537–61.

32. Campoy L, Read MR. Small animal regional anesthesia and analgesia. Ames (IA): Wiley-Blackwell; 2013.

33. Malhotra G, Abbasi A, Rhee M. Complications of transforaminal cervical epidural steroid injections. Spine (Phila Pa 1976) 2009;34(7):731–9.

34. Janssens L, Beosier Y, Daems R. Lumbosacral degenerative stenosis in the dog. The results of epidural infiltration with methylprednisolone acetate: a retrospective study. Vet Comp Orthop Traumatol 2009;22(6):486–91.

35. Kirksey MA, Haskins SC, Cheng J, et al. Local anesthetic peripheral nerve block adjuvants for prolongation of analgesia: a systematic qualitative review. PLoS One 2015;10(9):e0137312.

36. Williams BA, Ibinson JW, Mangione MP, et al. Research priorities regarding multimodal peripheral nerve blocks for postoperative analgesia and anesthesia based on hospital quality data extracted from over 1,300 cases (2011-2014). Pain Med 2015;16(1):7–12.

37. Leffler A, Frank G, Kistner K, et al. Local anesthetic-like inhibition of voltage-gated Na(+) channels by the partial mu-opioid receptor agonist buprenorphine. Anesthesiology 2012;116(6):1335–46.

38. Koppert W, Ihmsen H, Korber N, et al. Different profiles of buprenorphine-induced analgesia and antihyperalgesia in a human pain model. Pain 2005;118(1–2):15–22.

39. Brummett CM, Hong EK, Janda AM, et al. Perineural dexmedetomidine added to ropivacaine for sciatic nerve block in rats prolongs the duration of analgesia by blocking the hyperpolarization-activated cation current. Anesthesiology 2011;115(4):836–43.

40. Kroin JS, Buvanendran A, Beck DR, et al. Clonidine prolongation of lidocaine analgesia after sciatic nerve block in rats Is mediated via the

hyperpolarization-activated cation current, not by alpha-adrenoreceptors. Anesthesiology 2004;101(2):488–94.

41. Young GT, Emery EC, Mooney ER, et al. Inflammatory and neuropathic pain are rapidly suppressed by peripheral block of hyperpolarisation-activated cyclic nucleotide-gated ion channels. Pain 2014;155(9):1708–19.

42. Campoy L, Martin-Flores M, Ludders JW, et al. Comparison of bupivacaine femoral and sciatic nerve block versus bupivacaine and morphine epidural for stifle surgery in dogs. Vet Anaesth Analg 2012;39(1):91–8.

43. Li JY, Xie W, Strong JA, et al. Mechanical hypersensitivity, sympathetic sprouting, and glial activation are attenuated by local injection of corticosteroid near the lumbar ganglion in a rat model of neuropathic pain. Reg Anesth Pain Med 2011;36(1):56–62.

44. Vastani N, Seifert B, Spahn DR, et al. Sensitivities of rat primary sensory afferent nerves to magnesium: implications for differential nerve blocks. Eur J Anaesthesiol 2013;30(1):21–8.

45. Manchikanti KN, Pampati V, Damron KS, et al. A double-blind, controlled evaluation of the value of sarapin in neural blockade. Pain Physician 2004;7(1):59–62.

46. Manchikanti L, Pampati V, Rivera JJ, et al. Caudal epidural injections with sarapin or steroids in chronic low back pain. Pain Physician 2001;4(4):322–35.

47. Grimm KA, Lamont LA, Tranquilli WJ, et al, editors. Veterinary anesthesia and analgesia: the fifth edition of lumb and jones. Ames (IA): John Wiley & Sons, Inc.; 2015.

48. Kambadakone A, Thabet A, Gervais DA, et al. CT-guided celiac plexus neurolysis: a review of anatomy, indications, technique, and tips for successful treatment. Radiographics 2011;31(6):1599–621.

49. Koyyalagunta D, Engle MP, Yu J, et al. The effectiveness of alcohol versus phenol based splanchnic nerve neurolysis for the treatment of intra-abdominal cancer pain. Pain Physician 2016;19(4):281–92.

50. Waller A. Experiments on the section of the glossopharyngeal and hypoglossal nerves of the frog, and observations of the alterations produced thereby in the structure of their primitive fibres. Philos Trans R Soc Lond 1850;140:423–9.

51. Choi EJ, Choi YM, Jang EJ, et al. Neural ablation and regeneration in pain practice. Korean J Pain 2016;29(1):3–11.

52. Cornman-Homonoff J, Holzwanger DJ, Lee KS, et al. Celiac plexus block and neurolysis in the management of chronic upper abdominal pain. Semin Intervent Radiol 2017;34(4):376–86.

53. Cosman ER Jr, Cosman ER Sr. Electric and thermal field effects in tissue around radiofrequency electrodes. Pain Med 2005;6(6):405–24.

54. Ball RD. The science of conventional and water-cooled monopolar lumbar radiofrequency rhizotomy: an electrical engineering point of view. Pain Physician 2014; 17(2):E175–211.

55. Shealy CN. Percutaneous radiofrequency denervation of spinal facets. Treatment for chronic back pain and sciatica. J Neurosurg 1975;43(4):448–51.

56. Vatansever D, Tekin I, Tuglu I, et al. A comparison of the neuroablative effects of conventional and pulsed radiofrequency techniques. Clin J Pain 2008;24(8): 717–24.

57. Sunderland S. A classification of peripheral nerve injuries producing loss of function. Brain 1951;74(4):491–516.

58. Ilfeld BM, Preciado J, Trescot AM. Novel cryoneurolysis device for the treatment of sensory and motor peripheral nerves. Expert Rev Med Devices 2016;13(8): 713–25.

59. Govind J, King W, Bailey B, et al. Radiofrequency neurotomy for the treatment of third occipital headache. J Neurol Neurosurg Psychiatry 2003;74(1):88–93.
60. Manchikanti L, Kaye AD, Boswell MV, et al. A systematic review and best evidence synthesis of the effectiveness of therapeutic facet joint interventions in managing chronic spinal pain. Pain Physician 2015;18(4):E535–82.
61. Tang YZ, Jin D, Li XY, et al. Repeated CT-guided percutaneous radiofrequency thermocoagulation for recurrent trigeminal neuralgia. Eur Neurol 2014;72(1–2): 54–9.
62. Choi WJ, Hwang SJ, Song JG, et al. Radiofrequency treatment relieves chronic knee osteoarthritis pain: a double-blind randomized controlled trial. Pain 2011; 152(3):481–7.
63. Smith HP, McWhorter JM, Challa VR. Radiofrequency neurolysis in a clinical model. Neuropathological correlation. J Neurosurg 1981;55(2):246–53.
64. Erdine S, Bilir A, Cosman ER, et al. Ultrastructural changes in axons following exposure to pulsed radiofrequency fields. Pain Pract 2009;9(6):407–17.
65. Ren H, Jin H, Jia Z, et al. Pulsed radiofrequency applied to the sciatic nerve improves neuropathic pain by down-regulating the expression of calcitonin gene-related peptide in the dorsal root ganglion. Int J Med Sci 2018;15(2):153–60.
66. Higuchi Y, Nashold BS Jr, Sluijter M, et al. Exposure of the dorsal root ganglion in rats to pulsed radiofrequency currents activates dorsal horn lamina I and II neurons. Neurosurgery 2002;50(4):850–5 [discussion: 856].
67. Choi YH, Chang DJ, Hwang WS, et al. Ultrasonography-guided pulsed radiofrequency of sciatic nerve for the treatment of complex regional pain syndrome Type II. Saudi J Anaesth 2017;11(1):83–5.
68. Ke M, Yinghui F, Yi J, et al. Efficacy of pulsed radiofrequency in the treatment of thoracic postherpetic neuralgia from the angulus costae: a randomized, double-blinded, controlled trial. Pain Physician 2013;16(1):15–25.
69. Onofrio BM, Yaksh TL, Arnold PG. Continuous low-dose intrathecal morphine administration in the treatment of chronic pain of malignant origin. Mayo Clin Proc 1981;56(8):516–20.
70. Pope JE, Deer TR, Amirdelfan K, et al. The pharmacology of spinal opioids and ziconotide for the treatment of non-cancer pain. Curr Neuropharmacol 2017; 15(2):206–16.
71. Melzack R, Wall PD. Pain mechanisms: a new theory. Science 1965;150(3699): 971–9.
72. Dones I, Levi V. Spinal cord stimulation for neuropathic pain: current trends and future applications. Brain Sci 2018;8(8) [pii:E138].
73. Veizi E, Hayek SM. Spinal cord stimulation: implantation techniques. In: Diwan S, Staats P, editors. Atlas of pain medicine procedures. New York: McGraw Hill; 2015. p. 601–18.

Common Neurologic Problems

Impact on Patient Welfare, Caregiver Burden and Veterinarian Wellbeing

Julie M. Ducoté, DVM, MA, DACVIM (Neurology)

KEYWORDS

- Palliative care • Neuropalliative care • Caregiver burden • Veterinarian wellbeing

KEY POINTS

- Palliative care is a vital component of the treatment needed for companion animals with neurologic diseases.
- Clients with patients that have neurologic disease are likely to be uniquely affected by caregiver burden.
- Veterinarians treating patients with neurologic disease need to be proactive in building resilience, self-care, and establishing health boundaries, to maintain their own wellbeing.

INTRODUCTION

Despite advances in diagnostic capability and treatment options for patients with neurologic disease, most of these diseases are not curable. Long-term palliative management of symptoms is an essential component of the treatment plan for most of these syndromes. Depending on the underlying disease, the need for palliative care may be prolonged over months or years. Even when definitive therapy is possible, it is still necessary to manage symptoms with appropriate therapies, to help improve and maintain patient quality of life during treatment and recovery. In addition, humans are forming increasingly strong bonds with their pets, often considering their pets as members of their family, similar to human children.[1] This intense human-animal bond means that when faced with a pet that has a serious, life-altering or life-limiting neurologic disease, many clients will seek advanced treatment and pursue long-term nursing care for them.[1]

It is accepted that caregivers of human patients with serious or chronic neurologic diseases experience significant and unique stressors, described as caregiver

Disclosure Statement: The author has nothing to disclose.
Center for Veterinary Specialty + Emergency Care, 2700 Lake Vista Drive, Lewisville, TX 75067, USA
E-mail address: JDUCOTE@CVSECVET.COM

Vet Clin Small Anim 49 (2019) 463–476
https://doi.org/10.1016/j.cvsm.2019.01.012
0195-5616/19/© 2019 Elsevier Inc. All rights reserved.

vetsmall.theclinics.com

burden.[2–4] Recent reports have critically evaluated caregiver burden in clients caring for seriously or chronically ill pets,[5,6] and this phenomenon is explored in detail in this issue. Clinical signs or behaviors that are most strongly correlated with caregiver burden include weakness, appearing to have pain or discomfort, frequent urination, change in personality, and appearing depressed or anxious.[6] These are also the clinical signs associated with some of the most common neurologic problems in animals, such as seizures, vestibular syndromes, paralysis, cognitive dysfunction, neuropathies, and tumors of the nervous system. Owners and caregivers of pets with neurologic disease are likely to experience high levels of caregiver burden.

The more caregiver burden a client has, the more support they are likely to need and seek from the veterinarian and veterinary health care team.[5] Largely catalyzed by concern regarding suicide in the veterinary profession, recent attention has been focused on potential etiologies for poor wellbeing among veterinarians.[7–9] Demands of veterinary practice, including the role of client expectations, have been suggested as a possible contributor to poor wellbeing among veterinarians.[7] If clients of pets with serious neurologic problems have more caregiver burden, and thus need more support from their veterinarian, what affect might these needs and demands have on veterinarian wellbeing?

This article will discuss the unique needs for palliative interventions in patients with neurologic problems that are commonly seen in veterinary practice, and will propose a Neuropalliative Care Core Skill Set to aid veterinarians in identifying best practices in providing care for neurology patients and clients. The potential caregiver burden of clients with pets suffering from neurologic disorders will be reviewed. Comparisons will be made between issues common to companion animals and people with serious and chronic neurologic diseases, referencing the current literature available in groups of patients and their caregivers. Finally, the impact of caregiver burden on veterinarians who care for patients with neurologic disease will be explored, along with strategies for professionals to mitigate the emotional, physical, and moral stresses that are often associated with challenging neurology cases.

PARALYSIS/WEAKNESS

Many neurologic diseases may cause weakness or paralysis in companion animals. Some of the diseases most commonly encountered include intervertebral disc disease, caudal cervical spondylomyelopathy, degenerative myelopathy, spinal neoplasia, and peripheral neuropathies.

Intervertebral disc disease is the most common disease that leads to paralysis in dogs. Fortunately, this is also one of the most treatable and often, curable, neurologic diseases. Some dogs, however, experience irreversible spinal cord damage despite surgical intervention. Some owners elect not to pursue surgical intervention for financial, personal, or practical reasons. For some dogs, especially those with chronic spinal cord compression, surgery may have limited benefit because of pre-existing long-term spinal cord damage. In the most treatable cases— non-ambulatory chondrodystrophic dogs with acute nucleus pulposus extrusion, treated promptly with decompressive spinal surgery—the time to regaining the ability to walk independently is reported to be an average of 10 to 14 days after surgery.[10,11] Several patient and disease factors have been reported to be associated with a more prolonged or incomplete recovery, including body weight greater than 20 kg, having an annular protrusion rather than nucleus pulposus extrusion, advanced age, the presence of lower motor neuron signs, chronicity of spinal cord compression, and lack of deep pain perception.[11–15]

For patients in all of these groups, substantial nursing care and symptom management may be needed for weeks to months. For patients with a poor prognosis for recovery, lifelong nursing care will be needed. Even in patients that regain the ability to walk independently, adequate and appropriate nursing care may make the difference between a successful recovery and a patient that experiences serious or long-term complications. Caring for a dog that is unable to walk on its own is a completely unique experience for most owners. Lower coping scores have been reported in clients caring for dogs that were non-ambulatory compared with those that were ambulatory, suggesting that owners often suffer emotional distress when their dog becomes non-ambulatory.[16] Especially in situations where the dog's paralysis is very acute in onset, this may complicate the decision-making process. After the initial assessment is made, and there has been a preliminary discussion of treatment options, the next step is for the veterinarian to have a candid and compassionate conversation about the likely nursing care requirements for the patient going forward.

Providing support for walking is a central need for paralyzed patients and a major factor in quality of life. Patients that are able to use their thoracic limbs are more easily supported than those that are unable to use all 4 limbs. Understandably, patient size is also a major factor. Small dogs and cats can be carried, whereas larger dogs require much more support. Giant breeds may need multiple people to help support them when moving, doing physical therapy exercises, or attempting to walk. Mobility aids, such as slings, harnesses, and wheelchairs, can help improve patient quality of life, and make it easier for owners to care for their pets. It may also be helpful to encourage owners to make adjustments in their home, such as adding surfaces that provide traction when pets are trying to walk.

Patients that are non-ambulatory from spinal cord disease are likely to require manual bladder expression several times a day, at least on a temporary basis. Appropriate urinary bladder management prevents permanent damage to the detrusor muscle of the bladder, which can lead to long-term problems with urinary retention. Regular bladder expression also reduces the risk of urinary tract infection and urine scald. Manual bladder expression is routinely performed by experienced veterinary team members in the hospital setting. With adequate instruction and guidance, most owners are able to learn to do this for their dog at home. To enhance individual, in-person training for bladder expression, there are written instructions and online resources, with step-by-step photos and training videos available.[17–19]

Recumbency significantly increases the risk of pneumonia, particularly in larger dogs, those that are unable to use all 4 limbs, and those that are unable to maintain a sternal posture.[20] Rotating a patient's position every few hours and using pillows or padding to prop the patient in a more sternal position, may help decrease the chance of pneumonia. In addition to recumbency, the increased incidence of regurgitation and vomiting in patients with spinal cord disease can lead to pneumonia due to aspiration.[20] Brachycephalic breeds are particularly prone to aspiration if they vomit or regurgitate.[21] It should also be noted that many patients with spinal cord disease need to undergo general anesthesia for diagnostics and/or surgery, and may also receive opioid pain medications. Both general anesthesia and the use of opioid drugs increase the risk of regurgitation.[20] In patients with any of these risk factors, pre-emptive treatment with an antiemetic such as maropitant may help reduce the risk of regurgitation on anesthetic recovery.

Close attention must be paid to hygiene in dogs that are recumbent. Contact with urine or feces may lead to scalding and potential infection of the skin over the hindquarters, especially in the perineal area and medial thighs.[22] This kind of skin damage is a particular risk in large recumbent dogs and those with a long or thick hair coat. If patients in the hospital setting are receiving steroid medications or fluid therapy that may lead to increased frequency of urination, consideration should be given to placing an indwelling urinary catheter and collection system, for hygiene purposes and to help keep the urinary bladder empty. The risk of skin damage in recumbent patients is also increased by the pressure of body weight against the surfaces on which a patient is laying. Thick, soft bedding and frequent rotation of patients may help reduce the formation of decubital ulcers. These wounds are more common in dogs that are tetraparetic, those with increased body weight, and those with reduced muscle mass.[22] Wounds most often develop over pressure points, such as the elbows and hips. Extra padding at these anatomic areas may be helpful.

SEIZURES

Seizures are common in companion animals, particularly in dogs, in which there is a high incidence of idiopathic epilepsy.[23] Frequency of seizures has been found to be significantly associated with carer-perceived quality of life.[24] It is estimated that between 30% and 50% of epileptic dogs may continue to have frequent seizures, even when treated with medication.[23] Thus, it is important for the veterinarian to have a compassionate, yet honest conversation with owners of pets that are presented for seizures. This conversation should include a discussion of the nature of seizure events, what to expect during a typical seizure, counseling on when a seizure is considered an emergency, and what to do in an emergency. One of the most common owner concerns is whether or not seizures are painful to the patient. This should be addressed, as the perception that a dog is in pain is one of the most stressful clinical signs that owners report.[6] Evidence from human epileptic patients indicates that fewer than 2% of patients report pain associated with their seizures.[25,26] Veterinarians can reassure clients that in most dogs and cats with generalized seizures, the patient is not experiencing pain. It is reasonable to suppose that the seizure event is usually far more stressful to the person witnessing the episode than it is to the patient. Other important components of the conversation are the potential etiology of seizures, treatment options, goals of treatment, and prognosis.

Dogs receiving third-line anticonvulsants and those that experience adverse effects of anticonvulsant drugs are also judged to have lower quality of life by their owners.[24] Newer anticonvulsant drugs may fail to show improved efficacy over traditional anticonvulsant drugs, therefore drug side effects now often drive drug selection by the veterinarian, given the perceived impact of side effects on quality of life of the dog by the owner.[24] Nevertheless, because increased seizure frequency is correlated with reduced perceived quality of life, the potential benefits in reducing seizure frequency in comparison with the potential adverse effects of each drug, should be carefully weighed for each individual seizure patient. For example, although phenobarbital has a higher risk of side effects in most dogs, it has also been shown to be the most commonly prescribed first-line anticonvulsant drug in dogs, because it has the highest efficacy in reducing seizure frequency.[27] Levetiracetam has a very good safety profile in most dogs, but is reported to have a lower efficacy as a sole anticonvulsant drug when compared with phenobarbital.[27] When presented with an otherwise healthy, 2-year-old dog with idiopathic epilepsy characterized by frequent cluster seizures, phenobarbital would be a reasonable choice for first-line therapy. If presented with a geriatric patient for treatment of late-onset seizures, who also has pre-existing hepatobiliary disease and osteoarthritis, one might instead consider recommending levetiracetam for initial therapy, given its decreased risk of causing the side effects of sedation, ataxia, and hepatotoxicity.

Lack of control over events, unpredictability of events, sleep deprivation, and a feeling of helplessness are known factors in the development of stress in people.[28,29] Caring for a patient with seizures influences some, if not all, of these factors. Up to 50% of mothers are at risk of depression as a consequence of caring for an epileptic child.[30] Likewise, there is evidence that owners of epileptic dogs may suffer to some degree from depression or panic attacks, and may also describe feeling isolated as a result of caring for their dog.[24] Despite treatment, most epileptic dogs continue to have seizures, even if with a reduced frequency or severity.[23] Therefore, it is important to communicate clearly with owners to establish realistic expectations of results of treatment. Though there is no way to modify the inherent unpredictability of seizure events, outlining a plan for how the owners can manage a seizure event at home can help provide them a sense of more control and ease the feelings of helplessness when they witness a seizure. This "rescue" plan might include an additional medication the owner keeps at home for use during or after a seizure. Injectable diazepam may be given rectally, or injectable midazolam may be given intranasally.[31] Both of these drugs can be absorbed across mucous membranes and reach reasonable plasma concentrations within a few minutes. Another means of helping reduce the risk of cluster seizures is to prescribe an additional drug for use as pulse therapy following a seizure event. Levetiracetam has been described for this use in dogs, as its short half-life means that oral administration can provide reasonable plasma concentrations within a few days.[32] Finally, consideration can be given to using additional doses of a patient's usual daily anticonvulsant drug, given immediately after a seizure event, to temporarily increase the serum level and it is hoped to reduce the risk for cluster seizures.

COGNITIVE DYSFUNCTION AND DEMENTIA

Numerous neurologic diseases in companion animals are capable of leading to signs of cognitive dysfunction and dementia, which may include high levels of anxiety, whining, pacing, panting, circling, staring blankly into space, loss of learned commands and habits, restlessness and night time wakefulness, overall decreased activity, failure to recognize or acknowledge owners, or inappropriate urination and defecation.[6] Structural or inflammatory brain disease affecting the cerebral cortex may lead to cognitive impairment and symptoms of dementia. Cerebral neoplasia, disseminated or focal meningoencephalitis, cerebral ischemia/hypoxia, or traumatic brain injuries may have this effect. Several reports have also described a correlation between idiopathic epilepsy and behavioral disorders such as anxiety, ADHD-like behavior (including hyperactivity, impulsivity, inattention, and easy distraction), cognitive dysfunction, and dementia.[33–35] Neurodegenerative disease, most notably the Alzheimer's-like syndrome of canine cognitive dysfunction (CCD), is the most widely acknowledged disease that leads to cognitive impairment in dogs.[36,37] Even if definitive therapy is undertaken for diseases in which therapy is possible, attention should also be given to the coinciding stressors that the clinical signs of cognitive dysfunction are likely to have on patients and caregivers. Anxiety, sleep disturbances, and concern about their pet's discomfort are significantly correlated with caregiver burden in pet owners.[6] Thus, veterinary visits should openly address these concerns by asking the client how she or he is coping.

Therapy for cognitive impairment in dogs is supportive, with the goal of managing symptoms, maintaining quality of life, and slowing progression of clinical signs. In CCD specifically, therapy with seligiline (also known as L-deprenyl) is shown to improve clinical signs of cognitive impairment.[38] Antioxidants such as the amino acid S-adenosylmethionine, may also improve cognitive skills in dogs.[39] More recently, a diet high in medium chain triglycerides has shown promise in minimizing clinical signs of CCD.[35] A high-medium chain triglyceride diet may also reduce signs of ADHD-like behavior in epileptic patients.[40]

Behavioral and environmental modification are important components of support for dogs with cognitive impairment, regardless of the etiology. Clients should be reminded of the need for practical safety measures, such as avoiding swimming pools, stairs, or other dangerous areas without direct supervision. In dogs with restlessness and difficulty sleeping at night, encouraging a leash walk or other physical activity shortly before bed time may help reduce nighttime waking. Some patients respond well to a smaller physical environment, such as a smaller room or large kennel, rather than the open interior space of a large home. For others, confinement or restriction may increase agitation and anxiety. As in people with cognitive impairment, adherence to routines and maintaining familiar environments can be comforting and may minimize anxiety. If sleep disturbances or anxiety significantly impair quality of life for the dog or caregiver or both, then consideration should be given to use of sedative or anxiolytic drugs. Trazodone may be used for anxiety in dogs, and is usually well tolerated even in many patients, even those with significant metabolic disease.[41] The most common side effect is sedation, which makes it a good choice in patients with anxiety and difficulty sleeping.[41]

CAREGIVER BURDEN IN COMPANION ANIMAL NEUROLOGIC DISEASE

Caregiving for a patient with a serious or chronic neurologic disease has been strongly correlated with significant and unique stressors.[2] There are measurable adverse effects on mental health, physical health, and psychosocial wellbeing.[2] Caregivers of human patients with neurologic diseases are often faced with a diagnosis that is grim, with a short life expectancy. They may deal with the physical symptoms associated with loss of mobility and ability to perform tasks of daily living, as well as the cognitive and behavioral symptoms that usually accompany the diagnosis.[42,43] Caregivers of pets with neurologic disease are often required to support pets that have loss of mobility or incontinence. Seizures, cognitive impairment, and behavioral problems are common. In many cases, caregivers face the emotional and psychological effects of an uncertain or guarded prognosis for recovery. Anticipatory grief is likely experienced by many caregivers of animals with neurologic disease. As previously mentioned, lack of control over events, unpredictability of events, sleep deprivation, and a feeling of helplessness, are known factors in the development of stress in people; these factors are also believed to contribute to caregiver burden.[28,29] The nature of neurologic diseases is that their clinical signs may be unpredictable. When coupled with a guarded prognosis, the result may be feelings of helplessness, lack of control, anxiety, depression, and reduced caregiver quality of life.

During the course of treatment, it is important to acknowledge the potential impact of caregiver burden on clients. Asking clients how they are doing or how they are coping with their pet's illness demonstrates an understanding of the potential challenges they face, and provides a supportive environment for them to express their feelings and concerns. Veterinarians may discover some problems that can be modified with treatment changes. They may also have an opportunity to partner with, and encourage clients to accept support from other resources such as a Veterinary Social Worker or other mental health professional. Even when problems cannot be fixed or changed, acknowledging the reality of challenges inherent in these cases can help clients move toward acceptance and realism about their pet's disease and prognosis.

The human literature identifies building coping skills, such as using problem-focused strategies (defining the problem, seeking alternative solutions, choosing, and acting), acceptance, and social-emotional support, to be associated with improved outcomes for caregivers.[2] Negative outcomes are associated with wishful thinking, denial, and avoidance strategies.[2] It is also evident that caregiver burden may be increased by a sense of abandonment by health care providers, especially when the disease is complex, chronic, or unpredictable.[44] Through clear, compassionate communication and empathy, veterinarians can aid clients who are dealing with both the practical and emotional aspects of caring for patients with serious or chronic neurologic diseases. However, veterinarians are not trained to diagnose or treat mental health problems.

VETERINARY NEUROLOGISTS AS PALLIATIVE CARE PROVIDERS

Because many neurologic diseases are not curable and require either short- or long-term management of symptoms, veterinary neurologists are often palliative care providers. The role of neurologists as specialized palliative care providers has recently been described in human medicine.[45,46] It is important to acknowledge that, in veterinary medicine, clinicians are usually serving 2 stakeholders: the animal patient and the human client or caregiver. In developing a palliative care plan for patients, veterinary neurologists need to consider multiple patient factors: minimizing or preventing neurologic symptoms, minimizing adverse effects of any definitive treatment, and maintaining quality of life as much as possible for as long as possible. When considering the best approach for the client or caregiver, other considerations have significant impact. These include the role of the animal in that client's life, client background including cultural and spiritual values, client goals and expectations for, and fears related to, treatment, client's ability or willingness to pay for the financial costs of care, potential caregiver burden, and caregiver quality of life.

There is growing evidence that human patients with serious, chronic neurologic diseases receiving high-quality care continue to have unmet palliative needs.[46] There is growing support for incorporating palliative medicine into neurology practice.[45,46] A core palliative care skill set for veterinarians treating patients with neurologic disease includes the following: (1) effective communication of diagnosis, treatment options, and prognosis; (2) initiating and leading a Goals of Care conversation; (3) initiating and leading follow-up conversations pertaining to disease course and end-of-life planning; and (4) managing symptoms to optimize and maintain quality of life (**Box 1**). For veterinary neurologists, developing these Neuropalliative Care Core Skills and intentionally implementing them in daily practice may help optimize patient welfare. As the patient's disease progresses over time, practicing these skills has the potential to reduce caregiver burden, and might also lessen the stress on the veterinarian.

Communication and Goals of Care

The importance of clear, compassionate communication with clients and caregivers of pets with neurologic disease cannot be overstated. The initial conversation usually involves discussing the suspected or definitive diagnosis and its prognosis. Practical frameworks for having this conversation with clients have been outlined in previous sources[46–49] and are also explored in this issue. Even in emergency situations, it is helpful to first ask permission to discuss the diagnosis at the time of the consultation or phone call, thus inviting the client's agreement and participation in the discussion. This gaining of client consent to talk about something serious might sound like this: "Mrs. Jones, I'd like to talk to you about Fluffy's MRI results. Is this a good time for

---

Box. 1
Veterinary Neuropalliative Care Core Skill Set

1. Effectively communicate diagnosis, treatment options, and prognosis
    Breaking the news
        Gain consent from client to discuss difficult diagnosis.
        Ascertain how much awareness and knowledge client currently has.
    Communicate prognosis
        Estimates from literature
        Likely outcome with and without treatment
            Best case/worst case/most likely case scenarios
        Are client expectations of outcome realistic?
        Costs of care (caregiver burden)—financial and non-financial (time, energy, physical emotional)
    Manage uncertainty

2. Goals of Care conversation—elicit client preference accurately
    Role of animal in client's life
    Cultural, spiritual values
    Client goals and expectations for, and fears related to, treatment
    Client ability or willingness to pay for care
    Client willingness or ability to take on non-financial costs of care

3. Follow-up conversations
    Introduce health care team and clarify roles
    Disease course
    End-of-life planning
    Listen more than talk

4. Symptom management
    Physical symptoms (eg, weakness, urinary retention, seizures)
    Pain management
    Minimize adverse effects of any definitive treatment
    Anxiety, behavioral symptoms
    Nursing care needs
    Client psychological symptoms and existential distress

Adapted from Robinson MT, Holloway RG. Palliative care in neurology. Mayo Clin Proc 2017;92(10):1592–1601; with permission.

---

you?" Ascertaining the current level of knowledge or awareness a client has about the disease is also helpful. Questions such as "Are you familiar with the spinal problems that Dachshunds often develop?" can aid the neurologist in determining what level of medical information may need to be conveyed to the client during the conversation.

Goals of Care conversations are described as "those that focus on what is most important to people and their families as they face serious illness.[49,50] They are a core competency of palliative care providers, and the means by which patient (in human medicine) and client (in veterinary medicine) preferences, values, goals, and fears are elicited."[50] Once the diagnosis has been delivered, a Goals of Care conversation should ensue, either before or immediately following a discussion of treatment options. This Goals of Care conversation is the foundation of shared decision making between clients and clinicians.[49–51] In some situations, the conversation is initiated by the client, but when it is not, the veterinarian should introduce the discussion with empathy and compassion. Key components of the Goals of Care conversation in human medicine include sharing prognostic information, eliciting decision-making preferences, understanding fears and goals, exploring views on trade-offs and impaired function, and wishes for family involvement.[49] In veterinary medicine, one of the best ways to begin this conversation is by asking the client what is most important to them when considering their pet's treatment. This will usually clarify the client's values regarding their pet and their fears. The clinician can then place the known disease and treatment factors into context for the client. For example, if Mr. Smith says that his dog Spot's quality of life is of highest importance to him, and that he fears any adverse effects of treatment, then the neurologist can move the conversation to a detailed description of all possible adverse effects of each treatment option, thereby supporting Mr. Smith in making the most informed decision for Spot according to what he values most. Goals of Care conversations help align client goals and expectations with the reality of treatment outcomes and prognosis.[49] The conversation also helps to minimize patient suffering and may help reduce the stress that is associated with caregiver burden.

Modifiable versus Not Modifiable: Helping Clients Understand Limits

Given the uncertain outcome associated with many neurologic diseases, clients and caregivers may experience helplessness, lack of control, anxiety, depression, and reduced caregiver quality of life. Before and throughout treatment, efforts should be made to clarify the disease, including which care factors are modifiable and which are non-modifiable. For example, in the case of canine idiopathic epilepsy, the disease is not curable and most patients continue to be at risk for seizures throughout their lifetime. At this time, the lack of a cure is not a modifiable disease factor. Another factor that is rarely modifiable is that most caregivers are not able to provide 24-hour-a-day care for their pet by themselves. It is helpful to acknowledge these factors up front, because clients may experience varying degrees of difficulty in acceptance. In contrast, frequency and severity of seizures may be modifiable with anticonvulsant drug therapy. In these patients, neurologists commonly recommend caregivers maintain a log of all seizure events, including date and time of events, duration, severity, and any possible triggers. This information is often used to aid in decisions about the efficacy of current treatment and potential modification of treatment plans. Another benefit of the seizure log is that it provides caregivers with a sense of awareness and knowledge of their pet's epilepsy, as well as giving them a shared role in therapeutic monitoring and treatment decisions. This allows clients to have more of a sense of control and the capability to manage what they can about their pet's illness. At the same time, it may also help them to accept the parts of the disease that are not modifiable, such as lack of a cure or a terminal prognosis.

Interdisciplinary Team

Supporting clients or caregivers with seriously ill pets must be approached as a team. In a recent study of clients with dogs that had life-limiting cancer being treated at a tertiary care center, client expectations included: information being communicated in a forthright manner; in multiple formats; in understandable language; in an unrushed environment wherein staff took the time to listen, answer all questions, and repeat information when necessary; on a continuous basis, with 24-hour access to address questions or concerns; in a timely manner; with positivity; with compassion and empathy; with a non-judgmental attitude; and through staff with whom they had established relationships.[52] In light of this extensive list of client expectations, it is clear that no individual veterinarian can be available to support a client in all of these areas at all times. The veterinary neurologist should partner with the primary care veterinarian, and with skilled and experienced veterinary nurses, to help provide medical advice and practical support on an ongoing basis. Based on the typical needs and expectations of clients, it is helpful to introduce and clarify roles of all the members of the health care team to the client, and to outline a plan for follow-up, including how to handle any possible emergencies. The veterinary neurologist should also collaborate with a Veterinary Social Worker and other mental health professionals. Goldberg (2017) states that, "When distressed and poorly functioning clients are using veterinary services for their pets, the most important thing for veterinarians to do is to recognize that this type of client care is beyond their scope of practice, and know how to make a mental health referral."[50] Social workers are uniquely able to assess a client's emotional and psychosocial health, to determine if a mental health referral is needed, and to help facilitate that referral.[53,54]

Challenges in Neuropalliative Care

Significant challenges exist for veterinarians in the practice of neuropalliative care. For many neurologic diseases, the paucity of evidence in the scientific literature may lead to uncertainty about prognosis, especially in regards to different treatment options. Guiding clients in situations when faced with this uncertainty may prove difficult.

Another major challenge is the lack of outside resources for caregiver support for seriously or chronically ill animals with neurologic disease. For human family members, readily available options exist for: (1) hiring outside caregivers, (2) providing physical and occupational therapy either outpatient, or in the home, and (3) using residential rehabilitation centers particularly after neurosurgery, or other times when patients need significant support regaining mobility and independence with Activities of Daily Living. These resources are rarely, if ever, available for our veterinary patients and clients, placing the burden for care and support almost exclusively on the client and veterinary team.

As the need for neuropalliative care in veterinary medicine increases, so does the need for veterinary neurologists, veterinary nurses specializing in neurology, veterinary physical therapists, and veterinary social workers. Currently, the number of trained professionals in these areas, as well as trainees, is unlikely to be sufficient to meet the growing demand. It is also essential that these professionals receive focused training in neuropalliative care. Currently, this training is informal—usually gained through practical experience during clinical rotations, rather than a formal training program focused on development of a specific skill set. The Neuropalliative Care Core Skill Set described in this article provides an outline of focus areas for future professional development.

POTENTIAL IMPACT OF CAREGIVER BURDEN ON VETERINARIAN WELLBEING

In human medicine, it is known that caregivers use health care resources at a high rate, with elevated stress, anxiety, and attention-seeking behavior all predicting health care use.[5] Spitznagel (2017) proposes that "if burdened clients have difficulty separating their own distress from medically necessary and appropriate veterinary attention, service overuse may occur, such as greater communication demands, more frequent/ extended duration of office visits than is needed for the animal's health, contributing to longer hours for the veterinarian. In addition, a client's emotional distress could manifest as anger, such as expressions of disappointment or grievances, effectively transferring the client's burden to the provider."[5] It has also been demonstrated that pet owners who are emotionally attached to their pets are more likely to be conscientious and neurotic.[55] Neuroticism is a personality trait that is associated with higher levels of anxiety, depression, and hostility. In fact, a subset of these owners are more likely to display "anxious attachment."[55] Caregivers who have anxious attachment to their pets may be more attentive to their pets, and more sensitive to changes in their pet's behavior or health. However, they are also more likely to be concerned about physical or emotional states that are not harmful to the pet.[55] On the whole, it can be very stressful for veterinarians to communicate effectively and compassionately with clients who have seriously or chronically ill pets.[25]

It is crucial for veterinarians to recognize when clients are transferring their own emotional burden to the veterinarian.[50] Because veterinary neurologists are often palliative care providers, they should remain aware of the potential impact of their client's burden on their own wellbeing. All veterinarians should be proactive in building resilience, practicing self-care, and establishing clear boundaries, while remaining compassionate and empathetic to their client's and patient's needs.[50] Given the profound intensity of the human-animal bond, the need for veterinarians to learn and practice the skills that contribute positively to wellbeing may be the biggest professional challenge most of us will ever face.

SUMMARY

Palliative care is a vital component of the care needed for companion animals with serious or chronic neurologic disease. A Neuropalliative Care Core Skill Set includes multifaceted communication competencies as well as symptom management. Because some of the most common clinical signs of neurologic disease are also those associated with the stress of caregiving, veterinary neurologists should understand and acknowledge the unique potential for caregiver burden experienced by their clients. Veterinarians treating patients with neurologic disease must also, therefore, be proactive in building their own resilience to the occupational stress inherent in treating their patients and supporting their patients' caregivers.

REFERENCES

1. Lue TW, Pantenburg DP, Crawford PM. Impact of the owner-pet and client-veterinarian bond on the care that pets receive. J Am Vet Med Assoc 2008; 232:531–40.
2. Gilhooly KJ, Gilhooly ML, Sullivan MP, et al. A meta-review of stress, coping and interventions in dementia and dementia caregiving. BMC Geriatr 2016;16: 106–14.
3. Cooper C, Balamurali TB, Livingston G. A systematic review of the prevalence and covariates of anxiety in caregivers of people with dementia. Int Psychogeriatr 2007;19:175–95.
4. Mahoney R, Regan C, Katona C, et al. Anxiety and depression in family caregivers of people with Alzheimer disease: the LASER-AD study. Am J Geriatr Psychiatry 2005;13:795–801.
5. Spitznagel MB, Jacobson DM, Cox MD, et al. Caregiver burden in owners of a sick companion animal: a cross-sectional observational study. Vet Rec 2017; 181:321–7.
6. Spitznagel MB, Jacobson DM, Cox MD, et al. Predicting caregiver burden in general veterinary clients: contribution of companion animal signs and problem behaviors. Vet J 2018;236:23–30.
7. Nett RJ, Witte TK, Holzbauer SM, et al. Risk factors for suicide, attitudes toward mental illness, and practice-related stressors among U.S. veterinarians. J Am Vet Med Assoc 2015;247(8):945–55.
8. Bartram DJ, Baldwin DS. Veterinary surgeons and suicide: a structured review of possible influences on increased risk. Vet Rec 2010;166:388–97.

9. Griek OHV, Clark MA, Witte TK, et al. Development of a taxonomy of practice-related stressors experienced by veterinarians in the United States. J Am Vet Med Assoc 2018;252(2):227–33.

10. Langerhuus L, Miles J. Proportion recovery and times to ambulation for non-ambulatory dogs with thoracolumbar disc extrusions treated with hemilaminectomy or conservative treatment: a systematic review and meta-analysis of case-series studies. Vet J 2017;220:7–16.

11. Olby N, Levine J, Harris T, et al. Long-term functional outcome of dogs with severe injuries of the thoracolumbar spinal cord: 87 cases (1996–2001). J Am Vet Med Assoc 2003;222:762–9.

12. Macias C, McKee WM, May C, et al. Thoracolumbar disc disease in large dogs: a study of 99 cases. J Small Anim Pract 2002;43:439–46.

13. Cudia SP, Duval JM. Thoracolumbar intervertebral disk disease in large, non-chrondrodystrophic dogs: a retrospective study. J Am Anim Hosp Assoc 1997;33(5):456–60.

14. Ruddle TL, Allen DA, Schertel ER, et al. Outcome and prognostic factors in non-ambulatory Hansen Type I intervertebral disc extrusions: 308 cases. Vet Comp Orthop Traumatol 2006;19(1):29–34.

15. Dhupa S, Glickman NW, waters DJ. Functional outcome in dogs after surgical treatment of caudal lumbar intervertebral disk herniation. J Am Anim Hosp Assoc 1999;35(4):323–31.

16. Levine JM, Budke CM, Levine GJ, et al. Owner-perceived, weighted quality-of-life assessments in dogs with spinal cord injuries. J Am Vet Med Assoc 2008;233(6):931–5.

17. Available at: https://www.handicappedpets.com/blog/how-to-express-dog-bladder/. Accessed September 14, 2018.

18. Available at: https://www.handicappedpets.com/how-to-express-your-pets-bladder-general-information/. Accessed September 14, 2018.

19. Available at: http://www.dodgerslist.com/literature/Expressing.htm. Accessed September 14, 2018.

20. Java MA, Drobatz KJ, Gilley RS, et al. Incidence of and risk factors for postoperative pneumonia in dogs anesthetized for diagnosis or treatment of intervertebral disk disease. J Am Vet Med Assoc 2009;235(3):281–7.

21. Hoareau GL, Mellema MS, Silverstein DC. Indication, management, and outcome of brachycephalic dogs requiring mechanical ventilation. J Vet Emerg Crit Care (San Antonio) 2011;21(3):226–35.

22. Sharp NJH, Wheeler SJ. Postoperative care. In: Small animal spinal disorders: diagnosis and surgery. 2nd edition. London: Elsevier Limited; 2005. p. 339–62.

23. Montiero R, Adams V, Keys D, et al. Canine idiopathic epilepsy: prevalence, risk factors and outcome associated with cluster seizures and status epilepticus. J Small Anim Pract 2012;53(9):526–30.

24. Wessman A, Volk HA, Packer RM, et al. Quality-of-life aspects in idiopathic epilepsy in dogs. Vet Rec 2016;179(9):229.

25. Siess S, Marziliano A, Sarma EA, et al. Why psychology matters in veterinary medicine. Top Companion Anim Med 2015;30:43–7.

26. Siegel AM, Williamson PD, Roberts DW, et al. Localized pain associated with seizures originating in the parietal lobe. Epilepsia 1999;40(7):845–55.

27. Podell M, Volk HA, Berendt M, et al. 2015 ACVIM small animal consensus statement on seizure management in dogs. J Vet Intern Med 2016;30(2):477–90.

28. Henn FA, Vollmayr B. Stress models of depression: forming genetically vulnerable strains. Neurosci Biobehav Rev 2005;29(4–5):799–804.

29. Koolhaas JM, Bartolomucci A, Buwalda B, et al. Stress revisited: a critical evaluation of the stress concept. Neurosci Biobehav Rev 2011;35(5):1291–301.
30. Ferro MA, Speechley KN. Depressive symptoms among mothers of children with epilepsy: a review of prevalence, associated factors, and impact on children. Epilepsia 2009;50(11):2344–54.
31. Charalambous M, Bhatti SFM, Van Ham L, et al. Intranasal midazolam versus rectal diazepam for management of canine status epilepticus: a multicenter randomized parallel-group clinical trial. J Vet Intern Med 2017;31(4):1149–58.
32. Packer RM, Nye G, Porter SE, et al. Assessment into usage of levetiracetam in a canine epilepsy clinic. BMC Vet Res 2015;11:25.
33. Packer RM, McGreevy PD, Salvin HE, et al. Cognitive dysfunction in naturally occurring canine idiopathic epilepsy. PLoS One 2018;13(2):e0192182.
34. Shihab N, Bowen J, Volk HA. Behavioral changes in dogs associated with the development of idiopathic epilepsy. Epilepsy Behav 2011;21(2):160–7.
35. Packer RM, Law TH, Davies E, et al. Effects of a ketogenic diet on ADHD-like behavior in dogs with idiopathic epilepsy. Epilepsy Behav 2016;55:62–8.
36. Schutt T, Toft N, Berendt M. Cognitive function, progression of age-related behavioral changes, biomarkers, and survival in dogs more than 8 years old. J Vet Intern Med 2015;29:1569–77.
37. Rofina JE, van Ederen AM, Toussaint MJ, et al. Cognitive disturbances in old dogs suffering from the canine counterpart of Alzheimer's disease. Brain Res 2006;1069(1):216–26.
38. Landsberg G. Therapeutic agents for the treatment of cognitive dysfunction syndrome in senior dogs. Prog Neuropsychopharmacol Biol Psychiatry 2005;29: 471–9.
39. Reme CA, Dramard V, Kern L, et al. Effect of S-adenysylmethionine tablets on the reduction of age-related mental decline in dogs: a double-blinded, placebo-controlled trial. Vet Ther 2008;9(2):69–82.
40. Law TH, Davies ES, Pan Y, et al. A randomized trial of a medium-chain TAG diet as treatment for dogs with idiopathic epilepsy. Br J Nutr 2015;114(9):1438–47.
41. Gruen ME, Roe SC, Griffith E, et al. The use of trazodone to facilitate post-surgical confinement in dogs. J Am Vet Med Assoc 2014;245(3):296–301.
42. Zarit SH, Reever KE, Bach-Peterson J. Relatives of the impaired elderly: correlates of feelings of burden. Gerontologist 1980;20:649–55.
43. Petruzzi A, Finocchiaro CY, Lamperti E, et al. Living with a brain tumor: reaction profiles in patients and their caregivers. Support Care Cancer 2013;21:1105–11.
44. Boersma I, Miyasaki J, Kutner J, et al. Palliative care and neurology: time for a paradigm shift. Neurology 2014;83:561–7.
45. Creutzfeldt CJ, Robinson MT, Holloway RG. Neurologists as primary palliative care providers: communication and practice approaches. Neurol Clin Pract 2016;6:40–8.
46. Robinson MT, Holloway RG. Palliative care in neurology. Mayo Clin Proc 2017; 92(10):1592–601.
47. Baile WF, Buckman R, Lenzi R, et al. SPIKES: a six-step protocol for delivering bad news- application to the patient with cancer. Oncologist 2000;5:302–11.
48. Norton SA, Metzger M, DeLuca J, et al. Palliative care communication: linking patients' prognoses, values, and goals of care. Res Nurs Health 2013;36(6):582–90.
49. Bernacki RE, Block SD, American College of Physicians High Value Care Task Force. Communication about serious illness care goals: a review and synthesis of best practices. JAMA Intern Med 2014;174(12):1994–2003.

50. Goldberg KJ. Exploring caregiver burden within a veterinary setting. Vet Rec 2017;181:318–9.

51. Gwande A. Quantity and quality of life: duties of care in life-limiting illness. J Am Med Assoc 2016;315:267–9.

52. Stoewen DL, Coe JB, MacMartin C, et al. Qualitative study of the communication expectations of clients accessing oncology care at a tertiary referral center for dogs with life-limiting cancer. J Am Vet Med Assoc 2014;245(7):785–95.

53. Larkin M. For human needs, some veterinary clinics are turning to a professional: social workers see a place for themselves in veterinary practice. J Am Vet Med Assoc 2016;248(1):8–12.

54. Kahler SC. Moral stress the top trigger in veterinarians' compassion fatigue: veterinary social worker suggests redefining veterinarians' ethical responsibility. J Am Vet Med Assoc 2015;246(1):16–8.

55. Reevy GM, Delgado MM. Are emotionally attached companion animal caregivers conscientious and neurotic? Factors that affect the human companion animal relationship. J Appl Anim Welf Sci 2015;18:239–58.

Canine Cognitive Dysfunction

Pathophysiology, Diagnosis, and Treatment

Curtis Wells Dewey, DVM, MS, CTCVMP[a],*,
Emma S. Davies, BVSc, MSc[a], Huisheng Xie, DVM, MS, PhD, CTCVMP[b,c],
Joseph J. Wakshlag, DVM, PhD, CVA[b,d]

KEYWORDS

- Canine • Cognitive • Dysfunction • Dementia • β-Amyloid • Vascular
- Alzheimer disease

KEY POINTS

- Canine cognitive dysfunction (CCD) is the canine analog of human Alzheimer disease (AD).
- The pathophysiology of CCD/AD is multifaceted and involves brain vascular damage, deposition of toxic β-amyloid protein in the brain, oxidative brain injury, neuronal mitochondrial dysfunction, excitotoxic neuronal damage, and inflammation.
- CCD is common in aged (>8 years of age) dogs, affecting between 14% and 35% of the pet dog population.
- Apparent confusion, anxiety, disturbance of the sleep/wake cycle, and decreased interaction with owners are all common clinical signs of CCD.
- Although there is no cure for CCD, several proven effective therapeutic approaches are available for improving cognitive ability and maintaining a good quality of life; instituting such therapies early in the disease course is likely to have the greatest positive clinical effect.

INTRODUCTION

Canine cognitive dysfunction (CCD) is the canine analog of human Alzheimer disease (AD). CCD is common in older dogs, particularly those more than 8 years old. Slowly progressive signs of altered mentation and dementia characterize the disorder. The

Disclosure: The authors have nothing to disclose.
[a] Department of Clinical Sciences, College of Veterinary Medicine, Cornell University, C4 169 Clinical Programs Center, Ithaca, NY 14853, USA; [b] Department of Small Animal Clinical Sciences, College of Veterinary Medicine, University of Florida, Gainesville, FL, USA; [c] Department of Comparative, Diagnostic and Population Medicine, 9700 Highway 318 West, Reddick, FL 32686, USA; [d] Department of Comparative, Diagnostic and Population Medicine
* Corresponding author.
E-mail address: cwd27@cornell.edu

pathophysiology of CCD/AD involves brain vascular disease and accumulation of β-amyloid (Aβ) protein; these two processes are intertwined, each promoting the progression of the other. Aβ is a neurotoxic protein that accumulates in the brains of dogs with CCD and people with AD and forms plaques within the brain parenchyma. Accumulation of Aβ also contributes to cerebrovascular disease, referred to as cerebrovascular amyloid angiopathy (CAA).[1–6] Other pathologic processes that contribute to cognitive impairment in CCD/AD include oxidative brain damage, neuronal mitochondrial dysfunction, glutamate-mediated excitotoxic neuronal damage, impaired neuronal glucose metabolism, and proinflammatory processes that stem from abnormal microglial and astrocyte function.[1–11] The 3 most common misconceptions regarding CCD are that mild cognitive impairment reflects normal canine aging, CCD is not common, and that there are no effective treatments for the condition. Despite pathologic similarities between CCD and AD, dogs with CCD typically do not show the severe cognitive impairment that is experienced in patients with AD.[1,12] This article reviews the pathophysiology of CCD, as well as characteristic features and available treatment options. Most of the information in this article is based on currently available literature regarding CCD and AD, but the authors' collective clinical experience with CCD is also provided.

CLINICALLY RELEVANT PATHOPHYSIOLOGY AND GENERAL CONSIDERATIONS

CCD is an age-related disorder similar to AD in people that occurs in elderly dogs. Age-related cognitive dysfunction has been extensively studied in the dog, and this species seems to be the best naturally occurring animal model available for human AD. Estimates of the prevalence of CCD generally vary between 14% and 35% of the pet dog population. Many of the reported estimates of prevalence likely underestimate how common the disorder is. As with people with AD, the prevalence of CCD increases dramatically with age. In one study, the prevalence of CCD in dogs 11 to 12 years old was 28%, and 68% in dogs 15 to 16 years of age.[1,3,12–14] In a 2-year prospective longitudinal study of dogs more than 8 years of age, 33% of dogs with normal cognitive status progressed to mild cognitive impairment, and 22% of dogs with mild cognitive impairment progressed to CCD.[15]

There are pathologic similarities between the brains of people with AD and dogs with CCD (**Box 1**).

Cerebral vascular changes, meningeal thickening, gliosis, and ventricular dilatation occur in brains of both patients with AD and with CCD. More specifically, progressive

---

Box 1
Pathologic brain abnormalities identified in both people with Alzheimer disease and dogs with canine cognitive dysfunction

Cerebrovascular disease

Aβ accumulation

Oxidative brain damage

Neuronal mitochondrial dysfunction

Glutamate-mediated excitotoxic neuronal damage

Impaired neuronal glucose metabolism

Microglial dysfunction

Astrocyte dysfunction

accumulation of the neurotoxic protein Aβ in the brain (around neurons and blood vessels) is a consistent feature in both AD and CCD. These accumulations coalesce to form plaques (neuritic plaques) and are most prominent in the frontal cerebral cortex and hippocampus in both human and canine disorders. The most common form of insoluble Aβ found in brain tissue is a 42-amino-acid form, called Aβ42. In addition to this insoluble form of the protein, smaller soluble oligomeric forms of Aβ have been identified; these are highly toxic and interfere with synaptic function.[1–4,6,16–19] In both human and canine disorders, the degree of Aβ accumulation (Aβ load) has been correlated with the extent of cognitive impairment.[20] However, this is not uniformly accepted, and there is recent evidence that the relationship between Aβ load and cognitive impairment is tenuous at best. In one histopathologic study of dogs with CCD, cognitive impairment was associated with increased numbers of astrocytes and microglial cells, as well as increased ubiquitin protein levels, rather than with levels of Aβ.[21] In another histopathologic study, increasing Aβ load was a function of age rather than level of cognitive impairment; in this study, the type of Aβ plaques was similar to that seen in early stages of human AD.[11] In addition to the accumulation of neurotoxic Aβ protein in the aged canine brain, intraneuronal accumulation of a hyperphosphorylated microtubular-associated protein (tau protein) has also been shown. Tau protein is the precursor to neurofibrillary tangles (NFTs), another prominent histopathologic feature of human AD. The absence of mature NFTs in the brains of dogs with age-related cognitive dysfunction has been argued as evidence against the canine disorder being analogous to human AD. However, there are several potential explanations to account for the absence of NFTs in dogs with CCD. It is possible that dogs do not live long enough for the tau proteins to develop into NFTs as they do in people. Although the amino acid sequence of Aβ protein is identical in people and dogs, this is not the case for tau protein. Because the amino acid sequence of dog tau protein differs from that in people, this may affect the ability of tau protein to form NFTs in the former species. Other structural abnormalities (**Box 2**) found in the aging canine brain that are similar to those in humans include cerebral atrophy, ventricular enlargement, blood vessel wall fibrosis, amyloid deposition (meningeal and parenchymal), microhemorrhages (and occasionally macrohemorrhages) and infarcts, axonal degeneration with myelin loss, astroglial hypertrophy and hyperplasia, and intraneuronal accumulation of several substances (lipofuscin, polyglucosan bodies, and ubiquitin).[1,2,4–6,11,16–18,22]

The pathophysiology of CCD and AD is multifactorial and complex. In addition to Aβ deposition and vascular disease, numerous cellular and biochemical aberrations contribute to progressive cognitive decline. There is evidence in both diseases that

---

Box 2
Structural brain abnormalities identified grossly and on MRI in both people with Alzheimer disease and dogs with canine cognitive dysfunction

Cerebrovascular disease

Infarcts

Microhemorrhages and occasionally macrohemorrhages

Cerebral atrophy

Meningeal thickening

Ventricular dilatation

Gliosis

increased oxygen free radical–mediated cellular damage, decreased endogenous antioxidant defenses, decreased mitochondrial function, inflammation (from various processes), DNA damage, vascular compromise, and neurotransmitter imbalance are all interrelated processes that are involved in progressive cognitive impairment. Neurochemical changes occur in the aging brain that also contribute to progressive cognitive impairment. Age-associated decline in the brain neurotransmitter levels of acetylcholine, dopamine, norepinephrine, and gamma-aminobutyric acid (GABA) are documented in CCD and AD. Of these abnormalities, cholinergic dysfunction seems to have the highest and most consistent correlation with age-related cognitive impairment. Other neurochemical abnormalities identified in brains of patients with AD and with CCD include increased acetylcholinesterase levels (associated with cholinergic decline), increased monoamine oxidase B levels (catalyzes the breakdown of dopamine, with subsequent formation of free radicals), and increased cerebrospinal fluid (CSF) levels of lactate, pyruvate, and potassium.

Mitochondrial dysfunction is a central theme in the development and progression of AD/CCD. Mitochondria produce ATP via the electron transport chain and are responsible for providing most of the cellular energy requirements. In AD/CCD, mitochondria undergo both morphologic and functional changes (including mitochondrial gene expression), some of which are attributed to Aβ deposition. In general, mitochondrial function declines in AD/CCD. In addition to their role in cellular energy production in brain cells, the mitochondria have a proteostatic ability to decrease the toxic effect of Aβ on cellular function that diminishes as mitochondrial function declines. In addition, and related to, decreased mitochondrial ability to generate cellular energy, the CCD/AD brain has a diminished capacity to metabolize glucose. Glucose is the main energy substrate for neurons in the brain, and neurons affected by AD/CCD are impaired in both uptake and use of glucose.[1–11,23,24]

An imbalance in the levels of neuroexcitatory versus neuroinhibitory neurotransmission in the brain has been documented in animal models and patients with AD. Neuronal hyperexcitability is thought to contribute to cognitive decline in patients with AD. Excessive stimulation of glutamate receptors in AD/CCD contributes to neuronal excitotoxicity and death. In addition, there is evidence that impaired function of inhibitory interneurons is an important facet of abnormal neural networks in the AD brain. These abnormalities of synaptic plasticity have been correlated with Aβ deposition and mitochondrial dysfunction.[4,7,8]

As previously mentioned, there are several misconceptions regarding CCD that are often held by both dog owners and members of the veterinary community. These misconceptions likely contribute to misdiagnosis and delayed diagnosis of CCD, as well as undertreatment of the disorder. Pet owners often regard development of clinical signs of cognitive dysfunction, especially subtle early signs, as part of the normal aging process. CCD is a common disorder, and it often progresses from mild to more severe cognitive impairment. As cognitive ability progressively declines in patients with CCD, it is common for owners to assume that the outlook is hopeless and that nothing can be done. Although there are striking similarities between CCD and AD in terms of pathophysiologic characteristics and mechanisms, there are some important differences regarding disease severity, rate and extent of progression, and societal roles of the affected individual. Dogs with CCD tend to have less severe levels of Aβ-associated brain disorder than are observed in patients with AD, and are less likely to develop such severe impairment as occurs in people with AD.[1,11,14,15] Patients with CCD typically respond well to medical intervention, especially if instituted early in the disease process, and the interventions typically applied have little to no adverse effect. There is also evidence in both AD and CCD that preventive measures (eg, diet changes, environmental enrichment) can both delay the onset and slow the progression of cognitive decline.[1,3,24,25] Overall, successful management of patients with CCD entails prolongation of a good quality of life of the patient as an interactive family pet. Successful management of patients with AD is much more complex with respect to the patients retaining the same role in society as before the development of the disorder. Although it is useful to compare disease mechanistic processes between AD and CCD, veterinarians should also view CCD as a distinct disorder in its own right when considering treatment options and prognosis.

In consideration of the potential benefits of early intervention in CCD management, note that clinically inapparent cognitive decline has been documented to occur in some dogs before 8 years of age. Using specific behavioral testing tools, early cognitive impairment has been documented in beagles as young as 6 years old.[1,3,6,11–15] The same type of testing used in another study showed that young to middle-aged (1.5–7 years old) beagle dogs with increased CSF Aβ concentrations showed learning deficits, compared with dogs with low CSF Aβ concentrations.[25] Histopathologically observable brain Aβ deposits do not develop in dogs until age 8 or 9 years.[16,25] This information suggests that simple preventive measures against CCD (eg, dietary supplements, as discussed later) may be generally advisable in pet dogs as they near middle age.

SIGNALMENT, HISTORY, AND CLINICAL SIGNS

The typical scenario of CCD is an elderly dog (often >8 years of age) with slowly progressive cognitive decline, usually over a period of at least several months. In addition to advancing age, other reported risk factors for developing CCD include sex (females at highest risk, spayed/neutered at higher risk than intact dogs) and body size (smaller dogs at higher risk than larger dogs); however, other reports have not found associations between sex or body size and the likelihood of developing CCD.[1–4,6,11–14,24,26,27] One study found a significant association between idiopathic epilepsy and early-age onset of CCD in dogs; this is similar to people, in which there is an established relationship between temporal lobe epilepsy and early-onset AD.[28,29] The 4 main historical (ie, derived from the owner) clinical features of cognitive impairment are apparent confusion, anxiety, disturbance of the sleep/wake cycle (sleeping during the day, restless at night), and decreased interaction of the pet with the owners **Box 3**.[26]

In addition to these main features of CCD, historical complaints regarding the disorder are numerous and often nonspecific (**Box 4**). They include inattentiveness, inactivity, aimless wandering (often pacing at night), demented behavior, urinary and/or fecal incontinence (posturing normally, but voiding in inappropriate locations), difficulty navigating stairs, attempting to pass through narrow spaces (like the hinge region of a door), inability to locate dropped food, becoming lost in previously familiar environments, failure to recognize previously familiar people or animals, decreased interaction with family members, apparent hearing loss, and excessive vocalization

---

Box 3
Four main owner observations given in history

Apparent confusion

Anxiety

Disturbance of sleep/wake cycle

Decreased interaction of the pet with owners

Box 4
Other owner-reported behaviors commonly displayed by dogs with canine cognitive dysfunction

Inattentiveness

Inactivity

Compulsive wandering and pacing, especially at night

Demented behavior

Urinary and/or fecal incontinence (posture normally, but void inappropriately)

Difficulty navigating stairs

Attempting to pass through inappropriately narrow spaces

Unable to locate dropped food

Getting lost in familiar environments

Unable to recognize familiar people or animals

Decreased interaction with family

Apparent hearing loss

Excessive vocalization especially at night

Acting senile

(often at night). Owners of pets with CCD often describe their pets as acting senile.[1–4,6,12–15,26]

Dogs with CCD typically show evidence of forebrain dysfunction on clinical examination (**Box 5**). These patients have abnormal mentation and often respond inappropriately to their environment (dementia). Many dogs with CCD circle constantly in the examination room and either do not respond or respond inappropriately to visual and auditory stimuli. In the authors' experience, these dogs typically appear very anxious and tend to resist restraint. Also based on the authors' experience, dogs with suspected CCD occasionally show either transient central vestibular dysfunction or seizure activity of recent onset. Although not well described as a clinical feature of CCD, vestibulocerebellar dysfunction and seizures are reported as a potential consequence of AD in people.[4,30,31]

Box 5
Clinical signs associated with the forebrain that may be displayed by dogs with canine cognitive dysfunction

Anxiety

Abnormal mentation

Compulsive circling

Absent or inappropriate response to visual/auditory stimuli

Excessively resistant to even mild restraint

Transient vestibular episodes

Recent onset of possible seizure activity

DIAGNOSIS

In most cases, a CCD diagnosis is based on signalment, history, and clinical features that are all consistent with the diagnosis. Several useful and accurate behavioral tests have been developed that can objectively measure canine cognitive ability and deficits thereof in a laboratory setting. These tests include the delayed nonmatching to position (DNMP) memory task, and the attention task. The DNMP task evaluates short-term visuospatial memory, and the attention task tests selective attention.[1,3,4] Such tests have been, and remain, essential tools for CCD research but are not practical in a busy clinical setting. Other, more rapidly performed, cognitive tests (a food-searching [FS] task and problem-solving task) have been evaluated for clinical use, with the FS task showing the most promise.[32] Pivotal to a correct diagnosis of CCD is an accurate and comprehensive history from the pet owner. Clinicians must have a high index of suspicion for CCD in older dogs. In addition, specific questions regarding the patient's behavior need to be posed to the dog owner with suspected CCD. Owners often do not volunteer potentially useful historical behavioral observations, either because they do not associate them with the overall clinical picture or because they attribute them to signs of normal dog aging.

The only imaging modality of practical use for the diagnosis of CCD is MRI. Owners of dogs with CCD often elect not to pursue MRI, because of several factors. These factors include concerns over general anesthesia in a geriatric pet, costs associated with MRI, and the low likelihood that an MRI diagnosis will contribute meaningfully to the treatment plan. Because of this understandable reticence of owners to pursue MRI in dogs suspected of having CCD, the literature on MRI features of CCD is sparse compared with that available for AD. Brain imaging of patients with AD can be normal or may reveal brain atrophy, ventricular enlargement, and lesions in the medial temporal lobes of the cerebral cortex. Age-related changes appreciated on MRI of the brain in patients with CCD are primarily reflective of brain atrophy and include ventricular enlargement as well as widened and well-demarcated cerebral sulci. Although these are consistent findings associated with the aging brain, they can also be found in some older patients without evidence of CCD.[4] Periventricular white matter hyperintensities, also referred to as leukoaraiosis, are thought to be caused by vascular abnormalities of the arterioles in this region of the brain; in people, they have been associated with AD and other vascular brain disorders. Similar periventricular hyperintense regions have also been described in elderly dogs (**Fig. 1**).

In one report of 14 elderly dogs with suspected leukoaraiosis on MRI, a progressive decrease in interthalamic adhesion thickness was shown for 3 dogs for which serial

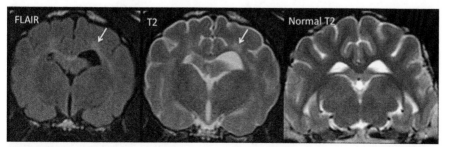

Fig. 1. Transverse fluid-attenuated inversion recovery (FLAIR) and T2-weighted (T2w) MRI of normal and affected brain showing bilateral hyperintense periventricular white matter lesions, referred to as leukoaraiosis (*white arrows*).

imaging was available.[33,34] The thickness of the interthalamic adhesion as measured on transaxial T1-weighted and T2-weighted MRI was significantly smaller in dogs with CCD compared with dogs without CCD; an interthalamic adhesion thickness of 5 mm or less was found to be consistent with a diagnosis of CCD (**Fig. 2**).[35]

A more recent study confirmed the diagnostic utility of measuring the thickness of the interthalamic adhesion in CCD; this study also found that the ratio of the interthalamic adhesion thickness to the brain height and the ratio of this number to the ratio of the lateral ventricle height to brain height were accurate predictors of CCD.[36]

Spontaneous intraparenchymal brain hemorrhage has been documented in both AD and CCD. Although MRI evidence of microhemorrhages is common in patients with AD, the prevalence of this finding in dogs with CCD has not been specifically investigated. The use of T2*-weighted MRI sequences has been shown to be useful in identifying hemorrhagic brain lesions in both people and dogs. In people with AD, MRI evidence of microhemorrhages on T2*-weighted imaging is common and is attributed to CAA. Occasionally, macrohemorrhages are also evident on T2*-weighted images in these patients.[5,37–43] In one large retrospective investigation of brain microhemorrhages in dogs that were imaged with T2*-weighted MRI sequences, older dogs of smaller breeds were significantly more represented. This study also found that these dogs were significantly more likely to present for vestibular dysfunction.[43] In the authors' experience, microhemorrhages are typically evident on T2*-weighted images of elderly dogs' brains that are imaged for recent onset of vestibular dysfunction, suspected seizure activity, and/or progressive behavioral abnormalities. We have also documented macrohemorrhages in several elderly dogs, with no obvious underlying metabolic cause for spontaneous intracranial bleeding (**Fig. 3**).

Laboratory findings are typically normal in dogs with cognitive dysfunction syndrome (CDS), unless there is an age-related concurrent disorder (eg, increased blood urea nitrogen/creatinine levels from chronic renal disease). In one study, plasma concentrations of $A\beta_{42}$ were significantly increased in dogs with CCD, compared with older dogs with either mild cognitive impairment or no cognitive impairment.[15] Because patients with suspected CCD are generally older, and the clinical features of CCD are numerous and often nonspecific, it is important to rule out geriatric

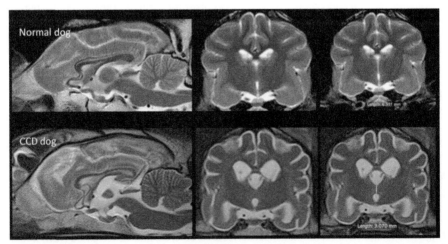

Fig. 2. Sagittal and transverse T2w MRI of normal and affected brain showing the reduced size and abnormal shape of the interthalamic adhesion.

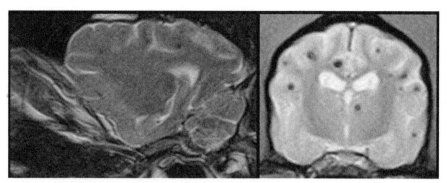

Fig. 3. Sagittal T2w and transverse T2*(fast field echo) MRI of affected brain showing multiple hypointense nonsymmetric bilateral punctate lesions affecting the forebrain.

disorders that may mimic signs of cognitive impairment. In particular, a differential diagnosis of a forebrain tumor is typically a top consideration in an elderly dog with behavioral changes. Organ dysfunction (eg, liver, kidneys) and pain may also lead to clinical signs that may be confused with cognitive impairment. In addition to confounding disease states that may mimic clinical features of cognitive impairment, it is important to know what drugs a patient is being administered, because some adverse drug effects may be misconstrued as signs of CCD.[1,4,44]

TREATMENT
Diet

In both human AD and CCD of dogs, diet and dietary supplements have a substantial impact on both the development and progression of cognitive decline. Both dietary risk factors and preventive factors have been identified for AD in people, and these are suspected to be similar in CCD (**Table 1**).[1,3,4,27,45-48]

For human AD prevention and treatment, general dietary recommendations include the following: high intake of plant-based foods, antioxidants (and foods high in these substances), probiotics, soy beans, omega-3 polyunsaturated fatty acids (and foods rich in these substances), whole grains, fruits, vegetables, nuts, food enriched with medium-chain triglycerides (MCTs), and fish. Dietary choices that are likely to increase the risk of cognitive decline include red meats, poultry, refined sugar, processed food, and high-fat dairy products.[45,46] In addition to the general dietary recommendations

Table 1	
Foods that have been identified to influence Alzheimer disease in people	
Likely to Prevent or Treat AD in People	**Likely to Increase Risk of AD in People**
High intake of plant-based foods	Red meat or poultry
Antioxidants	Refined sugar
Probiotics	Processed food
Soy beans	High-fat dairy products
Omega-3-polyunsaturated fatty acids	
Whole grains	
Fruits/vegetables/nuts	
Medium-chain triglyceride–rich foods	
Fish	

and supplements already mentioned, other nutrients are recommended for cognitively impaired patients (**Box 6**).

These nutrients are often deficient in such individuals and include B vitamins (eg, B_{12}), vitamin C, vitamin E, mitochondrial cofactors (eg, L-carnitine, DL-α-lipoic acid), and carotenoids from green leafy vegetables. The addition of carotenoids and flavonoids as natural antioxidants from fruits, and particularly vegetables, has been associated with improvements in CCD.[4,45,46,49–51] These antioxidants are much more than just antioxidant in their actions. They can also act as mitochondrial cofactors and increase cellular endogenous antioxidant upregulation.[52] Therapeutic approaches using MCTs and natural antioxidants with essential vitamins and minerals seem to be effective. The 2 commercial CCD diets with the most evidence of efficacy are Hills b/d and Purina One Vibrant Maturity 7+ formula in clinical trials of CCD. Hills b/d was a foundational dietary approach, demonstrating that laboratory dogs with CCD showed better learning in a laboratory environment using tasks designed to test special awareness and object recognition primarily.[49–51] In addition, a clinical study using client-owned dogs showed some behavioral improvements compared with a control population on a placebo food. This diet was enriched with carnitine, lipoic acid, long-chain omega-3 polyunsaturated fatty acids, vegetable-based carotenoids, vitamin E, and vitamin C.[53]

MCTs are recommended in dogs with CCD, either as part of a formulated diet or a supplement, for several reasons. The AD/CCD brain has an impaired ability to use glucose, the brain's main energy source; MCTs provide an alternative energy source for the brain in cognitively impaired patients. These ketone bodies are rapidly converted to glucose precursors through interactions of astrocytes and glial cells with the surrounding neurons. MCTs may also improve brain mitochondrial activity and decrease the level of brain amyloid precursor protein.[4,54] MCTs are commonly included in ketogenic diets for both people and dogs. In one study, a proprietary mix of MCTs was shown to improve cognitive function in aged beagle dogs when incorporated into commercial food at 5% of the dry matter.[55]

Although the underlying premise regarding MCTs generating alternative energy sources for neurons through astrocyte metabolic alteration holds validity in humans, the premise is suspect in dogs. In humans there is considerable generation of β-hydroxybutyrate during metabolism of MCTs, whereas in dogs the generation of β-hydroxybutyrate is obscure, being between 20% and 70% of what is observed in people.[55–57] The lack of consistent ketone generation suggests that other mechanisms may play a role and it has been shown that the individual medium-chain fatty acids that increase in the bloodstream of rodents and people can affect neuronal function. The MCTs generally discussed are decanoic acid (10 carbons long, also known as capric acid) and octanoic acid (8 carbons long, also known as caprylic acid). Decanoic acid has been shown to dampen or block seizure activity in rodents because of direct inhibition of the AMPA (α-amino-3-hydroxy-5-methyl-4-isoxazolepropionic acid) receptor, but more importantly may be involved in mitochondrial biogenesis

---

Box 6
Supplements recommended for people affected by Alzheimer disease

Vitamins B (B_{12}), C, and E

Mitochondrial cofactors (L-carnitine and DL-α-lipoic acid)

Carotenoids (green leafy vegetables)

through induction of PPARγ (peroxisome proliferator-activated receptor gamma), which may be important for neuronal survival.[58] Octanoic acid does not seem to have any action potential inhibitory activities from a neuronal perspective, but does seem to be easily metabolized by astrocytes, thereby allowing more local ketone production and promotion of the astrocyte lactate shuttle providing potential energy for neuronal metabolism.[58] Serum fatty acid derivatives of MCTs would be expected to increase from therapeutic trials; however, recent examination of food supplemented with 5% dry matter as a proprietary blend of MCTs that was proved to improve cognitive performance showed no increase in serum MCTs, whereas other less well-recognized fatty acid intermediates were enriched in the blood.[57] Foods rich in MCTs are limited, with only coconut and palm kernel oils being high enough to be used as sources of mainly lauric acid (12-carbon MCT) at nearly 50% of the triacylglycerols in these oils, with only 12% octanoic and decanoic acid in coconut oil and half this amount in palm kernel oil. Although coconut oil is used as the primary means of providing MCTs, it may not provide the appropriate MCTs; however, lauric acid, although not as well studied, does seem to have some antiinflammatory and antiamyloid properties as well.[59,60] To get the highest dose of MCTs, it may be best to purchase nutraceutical MCT oils, which are made from coconut and palm kernel oil but are pure MCTs at 100% of the oil. Proponents of using these oils suggest using them at approximately 5% of the dry matter in the diet initially by either providing as top dressing on a commercial food or providing primarily coconut oil as a fat source in a properly formulated home-prepared diet. This amount of coconut or MCT oil addition provides between 10% and 5% of the caloric content of the diet respectively. This additional oil can begin to create imbalance in the diet regimen, particularly if extra treats are being given as well. Therefore, addition of this oil should be conservative; **Table 2** shows relative quantities of MCT or coconut oil that can safely be provided, with consideration that these extra calories replace some of the calories consumed from the average commercial pet food. If home-prepared diets are warranted, it is best to have a board-certified veterinary nutritionist consulted to help formulate an appropriately balanced diet, particularly if a more ketogenic approach is desired.

Drugs and Nutraceuticals

In addition to dietary manipulation, there are numerous proposed therapeutic approaches to CCD, with variable evidence of efficacy in improving cognitive function and/or delaying progression of cognitive decline (**Box 7**).

Table 2
Calculated metabolizable energy for average elderly dog with potential amounts of coconut or medium-chain triglyceride oils that can be used to help with canine cognitive dysfunction

Dog Weight (kg)	ME (Kcal)[a]	10% ME Coconut Oil	5% ME MCT Oil	10% ME MCT Oil
5	335	1 tspn (35 kcal)	0.5 tspn (18 kcal)	1 tspn (35 kcal)
10	570	1.5 tspn (53 kcal)	0.75 tspn (27 kcal)	1.5 tspn (53 kcal)
20	950	3 tspn (105 kcal)	1.5 tspn (53 kcal)	3 tspn (105 kcal)
30	1280	3.5 tspn (123 kcal)	1.75 tspn (62 kcal)	3.5 tspn (123 kcal)
40	1590	4.5 tspn (158 kcal)	2.25 tspn (79 kcal)	4.5 tspn (158 kcal)
50	1880	5 tspn (175 kcal)	2.5 tspn (88 kcal)	5 tspn (175 kcal)

Abbreviations: ME, metabolizable energy; tspn, teaspoon.
[a] ME calculated from average ME for low-activity elderly dog – 100 (kg).$^{0.75}$

Box 7
Nutraceuticals and drugs used for treatment of canine cognitive dysfunction

Omega-3-polyunsaturated fatty acids

MCTs

Phytochemicals (curcumin, resveratrol, green tea catechins)

S-adenosylmethionine

Phosphatidylserine

L-Deprenyl oral (selegiline, Anipryl, Atapryl, Carbex, Eldepryl, Zelapar)

Levetiracetam

Antiinflammatory drugs (eg, carprofen)

Apoequorin

The use of omega-3 fatty acids and MCTs as supplements is discussed earlier. Several cholinesterase-inhibiting drugs are used in patients with AD, but these have shown limited and transient efficacy; they are often also associated with gastrointestinal side effects.[61,62] Dosage and safety information for these drugs in dogs is lacking. The use of oral L-deprenyl (selegiline; Anipryl, Atapryl, Carbex, Eldepryl, Zelapar), an irreversible inhibitor of monoamine oxidase B, has been purported to improve cognitive function and slow progression of the disease in most dogs with CCD. However, there is considerable variability in the degree of response achieved among patients. L-Deprenyl is thought to exert its beneficial effects in the brain by restoring dopaminergic balance as well as enhancing catecholamine levels and decreasing levels of damaging free radical species. Most patients show a positive response within the first month of therapy. Despite apparent positive responses of patients with CCD to selegiline, there is evidence that this drug does not have a significant effect on cognitive function in these patients or in people with AD. The clinical efficacy studies supporting selegiline use in CCD are based primarily on owner response to questionnaires rather than on standardized comparative cognitive testing procedures of treated and untreated patients. Because selegiline may produce nonspecific low-level hyperactivity by increasing brain catecholamine levels, the response observed by owners may not truly be representative of improved cognitive ability. Selegiline is not considered an effective drug for human AD because of variable responses and overall minimum improvement of cognitive function.[1,4,62–64] Recent evidence suggests that the anticonvulsant drug levetiracetam is effective in improving cognitive function and decreasing hyperexcitability in AD and animal models of AD; potential mechanisms of action include improved central nervous system mitochondrial function (and associated improved synaptic transmission) and inhibition of oligomeric Aβ-induced astrocyte glutamate release.[65–67] Behavioral changes (particularly anxiety) in patients with CCD may be alleviated with the use of GABAergic drugs, such as gabapentin or pregabalin. Because inflammatory changes have been identified in the brains of dogs with CCD, the use of antiinflammatory drugs (eg, carprofen) has also been proposed. Some naturally occurring phytochemicals (eg, curcumin, resveratrol, green tea catechins) may hold some promise as treatment options for CCD.[1,4] Oral S-adenosylmethionine (SAMe) was shown to be effective in improving clinical signs of mental decline in dogs with CCD in 1 randomized, placebo-controlled study.[68] Phosphatidylserine, a membrane phospholipid, showed some efficacy in improving cognitive function in patients with CCD in several clinical trials.[1,4,69,70] Apoequorin is a calcium-buffering protein

Box 8
Nutraceuticals and drugs used to suppress the clinical signs of canine cognitive dysfunction (anxiety and abnormal sleep-wake cycles)
Melatonin
Valerian root
Dog-appeasing pheromone

derived from jellyfish that has been shown experimentally to protect against ischemic neuronal cell death. Apoequorin has shown efficacy in improving cognition in older dogs and people, including people with mild cognitive impairment. A large number of complementary therapies have been suggested for the treatment of CCD, with the primary goals of calming the patient, reducing anxiety, and normalizing the sleep-wake cycle (**Box 8**). These therapies include melatonin, valerian root, dog-appeasing pheromone, docosahexaenoic acid(an omega 3 fatty acid), and various antioxidants and mitochondrial cofactors.[1,4,44]

Cognitive Enrichment

Cognitive enrichment, such as regular exercise, social interactions, and introduction of new toys, has been shown to improve cognitive function in dogs with CCD and prevent or delay cognitive decline in dogs as they age.[1,4,44,71] Similarly, cognitive enrichment has been proved to protect against cognitive decline and improve cognitive function in older people and human patients with AD, respectively. People who are more intellectually stimulated earlier in life (eg, education level, complexity level of work and/or leisure activity) and who exercise regularly are less likely to experience cognitive impairment in later years. This phenomenon has been shown even in older people with evidence of brain disorder. Instituting cognitive enrichment strategies such as regular physical exercise has been shown to improve cognitive function in people with AD.[71–73] Similar evidence has been accumulated in rodent AD experimental models.[71] Several mechanisms are thought to be involved in the beneficial effects of cognitive enrichment. These mechanisms include improved neuronal plasticity (with formation of new synapses) and decreased hippocampal neuronal loss. Related to these mechanisms is a concept of cognitive reserve. Cognitive reserve refers to a hypothesis that the brain can use available neural pathway networks as backup systems in case of brain disorder, as occurs with CCD/AD. This cognitive reserve is likely well developed in individuals who have experienced cognitive enrichment throughout early life but can also be developed to some extent in older patients showing signs of cognitive decline.[71,73]

Dog owners can provide cognitive enrichment to their pets in several ways. In addition to home-based methods (eg, regular walks, regular introduction to new toys), there are an increasing number of pet rehabilitation facilities available that can provide such enrichment on a recurring basis (**Fig. 4**).

Chinese Herbal Therapy

In recent years, Chinese herbal therapy has been investigated extensively in experimental (rodent) AD models, as well as in human AD clinical trials. There is evidence of efficacy for many single herbs, molecular compounds from such herbs, as well as herbal formulas. The mechanisms of action in improving cognitive function for many of the individual herbs or their chemical constituents have been elucidated.

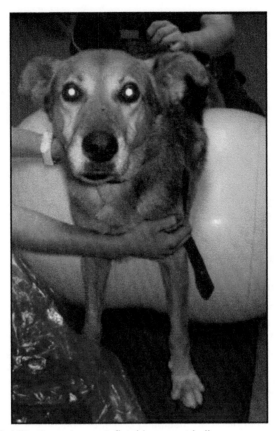

Fig. 4. Dog in rehabilitation using an inflatable peanut ball.

These mechanisms include dissolution of Aβ in the brain, inhibited generation of brain Aβ inclusions, reduction of brain acetylcholinesterase activity, antioxidant activity, protection of brain mitochondria from oxidative stress, protection against glutamate-mediated neurotoxicity, antiinflammatory activity, improvement in brain blood flow, improvement in neuronal glucose use, improvement in neuronal ATP production, and inhibition of neuronal apoptosis in the brain.[74–92] The list of individual Chinese herbs with evidence of efficacy for treating cognitive impairment is extensive. The most prominent such herbs in this category, in addition to their relevant molecular mechanisms of action, are summarized in **Table 3**.

In addition to single Chinese herbs, several herbal formulas have shown efficacy in the treatment of cognitive impairment in both experimental rodent models and people with AD. There are several studies showing efficacy of Liu Wei Di Huang (also known as Rehmannia 6) in the treatment of cognitive impairment.[88,90–92] Human clinical studies of Sai Luo Tong formula, which consists of the bioactive components of the 3 herbal extracts from *Panax ginseng*, *Ginkgo biloba*, and *Crocus sativa*, showed significant improvement in neurocognitive function, learning, and memory.[93,94] Other Chinese herbal formulas such as Fu Fang Dan Shen, Ba Wei Di Huang Wan, and Yi Gan San, have also shown encouraging data on treating cognitive and psychological symptoms in patients with dementia.[95–97]

Table 3
Individual Chinese herbs and their relevant molecular mechanisms

Latin and Chinese (in Parentheses) Herbal Name	Mechanism of Action
Ginkgo biloba (Bai Guo)	Antioxidant; antiapoptotic; antiinflammatory
Huperzia serrata (Qian Ceng Ta)	Procholinergic; antiglutamate (NMDA antagonism)
Curcuma longa (Yu Jin)	Inhibits Aβ production; antioxidant; antiinflammatory
Ginseng (Ren Shen)	Antioxidant; antiglutamate (NMDA antagonism); decrease Aβ
Coptis chinensis (Huang Lian)	Inhibits Aβ production; procholinergic; antioxidant; antiinflammatory
Polygala tenuifolia (Yuan Zhi)	Inhibits Aβ production; antiapoptotic
Salvia miltiorrhiza (Dan Shen)	Inhibits Aβ aggregation; antioxidant; antiinflammatory
Angelica sinsensis (Dang Gui)	Antioxidant; antiinflammatory
Crocus sativus (Zang Hong Hua)	Antioxidant; antiapoptotic
Gastrodia elata (Tian Ma)	Procholinergic; antioxidant
Rehmannia glutinosa (Shu Di Huang)	Procholinergic; antioxidant
Epimedium (Yin Yang Huo)	Antioxidant; antiapoptotic
Magnolia officinalis (Xin Yi Hua)	Procholinergic; antioxidant
Scutellaria baicalensis (Huang Qin)	Inhibits Aβ aggregation; antioxidant; antiinflammatory; antiapoptotic
Camellia sinensis (Cha Hua)	Reduces Aβ levels; antioxidant; antiinflammatory; antiapoptotic

Abbreviation: NMDA, *N*-methyl-ᴅ-aspartate.

Acupuncture

Although not yet clinically investigated as a therapeutic modality in dogs with CCD, there is considerable evidence in rodent AD models and human AD clinical trials supporting a beneficial role for acupuncture (particularly electroacupuncture) in the treatment of cognitive dysfunction.[98–101] Several likely mechanisms of action for the positive effects of acupuncture have been elucidated from experimental rodent AD models (**Box 9**).

These mechanisms include enhanced neuronal glucose use (as verified by PET scans), decreased accumulation of Aβ in the brain (via inhibition of the mTOR [mammalian target of rapamycin] pathway), increased production of neurotrophic factors (such as brain-derived neurotrophic factor [BDNF]) with subsequent proliferation of neuronal stem cells, and protection from or reversal of synaptic loss and dendritic atrophy in the hippocampus. Overall, the various mechanisms that have been uncovered experimentally are thought to enhance brain neuroplasticity and improve cognitive function.[98–100,102–108]

Electroacupuncture stimulation at Yin-tang and LI-20 significantly ameliorated the learning and memory deficits of AD mice (detected with maze tests) and was accompanied by increased BDNF and decreased amyloid formation of Aβ proteins (biomarker of CDS) in the brain. Acupuncture at GV-20, GV-14, and ST-36 increased expression of synaptophysin and neurotrophin in the hippocampal region; acupuncture at HT-7 and PC-6 promoted cholinergic neural transmission; acupuncture at

> **Box 9**
> **Mechanism of action for positive effects seen with acupuncture**
>
> Enhanced neuronal glucose use
>
> Decreased accumulation of Aβ in the brain
>
> Increased production of neurotrophic factors
>
> Proliferation of neuronal stem cells
>
> Protection or recovery from synaptic loss and dendritic atrophy in the hippocampus

GV-14, GV-20, CV-6, CV-12, CV-17, SP-10, ST-36, HT-9, KID-1, LU-11, PC-9, GB-34, and LIV-3 suppressed oxidative stress and attenuated apoptosis; acupuncture at GB-34, GV-20, LIV-3, SP-10, and ST-36 reduced the expression of microglia; and acupuncture at LI-4 and LIV-3 activated regions of the cerebrum responsible for memory and cognition.[109] A human clinical trial confirmed that acupuncture can enhance hippocampal activity in patients with AD. The study used 14 patients with AD and 14 healthy elders. Stimulation of acupoints LI-4 and LIV-3 was evaluated with functional MRI during baseline, resting, and after stimulation. In the resting state, several frontal and temporal regions (cognitive-related regions) showed decreased hippocampal connectivity in patients with AD relative to control subjects. Following acupuncture, patients with AD showed increased connectivity in most of the hippocampal-related regions.[110]

SUMMARY

CCD is a common neurodegenerative condition of aging dogs with many similarities to AD of people. The pathophysiology of CCD/AD is multifaceted, involving many interrelated biochemical aberrations. Central to the development of CCD/AD are compromised brain vasculature and the deposition in the brain parenchyma of a toxic protein called Aβ. These two central processes are intertwined, because each can promote progression of the other. Although dogs with CCD are typically recognized as showing cognitive impairment by 8 years or older, there is considerable evidence that the processes leading to this clinical state begin earlier in life. Pet owners and veterinarians should therefore consider preventive measures against the development of CCD when dogs are middle aged. Diagnosis of CCD often depends on an accurate history of the patient's clinical progression, derived from the dog owner. It is important for veterinarians to maintain a high index of suspicion for CCD and ask the right questions. It is important for dog owners and veterinarians to realize that cognitive impairment or senility should not be considered a normal part of the canine aging process. Because CCD-suspect dogs tend to be elderly, other disease processes that could mimic CCD need to be ruled out. Although not commonly pursued, brain MRI of dogs with CCD usually shows a small interthalamic adhesion thickness. Dogs with CCD usually do not reach the same level of disease severity as their human AD counterparts. These patients also usually respond well to therapeutic interventions and often have a good long-term quality of life. Several therapeutic approaches have been shown to be effective in treating CCD, principal among them being dietary modulations, a variety of nutraceutical supplements, and cognitive enrichment. The anticonvulsant drug levetiracetam has been shown to be effective in experimental models of AD as well as human AD clinical trials in improving cognitive function. This therapy should be considered for treatment of CCD as well. Recent literature in rodent AD models and human clinical AD trials suggests an important role for Chinese herbal therapy and acupuncture in the treatment and prevention of cognitive dysfunction.

REFERENCES

1. Landsberg GM, Nichol J, Araujo JA. Cognitive dysfunction syndrome: a disease of canine and feline brain aging. Vet Clin Small Anim 2012;42:749–68.
2. Vite CH, Head E. Aging in the canine and feline brain. Vet Clin Small Anim 2014; 44:1113–29.
3. Chapagain D, Range F, Huber L, et al. Cognitive aging in dogs. Gerontology 2018;64:165–71.
4. Dewey CW. Encephalopathies: disorders of the brain. In: Dewey CW, da Costa RC, editors. Practical guide to canine and feline neurology. 3rd edition. Ames (IA): Wiley-Blackwell; 2016. p. 141–236.
5. Van der Flier WM, Skoog I, Schneider JA, et al. Vascular cognitive impairment. Nat Rev Dis Primers 2018. https://doi.org/10.1038/nrdp2018.3.
6. Rofina JE, van Ederen AM, Toussaint MJM, et al. Cognitive disturbances in old dogs suffering from the canine counterpart of Alzheimer's disease. Brain Res 2006;1069:216–26.
7. Weinstein JD. A new direction for Alzheimer's research. Neural Regen Res 2018; 13:190–3.
8. Macdonald R, Barnes K, Hastings C, et al. Mitochondrial abnormalities in Parkinson's disease and Alzheimer's disease: can mitochondria be targeted therapeutically? Biochem Soc Trans 2018;46:891–909.
9. Ridge PG, Kauwe JSK. Mitochondria and Alzheimer's disease: the role of mitochondrial genetic variation. Curr Genet Med Rep 2018;6:1–10.
10. Mullins R, Reiter D, Kapogiannis D. Magnetic resonance spectroscopy reveals abnormalities of glucose metabolism in the Alzheimer's brain. Ann Clin Transl Neurol 2018;5:262–72.
11. Schutt T, Helboe L, Pedersen LO, et al. Dogs with cognitive dysfunction as a spontaneous model for early Alzheimer's disease: a translational study of neuropathological and inflammatory markers. J Alzheimers Dis 2016;52:433–49.
12. Salvin HE, McGreevy PD, Sachdev PS, et al. Under diagnosis of canine cognitive dysfunction: a cross-sectional survey of older companion dogs. Vet J 2010; 184:277–81.
13. Nielson JC, Hart BL, Cliff KD, et al. Prevalence of behavioral changes associated with age-related cognitive impairment in dogs. J Am Vet Med Assoc 2001;218:1787–91.
14. Azkona G, Garcia-Belenguer SG, Chacon G, et al. Prevalence and risk factors of behavioural changes associated with age-related cognitive impairment in geriatric dogs. J Small Anim Pract 2009;50:87–91.
15. Schutt T, Toft N, Berendt M. Cognitive dysfunction, progression of age-related behavioral changes, biomarkers, and survival in dogs more than 8 years old. J Vet Intern Med 2015;29:1569–77.
16. Head E, Pop V, Sarsoza F, et al. Amyloid β-peptide and oligomers in the brain and CSF of aged canines. J Alzheimers Dis 2010;20:637–46.
17. Borras D, Ferrer I, Pumarola M. Age-related changes in the brain of the dog. Vet Pathol 1999;36:202–11.
18. Tapp PD, Siwak CT, Gao FQ, et al. Frontal lobe volume, function, and β-amyloid pathology in a canine model of aging. J Neurosci 2004;24:8205–13.

19. Lee GS, Jeong YW, Kim JJ, et al. A canine model of Alzheimer's disease generated by overexpressing a mutated human amyloid precursor protein. Int J Mol Med 2014;33:1003–12.

20. Cummings BJ, Head E, Afagh AJ, et al. β-amyloid accumulation correlates with cognitive dysfunction in the aged canine. Neurobiol Learn Mem 1996;66:11–23.

21. Ozawa M, Chambers JK, Uchida K, et al. The relation between canine cognitive dysfunction and age-related brain lesions. Pathology 2016;78:997–1006.

22. Sanchez MP, Garcia-Cabrero AM, Sanchez-Elexpuru G, et al. Tau-induced pathology in epilepsy and dementia: notions from patients and animal models. Int J Mol Sci 2018. https://doi.org/10.3390/ijms19041092.

23. Sorrentino V, Romani M, Mouchiroud L, et al. Enhancing mitochondrial proteostasis reduces amyloid-β proteotoxicity. Nature 2017;552:187–93.

24. Cisternas P, Inestrosa NC. Brain glucose metabolism: role of Wnt signaling in the metabolic impairment in Alzheimer's disease. Neurosci Biobehav Rev 2017;80:316–28.

25. Borghys H, Van Broeck B, Dhuyvetter D, et al. Young to middle-aged dogs with high amyloid-β levels in cerebrospinal fluid are impaired on learning in standard cognition tests. J Alzheimers Dis 2017;56:763–74.

26. Fast R, Schutt T, Toft N, et al. An observational study with long-term follow-up of canine cognitive dysfunction: clinical characteristics, survival, and risk factors. J Vet Intern Med 2013;27:822–9.

27. Katina S, Farbakova J, Madari A, et al. Risk factors for canine cognitive dysfunction syndrome in Slovakia. Acta Vet Scand 2017. https://doi.org/10.1186/s13028-016-0196-5.

28. Vrinda M, Arun S, Srikumar BN, et al. Temporal lobe epilepsy-induced neurodegeneration and cognitive deficits: implications for aging. J Chem Neuroanat 2018. https://doi.org/10.1016/j.chemneu.2018.02.005.

29. Packer RMA, McGreevy PD, Salvin HE, et al. Cognitive dysfunction in naturally occurring canine epilepsy. PLoS One 2018. https://doi.org/10.1371/journal.pone.0192182.

30. Cretin B. Pharmacotherapeutic strategies for treating epilepsy in patients with Alzheimer's disease. Expert Opin Pharmacother 2018;11:1201–9.

31. Harun A, Oh ES, Bigelow RT, et al. Vestibular impairment in dementia. Oto Neurotol 2016;8:1137–42.

32. Gonzalez-Martinez A, Rosado B, Pesini P, et al. Effect of age and severity of cognitive dysfunction on two simple tasks in pet dogs. Vet J 2013;198:176–81.

33. Marek M, Horyniecki M, Fraczek M, et al. Leukoaraiosis-new concepts and modern imaging. Pol J Radiol 2018;83:e76–81.

34. Scarpante E, Cherubini GB, de Stefani A, et al. Magnetic resonance imaging features of leukoaraiosis in elderly dogs. Vet Radiol Ultrasound 2017;58:389–98.

35. Hasegawa D, Yayoshi N, Fujita Y, et al. Measurement of interthalamic adhesion thickness as a criteria for brain atrophy in dogs with and without cognitive dysfunction (dementia). Vet Radiol Ultrasound 2005;46:452–7.

36. Noh D, Choi S, Choi H, et al. Evaluation of interthalamic adhesion size as an indicator of brain atrophy in dogs with and without cognitive dysfunction. Vet Radiol Ultrasound 2017;58:581–7.

37. Charidimou A, Boulouis G, Gurol ME, et al. Emerging concepts in sporadic cerebral amyloid angiopathy. Brain 2017;140:1829–40.

38. Parkes I, Chintawar S, Cader MZ. Neurovascular dysfunction in dementia-human cellular models and molecular mechanisms. Clin Sci 2018;132:399–418.

39. Yamada M. Brain hemorrhages in cerebral amyloid angiopathy. Semin Thromb Hemost 2013;39:955–62.

40. Ungvari Z, Tarantini S, Kirkpatrick AC, et al. Cerebral microhemorrhages: mechanisms, consequences, and prevention. Am J Physiol Heart Circ Physiol 2017; 312:H1128–43.

41. Jakel L, Van Nostrand WE, Nicoll JAR, et al. Animal models of cerebral amyloid angiopathy. Clin Sci 2017;131:2469–88.

42. Hodshon AW, Hecht S, Thomas WB. Use of the T2*-weighted gradient recalled echo sequence for magnetic resonance imaging of the canine and feline brain. Vet Radiol Ultrasound 2014;55:599–606.

43. Kerwin SC, Levine JM, Budke CM, et al. Putative cerebral microbleeds in dogs undergoing magnetic resonance imaging of the head: a retrospective study of demographics, clinical associations, and relationship to case outcome. J Vet Intern Med 2017;31:1140–8.

44. Landsberg GM, DePorter T, Araujo JA. Clinical signs and management of anxiety, sleeplessness, and cognitive dysfunction in the senior pet. Vet Clin Small Anim 2011;41:565–90.

45. Solfrizzi V, Custodero C, Lozupone M, et al. Relationships of dietary patterns, foods, and micro-and macronutrients with Alzheimer's disease and late-life cognitive disorders: a systematic review. J Alzheimers Dis 2017;59:815–49.

46. Pistollato F, Iglesias RC, Ruiz R, et al. Nutritional patterns associated with the maintenance of neurocognitive functions and the risk of dementia and Alzheimer's disease: a focus on human studies. Pharmacol Res 2018;131:32–43.

47. Gandy S, Bartfai T, Lees GV, et al. Midlife interventions are critical in prevention, delay, or improvement of Alzheimer's disease and vascular cognitive impairment and dementia. F1000Res 2017. https://doi.org/10.12688/f1000research.11140.1.

48. Ravi SK, Narasingappa RB, Vincent B. Neuro-nutrients as anti-Alzheimer's disease agents: a critical review. Crit Rev Food Sci Nutr 2018. https://doi.org/10.1080/10408398.2018.1481012.

49. Milgram NW, Zicker SC, Head E, et al. Dietary enrichment counteracts age-associated cognitive dysfunction in canines. Neurobiol Aging 2002;23:737–45.

50. Milgram NW, Head E, Muggenburg B, et al. Landmark discrimination learning in the dog: effects of age, an antioxidant fortified food, and cognitive strategy. Neurosci Biobehav Rev 2002;26:679–95.

51. Milgram NW, Head E, Zicker SC, et al. Long-term treatment with antioxidants and a program of behavioral enrichment reduces age-dependent impairment in discrimination and reversal learning in beagle dogs. Exp Gerontol 2004;39: 753–65.

52. De Roos B, Duthie GG. Role of dietary pro-oxidants in the maintenance of health and resilience to oxidative stress. Mol Nutr Food Res 2015;59:1229–48.

53. Dodd CE, Zicker SC, Jewell DE, et al. Can a fortified food affect the behavioral manifestations of age-related cognitive decline in dogs? Vet Med 2003;98: 396–408.

54. Rebello CJ, Keller JN, Liu AG, et al. Pilot feasibility and safety study examining the effect of medium chain triglyceride supplementation in subjects with mild cognitive impairment: a randomized controlled trial. BBA Clin 2015;3:123–5.

55. Pan Y, Larson B, Araujo JA, et al. Dietary supplementation with medium-chain TAG has long-lasting cognition-enhancing effects in aged dogs. Br J Nutr 2010;103:1746–54.

56. Courchesne-Loyer A, St-Pierre V, Hennebelle M, et al. Ketogenic response to cotreatment with bezafibrate and medium chain triacylglycerolsin healthy humans. Nutrition 2015;31:1255–9.

57. Law TH, Volk HA, Pan Y, et al. Metabolic perturbations associated with the consumption of a ketogenic medium chain TAG diet in dogs with idiopathic epilepsy. Br J Nutr 2018;120:484–7.

58. Augustin K, Aziza K, Williams S, et al. Mechanism of action for medium-chain triglyceride ketogenic diets in neurological and metabolic disorders. Lancet Neurol 2018;17:84–93.

59. Nonaka Y, Takagi T, Inai M, et al. Lauric acid stimulates ketone body production in the KT-5 astrocyte cell line. J Oleo Sci 2016;65:693–9.

60. Nafar F, Clarke JP, Mearow KM. Coconut oil protects cortical neurons from amyloid beta toxicity by enhancing signaling of cell survival pathways. Neurochem Int 2017;105:64–79.

61. Liu K, Lin HH, Pi R, et al. Research and development of anti-Alzheimer's disease drugs: an update from the perspective of technology flows. Expert Opin Ther Pat 2018;28:341–50.

62. Evans JG, Wilcock G, Birks J. Evidence-based pharmacotherapy of Alzheimer's disease. Int J Neuropsychopharmacol 2004;7:351–69.

63. Milgram NW, Go I, Head E, et al. The effect of L-deprenyl on behavior, cognitive function, and biogenic amines in the dog. Neurochem Res 1993;18:1211–9.

64. Ebadi M, Brown-Borg H, Ren J, et al. Therapeutic efficacy of selegiline in neurodegenerative disorders and neurological diseases. Curr Drug Targets 2006;7: 1513–29.

65. Sanchez PE, Zhu L, Verret L, et al. Levetiracetam suppresses neuronal network dysfunction and reverses synaptic and cognitive deficits in an Alzheimer's disease model. Proc Natl Acad Sci U S A 2012. https://doi.org/10.1073/pnas. 1121081109.

66. Stockburger C, Miano D, Baeumlisberger M, et al. A mitochondrial role of SV2a protein in aging and Alzheimer's disease: studies with levetiracetam. J Alzheimers Dis 2016;50:201–15.

67. Sanz-Blasco S, Pina-Crespo JC, Zhang X, et al. Levetiracetam inhibits oligomeric Aβ-induced glutamate release from human astrocytes. Neuroreport 2016;27:705–9.

68. Reme CA, Dramard V, Kern L, et al. Effect of S-adenosylmethionine tablets on the reduction of age-related mental decline in dogs: a double-blinded, placebo-controlled trial. Vet Ther 2008;9:69–82.

69. Araujo JA, Landsberg GM, Milgram NW, et al. Improvement of short-term memory performance in aged beagles by a nutraceutical supplement containing phosphatidylserine, Ginkgo biloba, Vitamin E, and pyridoxine. Can Vet J 2008;49:379–85.

70. Heath SE, Barabas S, Craze BG. Nutritional supplementation in cases of canine cognitive dysfunction-a clinical trial. Appl Anim Behav Sci 2007;105:274–83.

71. Milgram NW, Siwak-Tapp CT, Araujo J, et al. Neuroprotective effects of cognitive enrichment. Ageing Res Rev 2006;5:354–69.

72. Guitar NA, Connelly D, Nagamatsu LS, et al. Ageing Res Rev 2018;47:159–67.

73. Sobol NA, Dall CH, Hogh P, et al. Change in fitness and the relation to change in cognition and neuropsychiatric symptoms after aerobic exercise in patients with mild Alzheimer's disease. J Alzheimers Dis 2018;65:137–45.

74. Fang J, Wang L, Wu T, et al. Network pharmacology-based study on the mechanism of action for herbal medicines in Alzheimer treatment. J Ethnopharmacol 2016. https://doi.org/10.1016/j.jep.2016.11.034.

75. Xu QQ, Shan CS, Wang Y, et al. Chinese herbal medicine for vascular dementia: a systematic review and meta-analysis of high-quality randomized controlled trials. J Alzheimers Dis 2018;62:429–56.

76. Howes MR, Fang R, Houghton PJ. Effect of Chinese herbal medicine on Alzheimer's disease. Int Rev Neurobiol 2017;135:29–56.

77. Dey A, Bhattacharya R, Mukherjee A, et al. Natural products against Alzheimer's disease: pharmaco-therapeutics and biotechnological interventions. Biotechnol Adv 2017;35:178–216.

78. Chang D, Liu J, Bilinski K, et al. Herbal medicine for the treatment of vascular dementia: an overview of scientific evidence. Evid Based Complement Alternat Med 2016. https://doi.org/10.1155/2016/7293626.

79. Wang ZY, Liu JG, Yang HM. Pharmacological effects of active components of Chinese herbal medicine in the treatment of Alzheimer's disease: a review. Am J Chin Med 2016;44:1525–41.

80. Tewari D, Stankiewicz AM, Mocan A, et al. Ethnopharmacological approaches for dementia therapy and significance of natural products and herbal drugs. Front Aging Neurosci 2018;10:1–24.

81. Jiang Y, Gao H, Turdu G. Traditional Chinese medicinal herbs as potential AChE inhibitors for anti-Alzheimer's disease: a review. Bioorg Chem 2017;75:50–61.

82. Zhou X, Cui G, Tseng HHL, et al. Vascular contributions to cognitive impairment and treatments with traditional Chinese medicine. Evid Based Complement Alternat Med 2016. https://doi.org/10.1155/2016/9627258.

83. Libro R, Giacoppo S, Rajan TS, et al. Natural phytochemicals in the treatment and prevention of dementia: an overview. Molecules 2016;21:518.

84. Wightman EL. Potential benefits of phytochemicals against Alzheimer's disease. Proc Nutr Soc 2017;76:106–12.

85. Hyde AJ, May BH, Dong L, et al. Herbal medicine for management of the behavioural and psychological symptoms of dementia (BPSD): a systematic review and meta-analysis. J Psychopharmacol 2016. https://doi.org/10.1177/0269881116675515.

86. Durairajan SSK, Chirasani VR, Shetty SG, et al. Decrease in the generation of amyloid-β due to salvianolic acid B by modulating BACE1 activity. Curr Alzheimer Res 2017;14:1229–37.

87. Lopresti AL. Salvia (sage): a review of its potential cognitive-enhancing and protective effects. Drugs R D 2017;17:53–64.

88. Pang XC, Kang D, Fang JS, et al. Network pharmacology-based analysis of Chinese herbal Naodesheng formula for application to Alzheimer's disease. Chin J Nat Med 2018;16:53–62.

89. Shi J, Ni J, Lu T, et al. Adding Chinese herbal medicine to conventional therapy brings benefits to patients with Alzheimer's disease: a retrospective analysis. BMC Complement Altern Med 2017;17:1–7.

90. Zhang Y, Lin C, Zhang L, et al. Cognitive improvement during treatment for mild Alzheimer's disease with a Chinese herbal formula: a randomized controlled trial. PLoS One 2015. https://doi.org/10.1371/journal.pone.0130353.

91. Wang JH, Lei X, Cheng XR, et al. LW-AFC, a new formula derived from Liuwei Dihuang decoction, ameliorates behavioral and pathological deterioration via modulating the neuroendocrine-immune system in PrP-hAβPPswe/PS1ΔE9

transgenic mice. Alzheimers Res Ther 2016. https://doi.org/10.1186/s13195-0226-6.

92. Huang Y, Zhang H, Yang S, et al. Liuwei Dihuang decoction facilitates the induction of long-term potentiation (LTP) in senescence accelerated mouse/prone 8 (SAMP8) hippocampal slices by inhibiting voltage-dependent calcium channels (VDDCs) and promoting N-methyl-D-aspartate receptor (NMDA) receptors. J Ethnopharmacol 2012;140:384–90.

93. Steiner GZ, Yeung A, Liu JX, et al. The effect of Sailuotong (SLT) on neurocognitive and cardiovascular function in healthy adults: a randomized, double-blind, placebo-controlled crossover pilot trial. BMC Complement Altern Med 2016. https://doi.org/10.1186/s12906-016-0989-0.

94. Liang J, Li F, Wei C, et al. Rationale and design of a multicenter, phase 2 clinical trial to investigate the efficacy of traditional Chinese medicine sailuotong in vascular dementia. J Stroke Cerebrovasc Dis 2014;23:2626–34.

95. Tian J, Shi J, Wei M, et al. The efficacy and safety of Fufangdanshen tablets (*Radix Salviae miltiorrrhizae* formula tablets) for mild to moderate vascular dementia: a study protocol for a randomized controlled trial. Trials 2016;17:281.

96. Iwasaki K, Kobayashi S, Chimura Y, et al. A randomized, double-blind, placebo-controlled clinical trial of the Chinese herbal medicine "ba wei di huang wan" in the treatment of dementia. J Am Geriatr Soc 2004;52:1518–21.

97. Iwasaki K, Satoh-Nakagawa T, Maruyama M, et al. A randomized, observer-blind, controlled trial of the traditional Chinese medicine Yi-Gan San for improvement of behavioral and psychological symptoms and activities of daily living in dementia patients. J Clin Psychiatry 2005;66:248–52.

98. Park S, Lee JH, Yang EJ. Effects of acupuncture on Alzheimer's disease in animal-based research. Evid Based Complement Alternat Med 2017. https://doi.org/10.1155/2017/6512520.

99. Zhou S, Dong L, He Y, et al. Acupuncture plus herbal medicine for Alzheimer's disease: a systematic review and meta-analysis. Am J Chin Med 2017;45:1327–44.

100. Lu YJ, Cai XW, Zhang GF, et al. Long-term acupuncture treatment has a multi-targeting regulation on multiple brain regions in rats with Alzheimer's disease: a positron emission tomography study. Neural Regen Res 2017;12:1159–65.

101. Jia Y, Zhang X, Yu J, et al. Acupuncture for patients with mild to moderate Alzheimer's disease: a randomized controlled trial. BMC Complement Altern Med 2017;17:556.

102. Liu W, Zhuo P, Li L, et al. Activation of brain glucose metabolism ameliorating cognitive impairment in APP/PS1 transgenic mice by electroacupuncture. Free Radic Biol Med 2017;112:174–90.

103. Shin HK, Lee SW, Choi BT. Modulation of neurogenesis via neurotrophic factors in acupuncture treatments for neurological diseases. Biochem Pharmacol 2017;141:132–42.

104. Kan BH, Yu JC, Zhao L, et al. Acupuncture improves dendritic structure and spatial learning and memory ability of Alzheimer's disease mice. Neural Regen Res 2018. https://doi.org/10.4103/1673-5374.235292.

105. Zheng W, Su Z, Liu X, et al. Modulation of functional activity and connectivity by acupuncture in patients with Alzheimer disease as measured by resting-state fMRI. PLoS One 2018. https://doi.org/10.1371/journal.pone.0196933.

106. Shan Y, Wang JJ, Wang ZQ, et al. Neuronal specificity of acupuncture in Alzheimer's disease and mild cognitive impairment patients: a functional MRI study.

Evid Based Complement Alternat Med 2018. https://doi.org/10.1155/2018/7619197.

107. Ye Y, Zhu W, Wang XR, et al. Mechanisms of acupuncture on vascular dementia–a review of animal studies. Neurochem Int 2017;107:204–10.

108. Xiao LY, Wang XR, Yang Y, et al. Applications of acupuncture therapy in modulating plasticity of central nervous system. Neuromodulation 2017. https://doi.org/10.1111/ner.12724.

109. Leung MC, Yip KK, Ho YS, et al. Mechanisms underlying the effect of acupuncture on cognitive improvement: a systematic review of animal studies. J Neuroimmune Pharmacol 2014;9:492–507.

110. Sutalangka C, Wattanathorn J, Muchimapura S, et al. Laser acupuncture improves memory impairment in an animal model of Alzheimer's disease. J Acupunct Meridian Stud 2013;6:247–51.

Perspectives on Feeding and Nutrition

Anthony J. Smith, DVM, MBA*

KEYWORDS

- Palliation • Hospice • Nutrition • Hydration • Benefits • Burdens

KEY POINTS

- Many pets develop symptoms of decreased consumption of food and water near the end of life, and there are many potential causes for such a decrease.
- In addition to the clinical and logistical issues, there are significant emotional and ethical concerns that must be addressed when developing treatment plans to address nutrition and hydration.
- When evaluating if, when, and how to provide assisted nutrition for pets in palliative care, one must carefully weigh the potential benefits of treatments against the burdens that such intervention might entail.
- Although some patients may derive benefit from assisted nutrition at the end of life, no strong evidence exists supporting the use of enteral/parenteral hydration/nutrition when near death.

INTRODUCTION

Hydration and nutrition are essential for the maintenance of life; however, many palliative care patients have reduced oral intake during their illness. The management of this symptom can have the aim of prolonging life, improving quality of life (QOL), or both. Yet, in patients at the end of life, managing inadequate intake through appetite stimulation and/or artificial hydration and nutrition can pose many clinical, ethical, and logistical dilemmas.

The provision of artificial or assisted feeding and hydration is one of the most controversial areas in end-of-life care for animal and human patients. This is in large measure because in addition to the clinical and logistical issues, there is also strong emotional and social symbolism associated with feeding those under our care. Feeding and the presence or absence of appetite/thirst in animal patients is a significant source of stress for caregivers who often ascribe excessive and incorrect meaning to their pet's eating and drinking when they are seriously ill and/or nearing the end

The author has nothing to disclose.
Rainbow Bridge Veterinary Services, Hercules, CA, USA
* 111 Caprice Circle, Hercules, CA 94547.
E-mail address: RainbowBridgeVet@gmail.com

Vet Clin Small Anim 49 (2019) 501–517
https://doi.org/10.1016/j.cvsm.2019.01.014
0195-5616/19/© 2019 Elsevier Inc. All rights reserved.

vetsmall.theclinics.com

of life. This is especially problematic in the terminal phase of life, when death is rapidly approaching.

There has been a good deal of information previously published regarding how to manage and treat reduced food intake in pets.[1–4] However, there has been little discussion in the veterinary literature regarding whether or not these treatments are actually of benefit to the terminally ill patient. How might one best navigate the options in the context of goals of care (GOC) and palliative care principles? If methods of artificial nutrition (eg, appetite stimulation, provision of parenteral hydration, feeding devices) are elected, what are the important considerations to keep in mind when managing this aspect of care for seriously ill and end-of-life patients?

This article aids the health care team in making appropriate recommendations regarding providing assisted nutrition and hydration for palliative care and/or terminally ill patients. It provides a decision-making framework, including an ethical approach to determining the appropriate use of assisted feeding and hydration methods in pets at the end of life. It also summarizes some of the clinical and logistical approaches to treating decreased food/water consumption, including potential benefits and burdens, should intervention be deemed to be appropriate.

EMOTIONAL AND ETHICAL ISSUES

There is a substantial amount of emotional baggage associated with a pet's ability and willingness to eat. For many caregivers, feeding is associated with nurturing and care. Many people express their love for others, including their animal companions, through food and equate food consumption with happiness and well-being. When an animal is not interested in food, caregivers may interpret this as a rejection of that love. Additionally, there is the common fear among caregivers that if their pet is not eating and/or drinking that she or he will "starve to death." Although this fear is not medically founded, it potentially engenders not only a concern that the pet is "suffering," but also feelings of guilt that the caregiver has not done everything possible. Another common emotion associated with a pet's lack of food consumption is helplessness. Often, caregivers have tried multiple ways, with varying success, to encourage eating (including novel food items, hand-feeding, offering treats), before even consulting the veterinary team. This is further complicated by the fact that most medications for pain relief or other symptom management are administered via the oral route. When an animal is not eating, this makes administration more difficult or impossible, furthering caregiver guilt and helplessness. These emotional factors all combine to contribute to a sense of frustration on the part of the family.

In this author's experience, and borne out by some published data,[5,6] if these emotions are not sufficiently addressed, the family may choose immediate euthanasia for the pet, even in situations where the remainder of the animal's QOL is good. Although there are multiple aspects to determining QOL in pets, caregivers frequently consider appetite as one of the most important determinants (along with pain and mobility issues).[7] Many clients share that they have been told that they will know "when it's time" for euthanasia, when their companion stops eating. Unfortunately, one cannot easily determine whether a pet has stopped eating as a result of its clinical condition, changes in hunger, or other factors. It is important to recognize that in human patients nearing the end of life, there is a natural decrease in appetite and thirst. People report that food loses its appeal and eating or drinking may cause discomfort as the body's ability to process nutrients (and eventually fluids) decreases. Providing assisted nutrition to these patients may potentially prolong life, but at the cost of QOL.[8]

In addition to the emotional aspects related to feeding, there are a host of ethical issues surrounding a decision of whether and how to intervene in providing assisted nutrition. Here are just a few of the specific concerns that might need to be addressed in the decision-making process:

- Because pets cannot directly communicate their wishes, how do we best respect their autonomy and interpret the patient's wishes with regard to their end-of-life experience?
- How can we ensure that a designated surrogate decision maker has the pet's best interests in mind, without undue influence of personal biases regarding their own care?
- When a patient is near death, some potential options for intervention might be considered to violate the principle of beneficence (obligation to promote benefit to the patient). How can we balance the ethical desire to help the pet against the need to avoid harm (nonmaleficence)?
- Can we justify decisions to intervene or not based on lack of family resources (eg, cost of medications or treatments, time required for care/maintenance of feeding tubes)?
- Is it ethical to allow a pet to pass naturally from its disease process without assisted nutrition and/or hydration?
- Should we advocate for euthanasia if we cannot address a patient's reduced food/water consumption?

ADDRESSING ETHICAL ISSUES

Before making decisions or recommendations about specific management of nutritional issues, it is important to frame the discussion with caregivers in an ethically considered context. Although the scholarly literature in veterinary medicine is lacking in this area, there is relevant exploration in human medicine[9–13] where legal considerations and clinical, logistical, and ethical issues persist. The consensus opinion in human medicine is that the medical administration of fluids and nutrition is an intervention subject to the same principles of decision making as all other medical interventions.[9]

Although there is minimal attention given to ethical consideration of feeding and nutrition in the end-of-life veterinary patient, there are a few general discussions of veterinary ethical considerations in palliative care,[14–16] and many excellent discussions in the human literature.[9,17–19] In the absence of veterinary-specific guidelines, an appropriate approach in this situation may be to adapt palliative care planning for veterinary patients using an approach recommended for human patients who lack decision-making capacity.[20] This is especially important for more aggressive methods of intervention, such as pharmacologic intervention or artificial nutrition (eg, feeding tubes, parenteral administration) and the option of nonintervention. The core principles of this approach include the following[20]:

- Structuring decision making as a consensus building process among caregivers, the health care team, and other family members.
- Achieving consensus about the diagnosis and prognosis, and the benefits and burdens of various available treatment options.
- Basing decisions on the best assessment of the patient's preferences and ability to relieve suffering and maximize QOL.

A suggested step-by-step method for implementing these principles is outlined in **Table 1**.

Table 1
Suggested steps to provide nutrition-related palliative care to pets

Step	Sample Statements
Identify the decision makers.	"We need to make decisions about [Pet]'s care. Who should be involved to help us think through what to do?"
Allow caregivers to describe the pet's symptoms.	"Can you tell me how [Pet]'s appetite has changed? How has that gone for you?" "How have you been dealing with this challenge?"
Educate decision makers about the expected course of the disease and how this might affect feeding/nutrition.	"[Pet] has an incurable and ultimately terminal disease. We can't predict how things might progress, but it's likely that she will decrease or even completely stop eating at some point."
Advocate for the pet's quality of life.	"We ought to care for [Pet] in a way that avoids any undue suffering." "If we can get [Pet] eating something, do you think that her quality of life would be good?"
Advocate for the pet's autonomy/agency.	"Do you think [Pet] would tolerate this treatment, if it meant that she could enjoy her food again?" "If [Pet] could talk to us, what do you think she would tell us that she wants?"
Offer guidance based on clinical experience and relevant evidence (repeat as needed for additional symptoms or potential treatments).	"For pets at [Pet]'s stage, feeding with a tube does not significantly improve quality of life or survival times." "For other pets with kidney failure, using an appetite stimulant may encourage eating, if only temporarily." "Based on my experience, providing periodic injections of fluid under the skin, may help her be more comfortable."

Adapted from Karlawish JHT, Quill T, Meier DE. A consensus-based approach to providing palliative care to patients who lack decision-making capacity. Ann Intern Med 1999;130(10):835.

DECISION MAKING

Managing decisions about feeding and nutrition in a palliative care situation requires making difficult choices that vary in complexity and perceived significance. There should be a thorough discussion with caregivers and other family members to determine what the expectations, hopes, fears, resources, and limitations are for the pet and family. As part of this discussion, family members need to be educated about the available options for intervention, including the benefits and burdens associated with each, and the costs and likely outcomes in relation to the pet and identified GOC. Furthermore, this discussion should include the option of nonintervention and how this might affect the pet, its QOL and quantity of life, clinical condition, and potential timing of euthanasia.

There is rarely a single correct approach or solution. Even given the same clinical condition in similar pets, the right plan can vary from one individual to another, depending on the particular circumstances of the family and specific patient.

Additionally, the right decision for a particular pet and family may evolve over time. Decision making is a process, rather than a one-time event; it must accommodate shifting facts and perceptions as a disease progresses and the pet approaches end of life.

INFORMATION GATHERING

Addressing nutrition and hydration in the palliative care patient should begin, like all aspects of palliative care consultation, with a discussion of the family's GOC for the pet, including preferences for specific treatments, the intensity of care, resource availability, and desires regarding potential euthanasia and its timing. These GOC then help guide the decision-making process regarding the implementation of a feeding/nutrition plan, in addition to other potential medical decisions. A more general assessment of GOC is found elsewhere,[21] but listed next are some specific items to address in evaluating concerns related to feeding and nutrition in the palliative care patient (adapted from Jonsen et al.[22]):

Clinical Considerations
- What is the patient's diagnosis, symptom burden, prognosis, and past history?
- What is the expected survival time?
- Is the pet actively dying?

QOL Considerations
- What other aspects of QOL are affected besides food and fluid intake?
- Would providing assisted nutrition improve QOL?
- How much detriment would result from treatment (or nontreatment)?
- What is the family's preference for the nature and timing of death (eg, euthanasia)?

Contextual Considerations
- Who are the caregivers and is there agreement in the family about treatment?
- What is the bond between the pet and family members?
- Are the caregivers interested in and capable of providing treatments?
- How do proposed treatments affect the caregiver's life (eg, financial, time)?

Patient Preferences
- Is eating important to the pet? Does the pet enjoy food/treats?
- How might the pet respond to various treatment options? What are the side effects of those options?
- How might the patient's individual personality affect treatment options?
- How might treatments affect the pet's sense of agency/autonomy?

Asking and addressing the previously mentioned questions helps to facilitate communication between the veterinary team and clients, allowing collaboration in developing a plan for addressing the patient's nutritional needs, while balancing these against the costs of intervention.

Information gathering should also include a thorough history and physical examination. Relevant questions to answer during this process should include the following:

- What is the current hydration and nutritional status?
- How much water is consumed (ideally with actual quantities measured)?
- What is the animal currently eating? Include main diet, treats, supplements, medications, and food used to administer medications.
- How much of each is consumed? How has this changed and when? Compare this amount with previous consumption.

- What steps has the caregiver already taken to address appetite changes?
- What is the caregiver's perception of the pet's appetite/thirst? Does the pet seem interested in food/water?
- Are there any physical limitations to eating/drinking? Is the gastrointestinal (GI) tract functional?
- What is the pet's weight? Ideally, this should be measured with an accurate scale, even in a home visit. How is this changing and at what rate?
- What is the Body Condition Score (using a standardized classification scale) and muscle mass?

Once this information has been collected, one can evaluate whether or not the food/water intake is appropriate. Calculation of nutrient requirements and water/electrolyte balance is beyond the scope of this article. However, there are excellent resources available to address this aspect of the evaluation.[3,4,23,24] If the pet's weight is stable, and Body Condition Score and hydration are normal, then the pet has adequate food/water consumption for its current needs, even if caregivers perceive a decreased appetite.

REASONS FOR DECREASED FOOD AND WATER CONSUMPTION

There are many potential causes, acting alone or in combination, for a decrease in food/water consumption at or near the end of life. Some of these causes may be obvious, such as physical limitations to eating (eg, oral masses, obstructions, dental disease) or a disease process causing reduced hunger (eg, liver or kidney disease). However, some causes may be more difficult to determine. Decreased interest in food may be the result of localized pain somewhere in the GI tract (eg, uremic oral ulceration in chronic kidney disease, intestinal neoplasia) or pain somewhere else in the body (eg, osteoarthritis or neuropathic pain). Any source of inflammation, especially that associated with some neoplastic processes, can cause altered neural control of appetite because of the release of inflammatory cytokines (interleukin-1, tumor necrosis factor-α). Many pets lose interest in food secondary to nausea caused by the primary disease process or to medications (eg, many antimicrobials). There may also be changes in GI motility secondary to a disease process or medications (eg, opioids). Another potential cause might be reduced taste or olfactory perception secondary to disorders of the mouth or nasal cavity or secondary to medications (eg, chemotherapeutics). Neurologic disease (brain tumors, vestibular disease) and cognitive disorders (canine cognitive disorder, dementia) might also lead to alterations in a pet's hunger levels or sense of taste and smell. Food aversions can also develop when pets associate discomfort or pain of illness with a particular food, or if food has been used to administer foul-tasting medications (eg, tramadol).[25] Dietary factors (palatability, texture, temperature, or smell), social interactions with family or other animals, stress, and generalized weakness may also play a role in decreased food consumption. Finally, in humans and animals, there is frequently a natural decrease in the body's energy requirements and a corresponding decrease in hunger/thirst during the dying process.[26,27]

MANAGING INADEQUATE FOOD INTAKE

Ideally, when approaching treatment of decreased food consumption, the underlying causes should be identified and managed appropriately. In a younger patient with a good prognosis for recovery, the benefits of intensive intervention might outweigh the temporary discomfort that might result from such treatment. However, in a setting where time is limited and/or patients are more fragile, comfort becomes much more critical and life-extending treatments may not be as important. As a result, one must often treat the patient symptomatically, rather than being able to address the root cause of a problem. Before considering how to intervene in a patient with reduced oral intake, one must address the patient as a whole, and consider what are the GOC. The way that one approaches an imminently dying pet is different from the approach to one who may be expected to live many more weeks or months.

BENEFIT VERSUS BURDEN

In palliative care provision, when deciding if, when, and how to intervene in a pet's nutritional management, it is especially important to weigh the potential benefit to the patient against the burden of providing the intervention. There are several different aspects to the burden of care for the patient and caregivers that should be identified and considered.[28,29]

For the caregiver, choosing certain interventions can have negative impacts on psychological, social, and/or physical health functioning. Caregivers are typically responsible for implementing whatever treatments are chosen, including obtaining and administering medications, caring for the patient, managing appointments with the health care team, and communicating with others about the treatment. Caregivers must frequently evaluate, monitor, and adjust any prescribed treatments. Managing all of these activities may require changes in work, living, and sleeping schedules, in addition to the stress that additional expenses may place on family resources. An additional area of burden involves the effort that is required to engage with other people in search of support, dealing with the emotions of caring for an ill pet, and managing the stress that this puts on relationships with other humans and pets inside and outside of the family unit.

For the patient, burdens of care include enduring the treatment (if uncomfortable), the side effects of any medications, and living with any treatment sequelae (eg, infection, GI upset) or change in QOL. Additionally, there is the potential that selected treatments may not be what the pet would have chosen for itself, if given an option.

As we consider each method of intervening to manage alterations in food/water intake, it is important to discuss several factors and how they fit with the defined GOC.

- Likelihood of response to treatment and how that response is defined
- Likely duration of survival with and without intervention
- Burdens of intervention (eg, side effects, discomfort of treatment)
- Duration of treatment
- If and how treatment can be provided (eg, at home vs hospitalization)
- Potential monetary and other resource costs
- What are the alternatives to the treatment

In situations where the proposed treatment has a potential for greater burden than benefit, nonbiased discussion should present the option of nonintervention, instead opting for comfort care or euthanasia, as viable alternatives.

METHODS FOR INCREASING FOOD CONSUMPTION

Generally speaking, nutritional concerns in pets at the end of life include dysrexia, hyporexia, and anorexia. Normally, regulation of food intake is a complex system, balancing energy intake and expenditure to maintain an animal at a stable body weight. The normal process is disrupted by a host of physical, psychological, and social factors. A detailed description of the regulation of food intake is beyond the scope of this article, but excellent reviews of that topic have been published.[30–32]

If the pet has the ability to eat, but has decreased or no food consumption, a potential first step is to ensure that there are minimal inhibitors in the environment. For example, one might remove barriers to eating, such as restrictive collars, food dishes that may be uncomfortable to reach, or competition with other animals in the household. Social cues may be used to encourage eating; some animals are more likely to eat if other pets are fed at the same time or if human family members are eating, whereas others do better with privacy. Many pets eat if offered food by hand or using a spoon, as opposed to eating directly from a food dish. Some pets prefer to eat from a flat plate, whereas others prefer a bowl. Food dish materials can also affect appetite; consider changing this to see if it encourages eating. Timing is also a factor. Altering the time of feeding in relation to light/dark, or proximity to treatments (eg, fluid or medication administration) might improve food consumption.

Changes to the food may also be a simple adjustment to implement. One can try offering the food at different temperatures. Although some pets prefer cold or room temperature food, gently warming and stirring the food can improve consumption either because of individual animal preferences, or by improving appetite via increasing the aroma of the offering. Changing consistency, moisture content, or texture of the diet can also improve consumption. Pets suffering with oral or GI pain may prefer food with a more liquid or stew-like consistency, whereas others may require or prefer food with a firmer consistency.

When considering changing from a commercial, nutritionally complete diet to home-cooked foods, there is more potential for adverse effects. Feeding only home prepared food or only things that the pet finds palatable may contribute to a nutritionally deficient diet with imbalances in the levels of the macronutrients: protein, fat, and carbohydrates, and/or lacking in particular vitamins, minerals, or other micronutrients. Additionally, these imbalances may potentially exacerbate certain underlying disease processes or comorbidities. This potential drawback must be carefully weighed against the many benefits that eating something palatable might provide. Ideally, consultation with a veterinary nutritionist can help minimize the adverse effects, but if a pet is very near the end of life, this becomes less of a concern. Some dietary changes that may improve food consumption include offering foods with a strong aroma, such as fish (especially in cats); adding palatability enhancers, such as fats or sweeteners; or offering "home-cooked" foods, such as chicken, beef, or broth. Other suggestions for diet change that may be effective in some cases include adding muscle, organ, or deli meats, or offering various flavors of baby food. Supplementing the main diet with liver powder, Bonita flakes, nutritional yeast, egg yolk, or other nutritional supplements have also been suggested.[33]

FOOD AVERSION

An important potential cause of a pet's reduced food consumption may be learned aversion to its regular diet or a particular food.[25] To prevent the development of food aversion do the following:

- Avoid using the pet's regular food to administer medications (at least until palatability of the medication has been determined).
- Schedule uncomfortable medical treatments, such as injections, at times distant from feeding regular meals and consider having a different person provide the regular food.

- If the patient has temporary vomiting or nausea, offer only a bland diet and avoid offering regular food or favored treats until the problem is resolved.

APPETITE STIMULANTS

Many different medications have been used as appetite stimulants with varying success. Thorough reviews on these drugs are found in the literature.[3,24,34] Although these medications are helpful in certain situations and with certain individuals, there are many limitations to their usefulness. In addition to unpredictable efficacy, most of these need to be administered orally, which is a challenge for caregivers with an anorexic animal, especially if needed long term. Forcing a patient to consume medication to increase appetite may be contrary to stated GOC, induce negative feelings toward the caregiver, and negatively impact the relationship with the pet. Additionally, caregivers may just not be comfortable with this type of intervention, especially if it requires them to perform the procedure at home. Furthermore, the reliance on appetite stimulants to artificially improve appetite may interfere with the ability to use appetite as an indicator of QOL, response to other treatments, or progression of disease. Finally, all appetite stimulants carry the potential for unwanted side-effects (especially in patients with end-stage disease) and interactions with other medications that may be needed for treatment of other symptoms. Because most appetite stimulants are metabolized in the liver and excreted by the kidneys, consider adjusting the dosage in patients suffering from hepatic or renal disease.

If use of an appetite stimulant is deemed to be warranted, there are several options. Mirtazapine, a tetracyclic antidepressant, has antiemetic and appetite stimulating effects. It has been shown to be effective at increasing body weight, and appetite, and reducing vomiting in cats suffering from chronic kidney disease.[35] At higher doses there may be more frequent incidence of side effects, such as hyperexcitability, tremors, and vocalization. One particular advantage to mirtazapine is that there is a newly approved feline transdermal formulation that can potentially be administered more easily to anorexic cats.[36]

Capromorelin is a newly approved appetite stimulant that directly stimulates the appetite by mimicking the hunger hormone ghrelin. Available as an oral solution, this selective ghrelin-receptor agonist has been shown to increase body weight and food intake in healthy dogs.[37,38] Another study demonstrated significant increase in owner-assessed food consumption in dogs with reduced appetite.[39] Commonly cited adverse effects include vomiting and diarrhea. Although not currently approved for use in cats, preliminary studies have shown safety and efficacy in this species.[40]

Cyproheptadine is an antihistamine that can stimulate appetite via inhibiting serotonin receptors in the hypothalamus. However, it has a variable bioavailability and may require 2 to 3 days to reach steady state concentrations. Potential side effects include sedation or paradoxic excitation and anticholinergic symptoms (eg, dry mucus membranes, tachycardia). Other historically used appetite stimulants, such as diazepam, oxazepam, and propofol, are generally no longer recommended, because of variable efficacy, side effects, and potential interaction with other medications.[1,41]

NAUSEA AND VOMITING

Nausea and/or vomiting are common symptoms of many conditions affecting pets near the end of life (eg, renal, hepatic, GI, vestibular diseases). It is important to treat these symptoms not only for the comfort of the patient, but also because if left untreated, they may result in a significant reduction in food and water consumption. Recognition of nausea in animals is not always simple, and it may be worthwhile to consider treating nausea when other causes of reduced appetite cannot be identified or remedied.

The cause and control of vomiting is complex, but excellent reviews are available.[42,43] In the palliative care patient, maropitant may be particularly useful. It is a selective neurokinin-1 receptor antagonist with good antiemetic effects in dogs and cats. There are oral and injectable formulations, which is helpful in situations where one or the other route is difficult because of administration challenges, patient concerns, or caregiver limitations. However, when considering benefits versus burdens of care, note that the injectable formulation is often painful on administration. This pain may be reduced by refrigerating maropitant before injection[44] or including the medication within a large volume of subcutaneous (SC) fluids. A study evaluating the use of maropitant in feline chronic kidney disease demonstrated significant reduction in vomiting, but no improvement in appetite or weight gain.[44] Although maropitant is labeled for use of less than 5 days, safety studies in dogs and cats have indicated minimal adverse effects when used longer term.[44,45]

Depending on the patient and individual circumstances, other medications, such as ondansetron, metoclopramide, mirtazapine, and H_2 receptor-antagonists, such as ranitidine or cimetidine, might be useful alone, or in combination, for treatment of nausea/vomiting.[43] Again, similar to appetite stimulants, each of these has potential side effects and interactions with other medications, so use must be carefully evaluated. A summary of the most useful medications for stimulating appetite and controlling nausea and vomiting is presented in **Table 2**.

ENTERAL NUTRITION

If none of the previously mentioned methods for increasing food consumption are effective, provision of artificial nutrition via feeding tube may be considered. However, it is important to recognize that the burdens associated with this type of intervention can be more significant than pharmacologic options for the patient and caregiving team. Again, one must carefully evaluate the potential benefits that might be achieved

Table 2
Summary of useful medications

Medication	Use	Dosage	Notes
Mirtazapine	Appetite stimulation, antiemetic	1.88 mg/cat PO q 24–48 h; 1.5-inch ribbon of ointment (~2 mg/cat)	Available in oral and transdermal formulations
Capromorelin	Appetite stimulation	3 mg/kg PO q 24 h for 4 d	Approved for 4 d, but seems to be safe longer term
Cyproheptadine	Appetite stimulation	1–4 mg/cat PO q 12–24 h	Cats only; higher doses more likely to have side effects
Maropitant	Antiemetic	1 mg/kg SC q 24 h; 1 mg/kg (cats) and 2 mg/kg (dogs) PO q 24 h	Labeled for use up to 5 d, but likely safe for longer term use
Ondansetron	Antiemetic	0.1–1 mg/kg PO, intravenous q 6–12 h	Particularly effective to control vomiting associated with chemotherapeutics

Data from Refs.[1–3,34–42,44–49]

versus the costs of instituting such a treatment and tailor the recommendation to the individual patient and particular circumstances.

Benefits to instituting artificial nutrition via feeding device include ability to bypass an obstruction, provision of calories needed for energy, reliable route for administration of medication and/or fluids, and potentially improved quantity or QOL. Artificial nutrition may also be able to provide temporary support for a particular condition or comorbidity in an individual patient.

Some of the potential burdens associated with artificial nutrition include the requirement for anesthesia and/or surgery for placement of a tube, ongoing monitoring, care and maintenance of access ports (along with potential for bleeding, tube blockage, infection, and pain at insertion site), increased mortality, cost (of procedure and food sources), increased chance of aspiration, and other adverse events (diarrhea, constipation, hyperglycemia, refeeding syndrome, and tube feeding syndrome).[50–54] It is also important to note that no studies have demonstrated an improved outcome (either in QOL or quantity of life) in human patients receiving enteral nutrition with advanced forms of cancer,[9–11,55] and it can reasonably be assumed that the same holds true for veterinary patients. Again, it is important to distinguish pets very near the end of life from those requiring palliation earlier in the course of a disease. Those very near death may have lost the ability to digest and process nutrients, making the use of enteral nutrition at this time not only ineffective, but actually detrimental to the patient's comfort.

If, after careful evaluation of the patient and caregiver needs, enteral nutrition is deemed appropriate, there are a variety of tube placements that may be considered. For short-term nutritional support of patients with a normal nasal cavity, pharynx, esophagus, and stomach, a nasoesophageal (NE) tube may be appropriate. One important advantage of the NE tube is that general anesthesia is not required for placement, although mild sedation may be required.[56] Major disadvantages to NE tubes are risk of aspiration, limited size of tube requiring a liquid diet, and careful monitoring, generally only available for hospitalized patients.

For long-term, at home nutritional support of patients with a normal pharynx, esophagus, and stomach, an esophagostomy tube may be considered. The main advantages of this type of tube are the ability to administer medications through the tube, and blended (vs liquid) food diets over the long-term. These tubes are well tolerated by many pets and are useful in cases where oral or nasal masses prevent an otherwise healthy pet from eating. Disadvantages include the need for anesthesia ± surgery for placement, and the potential for complications, such as infection and tube dislodgement. Tubes must also be bandaged and frequently monitored at home. In patients with oropharyngeal or esophageal disease, or where an esophagostomy tube is contraindicated, a percutaneous endoscopically guided gastrotomy tube may be considered. Advantages and disadvantages are similar to those described for the esophagostomy tube.

PARENTERAL NUTRITION

Under normal circumstances, the use of parenteral nutrition is a consideration when the patient cannot be fed orally or enterally. Caregivers often express concern that their anorexic pet will "starve to death," and may initially request that everything possible be done to keep their pet alive. However, for animal patients at the end of life, the requirement for hospitalization during administration in combination with the lack of demonstrated efficacy of artificial nutrition to improve QOL or survival time near death, tends to argue against the recommendation for parenteral nutrition in virtually all "end of life" veterinary patients. The use of artificial nutrition in the last days of life is not recommended in human medicine because of the lack of confirmed benefit and likelihood of adverse effects.[11,52]

FLUID THERAPY BENEFITS VERSUS BURDENS

Patients at the end of life frequently have reduced intake of water and reduced food intake leading to significant changes to the patient's hydration status. These changes are concerning to caregivers and palliative care providers, bringing along the same list of concerns as has been discussed for nutritional supplementation. Managing these changes should, again, begin with a consideration of GOC, along with a careful comparison of the benefits of treatment weighed against any burdens that the intervention might carry.

Similar to the situation previously described for enteral nutrition, there is considerable controversy regarding the benefits and efficacy of supplemental fluids for patients near the time of death. The prevailing practice in human hospice care holds that the provision of supplemental fluids does not improve the QOL or survival time.[8,13,57,58] Furthermore, providing supplemental fluids may increase discomfort or prolong suffering. In one study of human hospice patients with only weeks of life expectancy, a controlled trial of parenteral hydration found no benefit compared with control subjects.[10] Additional justification for nonintervention when voluntary drinking ceases, is that the resulting fluid deficit may be beneficial by decreasing the following[27]:

- Edema and ascites
- Pulmonary secretions, resulting in less dyspnea and coughing
- Saliva production resulting in less choking and drowning sensations
- Urine production resulting in less incontinence
- GI tract secretions resulting in less nausea and vomiting
- Level of consciousness leading to a decrease in the perception of suffering

A profound fluid deficit might also induce a level of general anesthesia, and increase the production of endogenous opioids, further reducing suffering.[27]

The disadvantages of instituting fluid supplementation include persistence of physiologic conditions that may be otherwise mitigated by allowing natural processes of fluid metabolism to proceed, and potentially negative psychosocial effects for caregivers. These include increasing distress at having to administer uncomfortable treatments, increasing treatment complexity, and fueling feelings of denial regarding a terminal pet's condition.[8,57,58]

However, some clinicians and researchers have challenged the practice of avoiding fluid supplementation, noting that some uncomfortable symptoms in the dying patient are ameliorated with careful fluid administration, including relief of thirst and constipation, decreased incidence of myoclonus and seizures, and decreased risk of pressure ulcer development.[12] Additionally, providing fluid supplementation can allow caregivers to be involved in efforts on behalf of their pet, although this "placebo effect" for veterinary clients is ethically suspect. In trying to decide a course of action using evidence-based medicine, note that in the human and veterinary literature, few good quality studies have been published on this topic.

PROVIDING FLUID SUPPLEMENTATION

In patients nearing death, the normal balance of fluid homeostasis maintained by complex interactions among the brain, kidneys, digestive tract, vascular, and endocrine systems is altered. This commonly results in underhydration or overhydration and electrolyte abnormalities that may result in fluid accumulations, weakness, fatigue, muscle twitching, discomfort, and further compromise of critical organ function.[12,59] Therefore, at any stage in the palliative care process, one should pay close attention to the patient's fluid status, constantly monitoring, reevaluating, and updating treatment plans as needed to maintain patient comfort and avoid symptoms of underhydration or overhydration.

Methods for delivering fluids might begin with attempts to increase oral intake. Ensuring that water bowls are clean and accessible or offering running water via a fountain may be helpful, especially in cats. Offering assistance via water-filled syringe or increasing water content of the pet's food are other simple methods for increasing fluid intake.

If these methods are insufficient, parenteral administration may be considered on a case-by-case basis. Although intravenous (IV) administration may be more effective or required in serious or emergent situations, this generally involves hospitalization and/or careful monitoring by trained personnel. In addition, IV administration tends to interrupt the ability of caregivers to closely interact with their pets. For these reasons, the IV route of fluid administration is less useful, especially late in the course of illness.

SC fluid administration is generally more useful, especially for home management, and many caregivers and patients can learn to accept this method of treatment well. Caregivers can be taught to administer SC fluids and maintain necessary supplies. Some pets may respond so well to the increased comfort provided by the treatment that they actively seek out fluid therapy. However, some patients may be distressed by the procedure, causing the pet to resent interaction with caregivers. If this is the case, QOL for patient and caregiver may be significantly decreased.

SUMMARY

Decreased food and/or water consumption is a frequent problem encountered in seriously ill pets at the end of life. This symptom is extremely concerning for pet families and health care professionals, and if not addressed, may be a trigger for euthanasia. The management of reduced food/water consumption has clinical, logistical, emotional, and ethical considerations that must be addressed. There are a variety of treatments available, including stimulation of appetite (via behavioral, social, practical, and pharmacologic methods), control of nausea/vomiting, and enteral supplementation using feeding tubes. Parenteral fluid supplementation is also frequently chosen as an intervention. Given that most research in terminally ill people has demonstrated a lack of efficacy in improving either QOL or quantity of life, the use of artificial nutrition/hydration in dying pet patients must be carefully evaluated. During the palliative care and/or end-of-life period, it is critical to carefully assess any potential treatment options with respect to identified GOC, potential benefits and burdens, ethical concerns, and patient status (especially regarding likely proximity to death).

REFERENCES

1. Agnew W, Korman R. Pharmacological appetite stimulation: rational choices in the inappetent cat. J Feline Med Surg 2014;16(9):749–56.

2. Delaney SJ. Management of anorexia in dogs and cats. Vet Clin North Am Small Anim Pract 2006;36(6):1243–9.

3. Chan DL. The inappetent hospitalised Cat: clinical approach to maximising nutritional support. J Feline Med Surg 2009;11(11):925–33.

4. Fascetti AJ, Delaney SJ. Applied veterinary clinical nutrition. Hoboken (NJ): Wiley-Blackwell; 2012. Available at: https://www.wiley.com/en-us/Applied+Veterinary+Clinical+Nutrition-p-9780813806570. Accessed August 31, 2018.

5. Spitznagel MB, Jacobson DM, Cox MD, et al. Predicting caregiver burden in general veterinary clients: contribution of companion animal clinical signs and problem behaviors. Vet J 2018;236:23–30.

6. Spitznagel MB, Jacobson DM, Cox MD, et al. Caregiver burden in owners of a sick companion animal: a cross-sectional observational study. Vet Rec 2017; 181(12):321.

7. Reynolds CA, Oyama MA, Rush JE, et al. Perceptions of quality of life and priorities of owners of cats with heart disease. J Vet Intern Med 2010;24(6):1421–6.

8. McCann RM, Hall WJ, Groth-Juncker A. Comfort care for terminally ill patients. The appropriate use of nutrition and hydration. JAMA 1994;272(16):1263–6. Available at: http://www.ncbi.nlm.nih.gov/pubmed/7523740. Accessed August 31, 2018.

9. Diekema DS, Botkin JR, Committee on Bioethics. Forgoing medically provided nutrition and hydration in children. Pediatrics 2009;124(2):813–22.

10. Hui D, Dev R, Bruera E. The last days of life: symptom burden and impact on nutrition and hydration in cancer patients. Curr Opin Support Palliat Care 2015; 9(4):346–54.

11. Dev R, Dalal S, Bruera E. Is there a role for parenteral nutrition or hydration at the end of life? Curr Opin Support Palliat Care 2012;6(3):365–70.

12. Huang ZB, Ahronheim JC. Nutrition and hydration in terminally ill patients: an update. Clin Geriatr Med 2000;16(2):313–25.

13. Dunphy K, Finlay I, Rathbone G, et al. Rehydration in palliative and terminal care: if not- why not? Palliat Med 1995;9(3):221–8.

14. Pierce J, Shanan A. Ethical decision making in animal hospice and palliative care. In: Shanan A, Pierce J, Shearer T, editors. Hospice and palliative care for companion animals. Hoboken (NJ): John Wiley & Sons, Inc.; 2017. p. 57–71.

15. Moore AS. Managing cats with cancer. J Feline Med Surg 2011;13(9):661–71.

16. Bishop G, Cooney K, Cox S, et al. 2016 AAHA/IAAHPC end-of-life care guidelines. J Am Anim Hosp Assoc 2016;52(6):341–56.

17. Levi BH. Withdrawing nutrition and hydration from children: legal, ethical, and professional issues. Clin Pediatr (Phila) 2003;42(2):139–45.

18. Annas GJ. "Culture of life" politics at the bedside—the case of Terri Schiavo. N Engl J Med 2005;352(16):1710–5.

19. Ganzini L. Artificial nutrition and hydration at the end of life: ethics and evidence. Palliat Support Care 2006;4(02):135–43.

20. Karlawish JHT, Quill T, Meier DE. A consensus-based approach to providing palliative care to patients who lack decision-making capacity. Ann Intern Med 1999; 130(10):835.

21. Carter B, Levetown M, Friebert S. Palliative care for infants, children, and adolescents: a practical handbook 2013. Available at: http://trafficlight.bitdefender.com/info?url=https%3A//www.researchgate.net/profile/William_Haley/publication/8366366_Family_Caregivers_of_Elderly_Patients_With_Cancer_Understanding_and_Minimizing_the_Burden_of_Care/links/59f28a46a6fdcc1dc7bb1b83/Family-Caregivers-of-Elderly-Patients-With-Cancer-Understanding-and-Minimizing-the-Burden-of-Care.pdf&language=en_US. Accessed September 6, 2018.

22. Jonsen AR, Siegler M, Winslade WJ. Clinical ethics: a practical approach to ethical decisions in clinical medicine. New York: McGraw-Hill, Health Professions Division; 1992. Available at: https://books.google.com/books/about/Clinical_Ethics.html?id=fydrAAAAMAAJ&source=kp_book_description. Accessed November 12, 2018.

23. Baldwin K, Bartges J, Buffington T, et al. AAHA nutritional assessment guidelines for dogs and cats. J Am Anim Hosp Assoc 2010;46(4):285–96.

24. Parker VJ. Nutritional management of hospitalised dogs and cats. Vet Nurse 2013;4(8):478–85.

25. Bernstein IL. Taste aversion learning: a contemporary perspective. Nutrition 1999; 15(3):229–34. Available at: http://www.ncbi.nlm.nih.gov/pubmed/10198919. Accessed August 31, 2018.

26. August K. Balancing efficacy of treatments against burdens of care. In: Shanan A, Pierce J, Shearer T, editors. Hospice and palliative care for companion animals. Hoboken (NJ): John Wiley & Sons, Inc.; 2017. p. 199–209. https://doi.org/10.1002/9781119036722.ch20.

27. Del Río MI, Shand B, Bonati P, et al. Hydration and nutrition at the end of life: a systematic review of emotional impact, perceptions, and decision-making among patients, family, and health care staff. Psychooncology 2012;21(9):913–21.

28. Oncol WH-JS, 2003 undefined. Family caregivers of elderly patients with cancer: understanding and minimizing the burden of care. Available at: researchgate.net http://trafficlight.bitdefender.com/info?url=https%3A//www.researchgate.net/profile/William_Haley/publication/8366366_Family_Caregivers_of_Elderly_Patients_With_Cancer_Understanding_and_Minimizing_the_Burden_of_Care/links/59f28a46a6fdcc1dc7bb1b83/Family-Caregivers-of-Elderly-Patients-With-Cancer-Understanding-and-Minimizing-the-Burden-of-Care.pdf&language=en_US. Accessed September 3, 2018.

29. Proot I, ... HA-... journal of caring, 2003 undefined. Vulnerability of family caregivers in terminal palliative care at home; balancing between burden and capacity. Wiley Online Libr. Available at: http://trafficlight.bitdefender.com/info?url=https%3A//onlinelibrary.wiley.com/doi/abs/10.1046/j.1471-6712.2003.00220.x&language=en_US. Accessed September 3, 2018.

30. Takeda H, Nakagawa K, Okubo N, et al. Pathophysiologic basis of anorexia: focus on the interaction between ghrelin dynamics and the serotonergic system. Biol Pharm Bull 2013;36(9):1401–5. Available at: http://www.ncbi.nlm.nih.gov/pubmed/23995649. Accessed August 31, 2018.

31. Woods SC, Benoit SC, Clegg DJ, et al. Regulation of energy homeostasis by peripheral signals. Best Pract Res Clin Endocrinol Metab 2004;18(4):497–515.

32. Woods SC, D'Alessio DA. Central control of body weight and appetite. J Clin Endocrinol Metab 2008;93(11_supplement_1):s37–50.

33. Pope G, Shanan A. Comfort care during active dying. In: Shanan A, Pierce J, Shearer T, editors. Hospice and palliative care for companion animals. Hoboken (NJ): John Wiley & Sons, Inc.; 2017. p. 231–49. https://doi.org/10.1002/9781119036722.ch22.

34. Cox S. Pharmacology interventions for symptom management. In: Hospice and palliative care for companion animals. Hoboken (NJ): John Wiley & Sons, Inc.; 2017. p. 165–80. https://doi.org/10.1002/9781119036722.ch18.

35. Quimby JM, Lunn KF. Mirtazapine as an appetite stimulant and anti-emetic in cats with chronic kidney disease: a masked placebo-controlled crossover clinical trial. Vet J 2013;197(3):651–5.

36. Buhles W, Quimby JM, Labelle D, et al. Single and multiple dose pharmacokinetics of a novel mirtazapine transdermal ointment in cats. J Vet Pharmacol Ther 2018;41(5):644–51.

37. Rhodes L, Zollers B, Wofford JA, et al. Capromorelin: a ghrelin receptor agonist and novel therapy for stimulation of appetite in dogs. Vet Med Sci 2018;4(1):3–16.

38. Zollers B, Rhodes L, Heinen E. Capromorelin oral solution (ENTYCE) increases food consumption and body weight when administered for 4 consecutive days

to healthy adult Beagle dogs in a randomized, masked, placebo controlled study. BMC Vet Res 2016;13(1):10.

39. Zollers B, Wofford JA, Heinen E, et al. A prospective, randomized, masked, placebo-controlled clinical study of capromorelin in dogs with reduced appetite. J Vet Intern Med 2016;30(6):1851–7.

40. Wofford JA, Zollers B, Rhodes L, et al. Evaluation of the safety of daily administration of capromorelin in cats. J Vet Pharmacol Ther 2018;41(2):324–33.

41. Johnson LN, Freeman LM. Recognizing, describing, and managing reduced food intake in dogs and cats. J Am Vet Med Assoc 2017;251(11):1260–6.

42. Kenward H, Elliott J, Lee T, et al. Anti-nausea effects and pharmacokinetics of ondansetron, maropitant and metoclopramide in a low-dose cisplatin model of nausea and vomiting in the dog: a blinded crossover study. BMC Vet Res 2017;13(1):244.

43. Trepanier L. Acute vomiting in cats. J Feline Med Surg 2010;12(3):225–30.

44. Quimby JM, Brock WT, Moses K, et al. Chronic use of maropitant for the management of vomiting and inappetence in cats with chronic kidney disease: a blinded, placebo-controlled clinical trial. J Feline Med Surg 2015;17(8):692–7.

45. Ramsey DS, Kincaid K, Watkins JA, et al. Safety and efficacy of injectable and oral maropitant, a selective neurokinin 1 receptor antagonist, in a randomized clinical trial for treatment of vomiting in dogs. J Vet Pharmacol Ther 2008;31(6): 538–43.

46. Benson KK, Zajic LB, Morgan PK, et al. Drug exposure and clinical effect of transdermal mirtazapine in healthy young cats: a pilot study. J Feline Med Surg 2017; 19(10). https://doi.org/10.1177/1098612X16667168.

47. Zollers B, Huebner M, Armintrout G, et al. Evaluation of the safety in dogs of long-term, daily oral administration of capromorelin, a novel drug for stimulation of appetite. J Vet Pharmacol Ther 2017;40(3):248–55.

48. de la Puente-Redondo VA, Siedek EM, Benchaoui HA, et al. The anti-emetic efficacy of maropitant (Cerenia) in the treatment of ongoing emesis caused by a wide range of underlying clinical aetiologies in canine patients in Europe. J Small Anim Pract 2007;48(2):93–8.

49. Quimby JM, Gustafson DL, Samber BJ, et al. Studies on the pharmacokinetics and pharmacodynamics of mirtazapine in healthy young cats. J Vet Pharmacol Ther 2011;34(4):388–96.

50. Bozzetti F, Arends J, Lundholm K, et al. ESPEN guidelines on parenteral nutrition: non-surgical oncology. Clin Nutr 2009;28(4):445–54.

51. van Schoor M. How to manage indwelling feeding tubes in critically ill dogs and cats. Vet Nurse 2015;6(2):118–23.

52. Queau Y, Larsen JA, Kass PH, et al. Factors associated with adverse outcomes during parenteral nutrition administration in dogs and cats. J Vet Intern Med 2011;25(3):446–52.

53. Arends J, Bodoky G, Bozzetti F, et al. ESPEN guidelines on enteral nutrition: non-surgical oncology. Clin Nutr 2006;25(2):245–59.

54. McClave SA, Chang W-K. Complications of enteral access. Gastrointest Endosc 2003;58(5):739–51. Available at: http://www.ncbi.nlm.nih.gov/pubmed/ 14595312. Accessed August 31, 2018.

55. Cox S, Goldberg ME. Nursing care for seriously ill animals: art and techniques. In: Shanan A, Pierce J, Shearer T, editors. Hospice and palliative care for companion animals. Hoboken (NJ): John Wiley & Sons, Inc.; 2017. p. 211–30. https://doi.org/ 10.1002/9781119036722.ch21.

56. DACVIM KDMDDvs. Enteral feeding in dogs and cats: indications, principles and techniques (Proceedings). dvm360.com. Available at: http://veterinarycalendar. dvm360.com/enteral-feeding-dogs-and-cats-indications-principles-and-techniqu es-proceedings. Accessed September 3, 2018.
57. Good P, Richard R, Syrmis W, et al. Medically assisted hydration for adult palliative care patients. Cochrane Database Syst Rev 2014;(4):CD006273.
58. Viola RA, Wells GA, Peterson J. The effects of fluid status and fluid therapy on the dying: a systematic review. J Palliat Care 1997;13(4):41–52. Available at: http:// www.ncbi.nlm.nih.gov/pubmed/9447811. Accessed August 31, 2018.
59. Bear AJ, Bukowy EA, Patel JJ. Artificial hydration at the end of life. Nutr Clin Pract 2017;32(5). https://doi.org/10.1177/0884533617724741.

Private Practice Oncology
Viewpoint on End-of-Life Decision-Making

Michael Kiselow, DVM

KEYWORDS

- Oncology • Private practice • Palliative care • Euthanasia • Neoplasia
- Comorbidities

KEY POINTS

- Treatment of veterinary oncology patients involves not only aggressive, anti-tumor modalities, but also ongoing palliative care during the transitional period between cessation of therapy and end-of-life.
- Along with treating neoplastic disease, the veterinary team must also consider comorbidities, which may influence the safety and efficacy of anti-tumor therapies.
- Before and after euthanasia of oncology patients, resources for grief management should be provided to family members.
- Successful management necessitates frequent communication among the pet owner, primary veterinarian, and oncologist.

INTRODUCTION

As the cultural view of companion animals continues to evolve, many people perceive pets to be members of their families, equal in importance to their human counterparts. As such, when it comes to the pursuit of health care—both preventive and for treatment of disease—there is a demand for high-quality veterinary services, including access to veterinarians specializing in individual areas of medical practice. In no other specialty has this change been as evident as in veterinary oncology, which has experienced rapid growth over the past 3 decades. From the early days of the first-established treatment protocols for canine patients with lymphoma in the 1980s,[1] there has been a constantly accelerating expansion of this particular discipline. Large-scale, funded, clinical trials are now commonplace in both veterinary teaching institutions and private practices, and multi-modality treatment regimens including combinations of surgery, radiation therapy, chemotherapy, and immunotherapy represent standard strategies in specialty facilities. Indeed, it is common for families to travel hundreds (in some cases, thousands) of miles to seek out the latest diagnostic

Disclosure Statement: The author has nothing to disclose.
Sage Centers for Veterinary Specialty and Emergency Care, 907 Dell Avenue, Campbell, CA 95008, USA
E-mail address: mkiselow@sagecenters.com

and therapeutic options. This behavior has been catalyzed by the concurrent development of Internet-based resources and social media communication tools, which provide instant access to information for owners seeking care for their pets.

In addition to the impact of technologic developments and resulting advanced care, veterinary medicine has also experienced a cultural revolution regarding end-of-life management for companion animals with terminal diseases. Whereas, in past generations, pets that failed to respond to prescribed therapies would commonly have treatment discontinued altogether, with no further intervention until the family elected to have them euthanized, today's pet owners often wish to maintain rigorous care during the transitional period between termination of aggressive treatment and death. Indeed, over the past 10 years, many veterinarians have shifted the focus of their practice toward providing end-of-life care; some are now exclusively dedicated to these services. This has been likened to hospice medicine in the human health care system, and often involves time-intensive, in-home visits to provide treatment recommendations that incorporate both symptom management and augmentations to the pet's individual environment. Although consistent, standardized definitions of the principles and guidelines under which hospice care should be provided in veterinary medicine are still being developed,[2] one common philosophy among practitioners is the need for a patient-centered transition to death, balanced with attention to the individual needs of a pet's family. This latter component can be multi-dimensional, including services such as pre-emptive and detailed discussions about a pet's final days and death, non-traditional arrangements for the pet's body after it is deceased, and provision of resources for grief management.

The impact of this trend on private referral oncology practice has been manifold. Primarily, it is evident in the expectations of clients as well as available options for palliative support beyond standard oncologic care. The role of the oncologist in providing emotional support to clients has also expanded, although no additional standardized training for veterinary oncologists exists to address how to perform this part of the job. This article will provide an overview of private practice oncology referral as it relates to end-of-life issues and decision-making. Its focus is patient care and dynamics between client, oncologist, and referring veterinarian, rather than treatment protocols or biologic behavior of disease. Its goal is to provide a framework for the medical aspects of care, which often dominate treatment planning and client communication.

THE ONCOLOGY REFERRAL

The professional relationship between veterinary specialists and general practitioners is one that continues to evolve as specialization becomes more common, and as the technologies for treating complex diseases become more advanced and readily available. Developing and fostering this partnership is essential for provision of the highest-quality care for veterinary patients, and is a responsibility that requires ongoing contributions from both parties.

Most cancers will be initially diagnosed by the primary veterinarian, who may subsequently arrange for referral to a specialty clinic for further diagnostic evaluation and treatment. Effective communication between veterinarians is of paramount importance for providing accurate client education, prompt referral once requested, and optimal management of complex diseases. It is therefore the duty of the specialty clinic to request all relevant case information for review before consultation, and the referring clinic to ensure that complete, concise medical records are submitted in a timely manner.

INITIAL ONCOLOGY CONSULTATION

As most cancers known to afflict veterinary patients have been well described in peer-reviewed literature, an essential part of the initial oncology consultation involves an assessment of the stage of disease within an individual pet. Not completely understanding this process, many pet owners—frightened by the diagnosis of cancer—will arrive at appointments with a list of questions pertaining to prognosis, clinical signs, and impact of the disease on quality of life. Although these questions are certainly relevant, and are ultimately influential for a client's decision-making process regarding therapy, performing additional staging diagnostic tests is necessary to provide the most accurate prognostic information.

Equally important is an understanding of comorbidities, which may have significant implications for progression of a specific case—not only for guiding diagnostic and therapeutic recommendations, but also for determining prognosis. Many clients arrive at appointments having already researched their pet's diagnosis, and therefore have preliminary notions of outcome. However, it is common for this information to be incomplete and/or incorrect, such that a thorough and clear description of the disease should be provided to rectify any misunderstandings. Furthermore, even if an individual pet's cancer is treatable, concurrent diseases may complicate—or in some instances completely preclude—anti-neoplastic therapy.

Based on findings from this initial assessment, clear, frank discussions may proceed outlining objectives for managing a pet's disease. Clarifying goals, which can be incongruent between pet owners and the veterinary team, is critical for cultivating trust and mutual understanding as diagnostic and treatment plans are formulated. In some cases, a client may have unrealistic expectations—such as avoiding all adverse effects from therapy, or ensuring a specific survival time. It is therefore essential to engage in honest, compassionate dialogue, so that both established facts and uncertainties of the case are reviewed openly, the client feels comfortable to ask additional questions, and that a mutually agreed upon action plan can be reached. As described previously, the Internet has afforded the current generation of pet owners a unique opportunity to easily research their pets' diagnoses before consulting with an oncologist. Unfortunately, the quality and reliability of sources that pet owners may encounter online are highly variable, ranging from peer-viewed, scientific literature and veterinarian-sponsored layperson education programs, to pet owner forums and individual blogs. The latter, although potentially helpful for allowing owners to connect and empathize over shared experiences navigating their pets' diseases, can also lead to the propagation of erroneous information in the form of misunderstanding of pathophysiology and adherence to anecdotal case outcomes that may not accurately reflect established, scientific knowledge.

It is also important to educate clients about the financial implications of working with a specialty hospital. Although monetary conversations can be awkward, especially in the emotionally charged context of a cancer diagnosis, the inevitable reality is that the provision of advanced, anti-neoplastic therapies for companion animals is expensive. Although utilization of veterinary health insurance has become more common in recent years, most owners still pay out-of-pocket for their pets' medical care. Certainly, the costs of therapy should never be a primary motivating factor for the veterinary medical team. However, it is still essential to be transparent and direct with pet owners regarding anticipated fees. Furthermore, discussions about finances must be guided by the veterinary care team in consideration of an individual patient's prognosis.

As is common in human oncology, some cancers in animals are diagnosed in advanced stages, and/or are known to be poorly responsive to treatment, such that efforts to control the disease can be futile. It is therefore of paramount importance that veterinarians provide honest and accurate prognostic information so that clients may be guided toward financially responsible decisions. Unfortunately, it is very common for owners to succumb to feelings of fear ("I cannot imagine losing him to this disease") or guilt ("I could not live with myself if I did not give her every possible chance"), which can result in expensive diagnostics and treatments being performed despite a low likelihood of clinical benefit. It is fairly common for pet owners to insist on therapies that are expected to be of little-to-no value to patients. The concept of medical futility is broadly debated in human medicine, particularly among hospice specialists, and is considered a crucial factor for quality of life scoring. In contrast, this concept receives minimal attention in veterinary curricula, and therefore represents an important educational opportunity for veterinarians, who—despite their medical training—are unprepared to navigate these emotionally complex conversations. In addition, the legal status of pets as personal property further complicates the matter, as owners feel entitled to demand specific treatments. Ultimately, if a pet owner's mind cannot be changed following discussion of the futile nature of a pet's disease, the veterinarian is not legally obligated to provide elective therapies, and has the option of declining care that s/he feels is medically inappropriate.

In contrast, occasionally the diagnosis of an early-stage disease, which may be associated with a favorable prognosis, will prompt the veterinary team to encourage owners to pursue aggressive therapy, or—perhaps subconsciously—to frame prognostic information in a more-positive light than would be presented for a patient with advanced disease. Such bias is a well-documented phenomenon.[3] However, some clients may not be inclined to pursue such treatment, and instead may elect conservative management, with a shift to less-intensive, palliative care as the disease progresses. In these instances, it is important to respect and support the owners' decisions, and to continue providing guidance as changes in the pet's status emerge.

THE TREATMENT PROTOCOL

Once a therapeutic plan is agreed on and enacted, the oncologist should communicate regularly with the patient's owners. This serves to continually advise them of achievements/progression of the process, as well as to maintain an open dialogue so that questions may be answered as needed. This frequent interaction can be empowering for family members—who may initially feel fearful and submissive to the direction of the doctor—and is therefore essential for building and maintaining trust. Furthermore, if the initial treatment protocol fails and disease progression is noted, the clients should again be educated in continued effort to support informed decision-making. Depending on the specifics of the individual case, this may involve reviewing basic information provided in the original consultation following a pet's initial diagnosis, outlining secondary ("rescue") therapies, or recommending the transition to less-aggressive, palliative care.

The oncologist should also provide frequent updates to the primary veterinarian, particularly when significant changes in patient status are identified (eg, remission, complications from therapy, disease progression). This not only fosters collaboration and professional courtesy, but also reduces the risk of medical errors if an unscheduled examination is required with the primary veterinarian, who may not have otherwise seen the patient in several weeks or months.

MANAGING COMORBIDITIES

As most veterinary oncology patients are adult-to-geriatric in age, many will present with one or more pre-existing medical conditions. Although usually unrelated to their oncologic diagnosis, these comorbidities may influence diagnostic and/or therapeutic options for their cancers. For example, a cat with an injection-associated fibrosarcoma and chronic renal failure may be at risk for exacerbation of azotemia when anesthetized for a staging computed tomography scan (which typically involves administration of potentially nephrotoxic contrast agents); an obese, arthritic dog with appendicular osteosarcoma may be a poor candidate for amputation because of expected difficulties with ambulation following surgery; a canine patient with lymphoma and pre-existing cardiomyopathy may not be able to safely receive doxorubicin chemotherapy because of its known cardiotoxic effects.

Fortunately, it is uncommon for concurrent diseases to completely impede treatment of cancer. Nevertheless, it is the responsibility of the managing oncologist to work collaboratively with the primary veterinarian, and with other specialists, to ensure all relevant diseases are considered appropriately. Indeed, management of oncology patients in a specialty facility typically allows for rapid, in-house consultation among doctors to augment treatment regimens regularly for continual refinement of care. These strategies must also be clearly conveyed to the pet owners, who should be aware of not only the potential complications of treating multiple diseases, but also of the additional logistical and financial implications.

END-OF-LIFE CARE IN ONCOLOGY PRACTICE

In the context of veterinary oncology, many patients' diseases will ultimately result in their death, even with aggressive treatment efforts. As such, discussions regarding end-of-life care can be just as important as those outlining complex treatments focused on trying to control progression of cancer. Indeed, on learning of cancer diagnosis, many pet owners will decline anti-tumor therapy, and will instead focus efforts on conservative, palliative strategies. Furthermore, even when clients initially elect aggressive therapies, many still request information about prognosis and end-of-life management to prepare themselves logistically and emotionally for their eventual loss. Such conversations may certainly be guided by the primary veterinarian. However, some clients—and even some veterinarians—still prefer referral to an oncologist to ensure that all information regarding the biologic behavior of a particular disease and treatment options are understood, including options for palliative care.

Many oncology patients will eventually develop clinical signs that significantly affect quality of life. It is common for owners to not understand the severity of their pets' decline and clinical signs. It is therefore incumbent on the veterinary care team to serve as the patient's advocate and to guide clients toward palliative therapies, including euthanasia if deemed medically appropriate and in the patient's best interests. If primary, anti-neoplastic therapy is discontinued (due to exhaustion of options, severity of clinical signs, and/or client decision), strategies for palliative care should be considered. These will vary depending on type/stage of cancer, as well as the specific signs experienced by an individual patient. Treatments may include, but are not limited to, anti-emetic/anti-diarrheal medications, analgesics, diuretics, anti-tussives, antibiotics, acupuncture, and physical therapy. Palliative measures are also provided by oncologists along with targeted, curative therapies throughout the treatment trajectory.

Palliative therapies may include strategies that are more technologically and logistically involved, yet are still primarily focused on mitigating clinical signs of a disease. Examples include placement of urethral stents to alleviate obstruction from transitional cell carcinoma[4]; application of brief courses of radiation therapy for curbing epistaxis from intra-nasal tumors[5]; administration of bisphosphonates for reducing pain associated with primary and metastatic bone tumors.[6] Although some of these modalities may certainly slow the progression of cancer, their principal goal is palliative, not life-prolonging in nature, and the intensity of treatment may be attenuated to minimize adverse effects.

Euthanasia in Oncology Practice

Traditionally, euthanasia for companion animals has been performed in the veterinary clinic. Families would occasionally inquire about the possibility of having it done at home, but this service was largely unavailable. However, this model has shifted over the past decade, and in-home, end-of-life care is now commonplace. In this author's experience, pet owners' responses to this option are variable: some are relieved to know their pet does not need to endure the stress of a car ride before euthanasia. In contrast, others quickly express discomfort with the prospect of seeing their deceased pet in their home. Nevertheless, all appreciate learning of the option. It is therefore important for both primary and specialty veterinarians to be familiar with these services, and to develop professional relationships with in-home providers to facilitate referrals for euthanasia when requested.

Whether euthanasia is performed in the veterinary clinic or in a pet owner's home, the experience should be conducted to help the family feel as comfortable as possible. In addition to honing the medical and technical aspects of euthanasia, attention to interpersonal relationships can help to transform what may be perceived as an abrupt, one-dimensional procedure into a shared, human experience between family and veterinarian. Indeed, this may help to diffuse emotional tension not only for the grieving family, but also for the veterinary team, which also often feels personally invested in the patient after having provided long-term care.

Continuous support of the primary veterinarian is of paramount importance when managing animals that are referred to an oncologist following a diagnosis of cancer. This includes the need for immediate notification following the euthanasia of a mutual patient. Not only does this allow for the primary veterinary clinic staff to extend its sympathy, but also helps to avoid the potentially awkward scenario in which the veterinarian unknowingly contacts the client for a status update and inadvertently upsets members of the family.

Human Support in Oncology Practice

Although euthanasia often represents the final step in relief of suffering associated with the progression of a patient's cancer, further attention to the pet's family members is also warranted, as clients' grief typically continues long after the final encounter with the veterinary team. Along with the extension of simple, yet meaningful, gestures such as sympathy cards and flowers, veterinarians should also provide pet owners with information regarding options for grief support. Although compassionate euthanasia practices are likely to minimize complicated grief, many clients will still benefit from additional and ongoing emotional support. This requires both time commitment and professional training beyond veterinarians' scope of practice. Fortunately, social workers are being integrated into more veterinary practices, and there are numerous resources that are readily accessible by phone and the Internet.[7] Furthermore, as the concepts of professional burnout, moral distress, and compassion fatigue continue to be defined and evaluated within the veterinary profession, licensed mental health support services are being extended to the veterinary care team in addition to clients.[8]

Currently, the author's organization (comprised of 4 clinics within a 70-mile radius) employs a Licensed Marriage and Family Therapist who is also a certified pet loss and bereavement counselor. She provides free services to people in various stages of emotional distress associated with their pets' illnesses. These occur as anonymous telephone conversations, and as group meetings with multiple families (rotating among facilities). Both opportunities are used regularly, and have been very well received by our clientele. In addition, in an effort to support the veterinary staff, this counselor leads sessions intended to define common workplace stressors and to brainstorm solutions for lessening their impact on wellbeing.

Accompanying the positive feedback related to this service has been the realization that it needs to be expanded to provide broader access—for clients and for employees. Indeed, the psychological needs of people facing the impending loss of their pet often exceed the availability and professional training of the veterinary staff. As such, supporting dedicated, on-site, mental health professionals is an area of active development, not only in our organization, but also within many veterinary teaching institutions and private specialty hospitals.

UNIQUE END-OF-LIFE CARE EXPERIENCES IN ONCOLOGY PRACTICE

Veterinary oncologists engage in conversations about death—and provide euthanasia—on a frequent basis. Nevertheless, it is important to remain present and open-minded for each family, as needs can vary. In this author's experience, following descriptions of routine end-of-life options, most owners elect for euthanasia to occur in the veterinary clinic. This often takes place in the specialty hospital, although some people decide to return to their primary veterinarian. Occasionally, unique requests are made based on an individual family's beliefs and/or specific end-of-life plan for the pet. As long as these do not negatively affect the patient, every effort is made to accommodate these final wishes. Examples have included.

Having Other Family Pets Present

Some people express concern about the emotional impact of the loss of one pet on other animals in the home. They therefore bring these housemates to witness the act of euthanasia in effort to provide them with the opportunity to recognize the loss.

Witnessing Sedation Only

In the author's clinic, barbiturate administration is preceded by heavy sedation (typically Propofol). Although most family members remain present until their pet is pronounced dead, some will ask to leave between medications (ie, following sedation, but before barbiturate).

Not Being Present

Rarely, pet owners decline being present for euthanasia, and instead elect to leave the clinic before the pet is deceased. Similar situations have occurred for patients that are hospitalized for several days, wherein the election of euthanasia is made over the phone, and the family decides to not return to the clinic. These instances have been particularly challenging for the veterinary staff, who are emotionally invested in the patients, and who—although usually in support of the decision to euthanize—will commonly express their dismay at the notion of the patient not having family present for its final moments. Once confirmed (verbal authorization for euthanasia involves pet owners sharing their decision with 2 doctors for documentation), euthanasia is performed immediately. Afterward, this author invites feedback from the nursing team to provide an opportunity for case debriefing and sharing of any concerns.

Request for "Natural" Death

Occasionally, people express an intention to never euthanize their pet, often citing religious or other personal beliefs. This decision has the potential to elicit criticism from the veterinary staff. Indeed, this is a product of the culture of modern veterinary medicine, wherein the unofficial dogma states that pets should ultimately die from chemical intervention. This is an intriguing contrast to human medicine, in which doctor-facilitated death has only recently started to gain societal acceptance. Nevertheless, it is important to foster a direct, respectful conversation, involving an explanation of the reasons for this choice, as well as an understanding of the family's alternative end-of-life plan for their pet. In this author's experience, many pet owners change their minds after understanding the anticipated clinical signs associated with progression of their pets' diseases, and ultimately elect euthanasia. However, for those whose minds are unwavering, it is essential that the veterinary team remains actively involved to provide both guidance and continued, non-lethal medical treatments to minimize pain, anxiety, and any other clinical signs observed during a pet's dying process.

Request for Cloning

Among the myriad commercial services that have accompanied the evolution of biotechnology over the past 20 years are options for pet owners to replicate their deceased pets. These products are marketed directly to pet owners, and only involve veterinarians for the step of sample retrieval. Owners purchase "kits," which include vials of preservation media for patient tissues (typically multiple skin biopsies, collected immediately post-mortem), that are returned to the companies by the pet's family. In this author's experience, cloning requests are often met by the staff with skepticism, but have rarely been decried as ethically objectionable.

Overall, these experiences have served as profound educational moments, such that end-of-life plans do not—and should not—always proceed according to a single, rigid protocol. Quite the contrary; in this era when pets are considered family members, it is essential that every [medically sound] effort be made to grant clients' final wishes to optimize healthy grieving following the loss of their animal.

Finally, it is common for oncology patients treated in private specialty hospitals to have been managed by a variety of doctors within different departments. As such, the emotional impact of patient death is often felt by several members of the doctor and nursing staff. Therefore, along with providing logistical and grief-related support for the pet's family, it is important to acknowledge the shared sense of loss among the medical team. This occurs both formally and informally in this author's clinic, from impromptu debriefings and collegial support, to official morbidity and mortality rounds, wherein cases are reviewed extensively to identify and learn from unique/unexpected challenges encountered before death.

SUMMARY

Despite the many advances achieved over the past 30 years within the specialty of veterinary oncology, many patients still ultimately succumb to their disease. Therefore, as clinical research continues and new therapies are developed, concurrent effort must also be lent to the ongoing education of veterinarians and pet owners regarding the many available treatment options for patients with terminal disease, as well as when and whether to use them. As outlined herein, this involves not only an understanding of pathophysiology and mechanisms of palliative therapies, but also an awareness of the emotional and psychological needs of pet owners as they proceed through their grieving process. Finally, a commitment to supporting clients through end-of-life management of their pets can also help the veterinary care team achieve personal closure following the loss of patients.

REFERENCES

1. Vail DM, Pinkerton ME, Young KM. Hematopoietic tumors. In: Withrow SJ, Vail DM, Page RL, editors. Withrow & MacEwen's small animal clinical oncology. 5th edition. St Louis (MO): Elsevier Saunders; 2013. p. 608–38.
2. Goldberg K. Veterinary hospice and palliative care: a comprehensive review of the literature. Vet Rec 2016;178:369–74.
3. Groopman J. In service of the soul. In: How doctors think. Boston: Houghton Mifflin; 2007. p. 234–59.
4. Blackburn A, Berent AC, Weisse CW, et al. Evaluation of outcome following urethral stent placement for the treatment of obstructive carcinoma of the urethra in dogs: 42 cases (2004-2008). J Am Vet Med Assoc 2013;242:59–68.
5. Gieger T, Rassnick K, Siegel S, et al. Palliation of clinical signs in 48 dogs with nasal carcinoma treated with coarse-fraction radiation therapy. J Am Anim Hosp Assoc 2008;44:116–23.
6. Fan T, de Lorimier L, Garrett L, et al. The bone biologic effects of zoledronate in healthy dogs and dogs with malignant osteolysis. J Vet Intern Med 2008;22:380–7.
7. Argus Institute Counseling and Support Services. Available at: http://csu-cvmbs. colostate.edu/vth/diagnostic-and-support/argus/Pages/default.aspx. Accessed September 23, 2018.
8. Kahler S. Moral stress the top trigger in veterinarians' compassion fatigue: veterinary social worker suggests redefining veterinarians' ethical responsibility. J Am Vet Med Assoc 2015;246:16–8.

Palliative Care Services at Home

Viewpoint from a Multidoctor Practice

Courtney Bennett, DVM[1], Nathaniel Cook, DVM*

KEYWORDS

- Mobile veterinary practice • Severe illness • Terminal illness • Palliative care
- Hospice care • End-of-life care • In-home euthanasia
- Hospice-assisted natural death

KEY POINTS

- Although veterinary hospice and palliative care are still in the early stages of growth and development, demand for these services among families with pets is increasing.
- All patients with chronic debilitating conditions and/or serious or terminal illness should be offered hospice and palliative care services, even if the plan is still to pursue curative therapy.
- Earlier referral and implementation of hospice and palliative care services is one of the most significant issues being faced.
- Frequent, in-depth communication and regular appointments for patient reassessment are critical in providing hospice and palliative care services that support both patients and caregivers.
- Strengthening collaboration between hospice and palliative care providers and primary/specialty care veterinarians has the potential to streamline patient care and optimize convenience for the patients and their families.

INTRODUCTION

The availability of veterinary care services focused on palliative, hospice, and end-of-life (EOL) care is a fairly new option for families with pets. Companion animals are living longer lives, and likewise families want to make sure that their pets are comfortable and well cared for in their senior and geriatric years. In addition, there has been an increase in the demand for more advanced and specialized care for pets with serious illness and/or chronic illness. Although use of mobile euthanasia services is well accepted and available in veterinary medicine, services focused on all forms of

Disclosure: The authors have nothing to disclose.
Heart's Ease Veterinary Care, Louisville, KY, USA
[1] 1437 Story Avenue, Louisville KY 40206.
* Corresponding author. 1437 Story Avenue, Louisville, KY 40206.
E-mail address: ncook@heartseasevet.com

Vet Clin Small Anim 49 (2019) 529–551
https://doi.org/10.1016/j.cvsm.2019.01.018
0195-5616/19/© 2019 Elsevier Inc. All rights reserved.

palliative medicine (palliative, hospice, and EOL care) remain unavailable in many areas. In addition, awareness of comprehensive hospice and palliative care (HPC) services for animals is still limited within both the pet-owning public and the veterinary profession. This article describes the patient population of a growing, multidoctor, mobile palliative care practice with services exclusively dedicated to palliative medicine, hospice, and EOL care in Louisville, Kentucky.

THE PHILOSOPHY OF HOSPICE AND CRITERIA FOR PATIENT ENTRY

Hospice is not a specific place or therapy, but instead a philosophy of care. The terms palliative medicine, palliative care, hospice care, and EOL care describe supports and interventions that are aligned with hospice philosophy but represent distinct aspects of care. This article uses the term hospice and palliative medicine (HPM) to describe medical interventions (including EOL care, such as in-home euthanasia) that are associated with the broader term of HPC. The philosophy of hospice prioritizes comfort and quality of life (QOL) for patients with chronic and debilitating conditions, and severe or terminal illness, and any patient in the final stages of life. There is a shift away from the predominant medical goal of prioritizing QOL above all by pursuing curative therapies. For some medical conditions there is no cure, and, for others, pursuing a cure might involve therapies that are undesirable or unavailable for veterinary patients. In these cases, it is still possible to improve a patient's comfort and QOL by implementing an HPM program; this may also give the patient's family more time with their pet. HPM services generally involve managing symptoms (especially pain, nausea, and anxiety) for the patient and providing compassionate communication, education on caregiving, and counseling services to help support the patient's family and other caregivers.

In veterinary medicine, as in human medicine, it is at the request of the family and/or advice of the primary care and/or specialty care veterinarians that HPM services are pursued. Unlike in human medicine, where dependence on health insurance often defines the path of medical care, there are currently no specific eligibility criteria for HPM services in veterinary medicine. In addition, there is no real consensus among families with pets or the veterinary community at large regarding when HPM should formally begin or referral should be provided.

This article considers EOL services as a segment of HPM in veterinary medicine, which includes euthanasia, hospice-assisted death without euthanasia, death without any medical intervention, and provision or coordination of aftercare arrangements such as burial or cremation with any of these outcomes; this constitutes an important difference between veterinary and human medicine because EOL services in veterinary medicine may include euthanasia. Although veterinary euthanasia is legal and has widespread acceptance, defining criteria for when euthanasia should be recommended, provided, or even allowed is a complex issue. Just as euthanasia is accepted as a means of providing a gentle death in veterinary medicine, it is important to understand that some families hope to support their pets through the dying process without euthanasia. Although the authors have had many families express interest in avoiding euthanasia if possible, we have found that most families do not maintain this position if there is a prolonged period of impaired QOL requiring intensive caretaking or complete loss of QOL requiring palliative sedation. A complete discussion of the ethics of euthanasia is beyond the scope of this article. Euthanasia is defined and understood in this article as a medical procedure that can be used to help pets when there is no longer the opportunity to prevent suffering, and/or a poor QOL persists, even with provision of the elected veterinary (and other) care services.

Although it is important to increase awareness, understanding, and availability of HPM services in veterinary medicine within the profession, the autonomy of veterinarians and veterinary clients to decide whether and when HPM services will be recommended and/or pursued also needs to be respected. To aid in navigating this process, at our clinic, we have defined the levels of care described in **Table 1** to indicate patient criteria for enrollment in HPM and also requirements to maintain care in terms of minimal communication and appointments. Because HPM is very much a hands-on form of medicine, regular communication and appointments to discuss and identify changes in patient and family/caregiver conditions and concerns is of vital importance to providing effective care. By defining these levels of care, it is also our goal to help guide families about what care is needed based on the pet's current condition.

CHALLENGES AND BENEFITS OF A MOBILE PALLIATIVE MEDICINE PRACTICE

The challenges and benefits of a mobile clinic offering HPM services are not mutually exclusive, which means that many of the challenges of providing this type of care also provide a benefit to one or more stakeholders. It is also important to note that most of

Table 1
Levels of care in hospice and palliative care

Level of Care	Communication	Ongoing Care Appointments
Palliative care	Every 2–4 wk	Every 1–3 mo

- Patients who are stable and either have not been diagnosed with a terminal diagnosis or are in the early stages of a slowly progressive terminal diagnosis, and/or have 1 or more chronic and debilitating health conditions
- Unlikely to require emergency care, significantly deteriorate, die, or be euthanized within 1–3 mo
- Examples:
  - Chronic pain conditions, such as DJD/osteoarthritis
  - Early-stage organ failure, such as IRIS stage 1/2 CKD
  - Early stages of some cancer types, such as hepatocellular carcinoma

Early Hospice Care	Every 1–2 wk	Every 2–4 wk

- Patients who are relatively stable but have been diagnosed with a terminal illness, and/or have 1 or more chronic and debilitating health conditions
- May require emergency care from time to time, and/or may significantly deteriorate, die, or be euthanized within 1–2 mo
- Examples:
  - Later stages of organ failure (most CHF, IRIS stage 3/4 CKD)
  - Most patients with cancer

Advanced Hospice Care	Every 1–7 d	Daily Every 2 wk

- Patients with any terminal diagnosis or severe illness who are unstable and any patient who is already in the process of dying
- Likely to need emergency care, and/or may significantly deteriorate, die, or be euthanized at any time
- Examples:
  - Patient with splenic/metastatic hemangiosarcoma who has had a bleeding event and who may or may not recompensate
  - All patients receiving care for hospice-assisted natural death

Abbreviations: CHF; congestive heart failure; CKD, chronic kidney disease; DJD, degenerative joint disease; IRIS, International Renal Interest Society.

these challenges are present to some degree for all veterinarians and clinics, whether mobile or not, and whether offering HPM (including EOL services such as euthanasia) or not. These challenges include:

- Cost of care
- Patient and family compliance
- Effective and timely communication
- Scheduling and availability
- Appointment preparations
- Managing veterinarians and staff

This article discusses many of the challenges and benefits commonly faced in the provision of mobile HPM, using examples from our practice.

Cost of Care, Compliance, and Communication

These 3 Cs represent 3 of the most common challenges of providing excellent veterinary medicine services. All veterinarians must work through the difficulties of the cost of care, compliance (both from the patients and the families), and ways to communicate effectively. When good solutions or compromises are found that maintain patient care and also are affordable, improve compliance, and promote effective communication, everyone benefits. For example, sometimes a less expensive medication can be used, an easier method of delivering medication to the patient can be found, or a more convenient mode of communication (such as email) can be used.

Cost of care

In contrast with in-clinic veterinary care, the primary costs to families for mobile HPM services are usually appointment and travel fees rather than procedures, diagnostic testing, and medications/treatments. In mobile HPM, appointments are much longer than most in-clinic appointments for several reasons, but the 2 most important are the time needed to travel to and from the appointment and the longer appointment time needed to adequately communicate based on the complexity of caring for HPM patients. For some patients, medications/therapies do become a significant cost, and, for patients with a finicky or poor appetite, food costs can also be very high. Of course, operating costs, including doctors' salaries, have to be balanced with the ability of families to afford care, and this means that mobile services for HPM are likely to be at the higher end of the spectrum of cost for veterinary services overall.

Compliance

Most families who seek HPM services for their pets are highly motivated caregivers, and try hard to adhere to the recommended care plan. In cases in which there is a lack of compliance, the authors have found that one or more of the following is often at play:

- Lack of patient compliance, meaning they might not allow or might object to the therapy (such as not taking medications reliably)
- Disagreement within the family about what care is needed/desired
- Breakdown in communication, such as the cost being too high, but not communicating this to the veterinarian

One of the greatest benefits of in-home HPM is an improved ability to reduce stress for the patients and understand individual concerns, which often also helps to improve compliance.

It is the responsibility of the veterinarian and staff to advocate for the patient first, meaning that, if the patient's QOL is deteriorating, changes in the care plan are needed.

Communication

It is well recognized that effective, in-depth, and ongoing communication is a tenet of HPM. Excellent communication skills are important for all veterinarians and are essential in providing HPM services. The following are some of the most important considerations for effective communication in HPM:

- Veterinarians' and staff's ability to communicate effectively with families in a difficult and emotional time and provide education around patient care
- Family's ability and willingness to communicate effectively with the veterinarian and staff
- Family's ability and willingness to communicate effectively with each other
- Family's ability to make decisions when time dependent/urgent

The authors have found that the communication that takes place in the family/patient's home during mobile HPM consultations is often much more comfortable and less intimidating than trying to have these discussions in a clinical setting. It is particularly helpful for all family members who are participating in the patient's care to be present during appointments. Veterinarians with a calm, patient demeanor, who are good listeners, and who can explain complex medical topics in a clear and concise way are particularly adept at providing HPM services.

Sometimes though, especially for ongoing communications about particularly emotional topics, email and forms of indirect communication can be less intimidating and therefore more effective. Examples of indirect communication include handouts, surveys, and questionnaires. The authors have found email to be an invaluable part of ongoing communication in HPM services, and also frequently use questionnaires, handouts, and surveys. These materials can be particularly helpful for topics that are difficult to discuss and/or require a lot of thought and consideration. **Fig. 1** is a preplanning questionnaire about planning ahead for EOL services. Our QOL scale (**Fig. 2**) is another questionnaire we developed as a tool to help families in monitoring their pets' QOL. We developed this scale in order to help families monitor their pets' QOL with a quick daily exercise, designed to take no more than 3 to 5 min/d. Our scale is loosely based on the HHHHHMM (hurt, hunger, hydration, hygiene, happiness, mobility and more good days than bad days) QOL scale first presented by Dr Alice Villalobos.[1] Our goal with questionnaires such as these is to find a way to make it easier to start and/or maintain difficult conversations. These conversations, difficult as they may be, are even harder if they are attempted at the last minute or in an emergency situation. In addition, patient care will almost certainly be affected negatively if these conversations are neglected.

Scheduling and Availability

Day-to-day appointment scheduling and maintaining the ability to provide urgent and emergency appointments are some of the most challenging aspects of a mobile veterinary HPM clinic. Although overbooked schedules are common in all veterinary clinics, scheduling for mobile clinics is particularly challenging for 3 reasons:

- Longer appointment times needed for in-depth discussion and care
- Inability to multitask between patients
- Travel between locations

Planning Ahead

Please take some time to consider these difficult but important questions so that we can work together to provide the end of life care best for your pet. When you are ready, please share your plans with us so that we may help carry out your wishes (it is ok to email or fax this page to us).

Your Pet's Name: _____ **Date:** _____

❖ Are there experiences and/or activities you want to enjoy with or provide for your pet before you say good – bye (car rides, favorite meals, photo shoot, videos, party with friends, etc.)?
  ◆ *You could also think of this as a "bucket list".*

❖ Are there things you want to avoid during this stage of your pet's life?
  ◆ *This might include things like hospitalization, invasive therapies, and stressful events.*

❖ Do you have specific questions or concerns about making the decision for end of life care?
  ◆ *Past experiences may have shown you what you do or do not want for your pet.*
  ◆ *This also includes considerations surrounding your belief system and whether you consider euthanasia to be a potential option to help your pet (see page 5).*

❖ What do you consider to be the stopping points for your pet's care?
  ◆ *Please also consider any limitations (physical, emotional, financial, etc.) of how much are you willing/able to go through for the possibility of more time together.*

❖ Do you have specific wishes during your pet's end of life care appointment?
  ◆ *This might include things like location (such as being at home—and in a favorite place), having friends & family present, special foods or treats, music, candles, and readings.*

❖ What aftercare arrangements would you prefer?
  ◆ *For cremation, would you like to have ashes returned, or for burial, have you chosen a location?*
  ◆ *Would you like to have memorial keepsakes (eg, paw prints, fur clippings, urns, etc.).*

Heart's Ease Veterinary Care, ©2018 ·

Fig. 1. Planning ahead.

We find that our schedule varies considerably seasonally, week to week, and even day to day. Careful planning, attention to travel time between appointments, reserving space for emergencies, and setting realistic expectations with families regarding availability of emergency care (and cost) are all critical to managing the schedule. Flexibility

PATIENT NAME: _____   QOL (Quality of Life) Evaluation Scale

MO: ___	MON	TUES	WED	THURS	FRI	SAT	SUN	WEEKLY TOTAL
1 Ease of Breathing	/3	/3	/3	/3	/3	/3	/3	
Ability to breathe freely and easily with normal effort and a normal respiratory rate. **THIS IS THE TOP PRIORITY. ANY SCORE LESS THAN "3" NEEDS TO BE ADDRESSED IMMEDIATELY.**								/ 21
2 Pain Control	/3	/3	/3	/3	/3	/3	/3	
Ability to feel comfortable and pain-free (with prescribed medications, supplements, and physical therapies).								/ 21
3 Basic Faculties	/3	/3	/3	/3	/3	/3	/3	
Ability to eat & maintain body condition, drink & maintain hydration, and eliminate (urinate & defecate) comfortably.								/ 21
4 Mobility & Activity	/3	/3	/3	/3	/3	/3	/3	
Ability to accomplish needed/desired activities with an acceptable amount of help.								/ 21
5 Cleanliness & Hygiene	/3	/3	/3	/3	/3	/3	/3	
Ability to keep clean & maintain hygiene (including oral hygiene) with an acceptable amount of help.								/ 21
6 Your Pet's Happiness	/3	/3	/3	/3	/3	/3	/3	
Your pet's ability to participate in life and the current care plan while maintaining comfort, contentment, and enjoyment of life. **Includes that none of the current treatments are causing undue emotional or physical stress to your pet.**								/ 21
7 Your Family's Happiness	/3	/3	/3	/3	/3	/3	/3	
Your family's ability to participate in the current care plan for your pet as well as comfort and understanding of the care being provided. **Includes that none of the current treatments are causing undue emotional or physical stress to the family.**								/ 21
DAILY TOTAL	/ 21	/ 21	/ 21	/ 21	/ 21	/ 21	/ 21	/ 147
0: Unacceptable/Absent 1: So – So/Needs Improvement 2: Acceptable/Decent 3: No Concerns								
Please call or email to discuss if: A score of "0" for any category, a daily total < 14 / 21, or a weekly total of < 98 / 147.								
Based on the HHHHHMM Scale developed by Dr. Alice Villalobos (www.pawspice.com).								

© Heart's Ease Veterinary Care, 2017

Fig. 2. QOL scale.

on the part of the veterinarians and staff is absolutely required but maintaining work-life balance and setting boundaries are essential for sustainability.

A great help in scheduling can be to define the types of appointments offered, meaning what they entail and how much time is allotted. Defining appointment types (**Table 2**) helps the veterinarian (and clinic staff) to prepare for the appointment in advance and can also help to guide expectations of families. Although an excessive number of appointment types may be burdensome to manage, the authors have found that some delineation is extremely helpful. For example, although an initial consultation and QOL evaluation consultation have the potential to have the same outcome of enrolling a patient in HPM, there is the critical difference that the materials need to be ready for EOL services, such as in-home euthanasia, for QOL evaluation consultations. It is the veterinarian's responsibility to manage time during the appointment to adhere to recommended time frames as much as possible. It is inevitable that extenuating circumstances arise frequently, such as unexpected examination findings causing the need for additional treatments and therapies and/or more extensive explanations and discussion.

In managing a mobile clinic for HPM services, it is not possible to only travel to certain areas each day, as is common for many mobile primary care practices. Therefore, defining a realistic service area is essential. This point is of particular importance when traveling between appointments and on days when urgent care and emergency appointments are needed. The authors have defined our regular travel area as a 48-km (30-mile)/45-min radius, but this needs to be tailored to meet the specifics of each locale. We also frequently see patients in an extended service area when possible, especially for EOL services if local resources for mobile HPM services are less available.

Although there is an ebb and flow in requests for appointments for new patients, it is often a challenge to be available for urgent care requests in a timely manner, and at a

Table 2
Appointment types in hospice and palliative medicine

Appointment Types	Time	Goals of Appointment
Initial consultation for palliative/ hospice care	≥2 h	• Discuss history and current conditions • Discuss patient and family goals • Implement initial care plan
QOL evaluation consultation (includes option for in-home euthanasia on same appointment)	≥2 h	• Discuss history and current conditions • Discuss patient and family goals • QOL evaluation using QOL scale • Decide on euthanasia vs initiating palliative/hospice care
Ongoing care consultations	45–60 min	• Physical examination and reassess patient status • Discuss recommendations with family • Adjust treatments and care plan
Treatment and service visits	30–45 min	• Brief examination and consultation • Provide specific services, such as diagnostic testing, minor procedures, or therapeutic treatments
In-home euthanasia	1 h	• Greet family and pet to establish trust and a stress/fear-free environment • If needed, give pain medication immediately • Carefully discuss options for procedure, aftercare, and keepsakes • Provide gentle euthanasia services • Provide dignified aftercare services
Deceased pet services	1 h	• Confirm death and counsel family on possible cause of death if desired • Carefully discuss options for aftercare and keepsakes • Provide dignified aftercare services

time that is preferable or needed for the family/patient. In many cases we are contacted for same-day appointments, which can be difficult to coordinate because of the scheduling considerations already mentioned. In these cases, patient triage and screening are needed before making schedule changes. Our general triage procedure includes the following:

- Responding and providing information as quickly as possible (usually within 1–3 hours, always within 1 business day)
- Clearly discussing availability and additional costs (if any)
- Prioritizing less stable patients
- Prioritizing direct referrals from veterinarians
- Requiring initial paperwork to be completed before scheduling to assess the family's commitment to care

If we are not able to provide care because of scheduling limitations, we provide a list of additional mobile veterinarians in the area who may be able to help.

Our top scheduling priority is to be available for our current HPM patients, especially for urgent care and emergency appointments (during regular clinic hours and also afterhours on-call times). This priority is of the utmost importance, because one of the most common reasons that families seek out our care is to avoid having to stress their pets by leaving home, especially to go to the emergency clinic. Occasionally, we have to postpone or delay care for a stable patient in order to be available on emergency for a current HPM patient, and we have found that this is usually well accepted because families know that it means we would do the same for them. Note that we also try very hard to prevent emergencies for our patients through careful planning; emergencies are stressful for everyone and should always be avoided or prevented if possible. We carefully discuss emergency planning, expectations, and procedures at every patient's initial consultation appointment (and review during ongoing care as needed). Our general stated goal is to be available by phone within 1 to 3 hours at most, and to be available for an emergency appointment within 1 to 6 hours at most. We also provide a variety of handouts to assist with urgent and emergency care considerations and develop an emergency plan for every patient, including provision of a comfort care kit with emergency medications/therapies as deemed appropriate and agreed on by the family.

Appointment Safety and Preparations

A feature of all mobile veterinary care is that thoughtful preparation for appointments can make all the difference in having the materials needed to attend to individual patient needs. First and foremost, though, is to follow general safety precautions:

- Keep a record of where you plan to be at all times
- Keep up with regular vehicle maintenance and have a roadside assistance plan
- Carry a mobile phone with GPS (global positioning system) and charger
- Carry a first-aid and vehicle emergency kit

Obtaining and reviewing a new patient's previous medical records and a new patient form/questionnaire in advance can be a great help. For record keeping, we have found cloud-based veterinary software to be ideal because it can be used over WI-FI or cellular networks. We also use several custom-printed carbonless (2-part) forms, such as our consultation and care notes form (**Fig. 3**), so that we can leave a copy for the family and also retain a copy for the patient's medical record. A summary of materials that we generally bring to every appointment versus materials we bring based on specific patient needs or specific appointment types is presented in **Table 3**. We have found it to be particularly helpful to use small duffle bags or backpacks and tackle boxes to organize materials both so that they are easy to restock and also so that they can be ready at any time based on daily appointments. Unless needed immediately, medications and other care supplies can either be picked up from the clinic's office location or obtained from other sources, such as human pharmacies and online. When needed, nurse/technician assistance, such as for specimen collection for diagnostic testing, needs to be prearranged.

Managing Veterinarians and Staff

Mobile veterinary practices are generally small clinics, often with only 1 doctor and limited support staff. Although this may be a benefit in terms of reducing overheads, requiring fewer management duties, and preserving the private nature of in-home appointments, it also poses significant challenges. Before working together, both doctors in our clinic had previously managed single-doctor mobile clinics with services

Consultation & Care Notes

Patient Name: _____   Weight: _____   Date: _____

❖ Diet & Hydration:

_____

_____

❖ Treatments, Medications, & Supplements:

_____

_____

_____

_____

_____

_____

_____

_____

_____

_____

_____

_____

_____

_____

_____

_____

❖ Monitoring & Special Handling:

_____

_____

_____

_____

❖ Diagnostic Testing & Referrals:

_____

❖ Plan for On-Going Care & Communications:

Progress Report: _____   Appointment: _____

© Heart's Ease Veterinary Care, 2017 ·

Fig. 3. Consultation and care notes.

limited to HPM. The following are some of the most important benefits of a multidoctor practice that we have experienced:

- Collaborative discussions
  - Patient rounds to learn from each other's individual approaches to patient care and to keep up with all patients in practice
  - Journal club to keep up with new advances and topics
  - Division of patient population and therapeutic modalities by doctor preferences and special interests (such as specific type of animals and traditional Chinese veterinary medicine/acupuncture)

Table 3
Materials and supplies needed for hospice and palliative medicine appointments

Every Appointment	Based on Appointment
Record keeping and client education: • Laptop or tablet (with keyboard) • Pens, clipboard and lined paper • Carbonless forms (eg, patient care notes, emergency meds/comfort care kit, clinic policies) • Handouts and educational materials	Laboratory specimen collection kit: • Glucometer • Syringes, needles, and butterfly catheters • Tourniquet • Preassembled specimen collection kits for sample submission to reference laboratory • Small cooler
Physical examination supplies bag: • Stethoscope • Otoscope and ophthalmoscope • Wristwatch or stopwatch • Portable scales (large and small) • Cordless clippers • Medical grooming and hygiene supplies (eg, gloves, cordless clippers, nail trimmers, baby wipes)	Minor procedure kits: • Electrocardiogram and blood pressure • Bandaging • Eye examination and tonometry • Mobility devices (eg, harnesses, slings) • Thoracocentesis/abdominocentesis • Urinary catheterization and enema • Nebulizer ± oxygen • Acupuncture/other special services
Mobile pharmacy bag: • Medications/therapies for immediate care (eg, subcutaneous fluids, syringes/needles, injectable medications)[a] • Small mobile pharmacy of commonly dispensed medications[a] • Prescription vials and labels • Prescription pad	In-home euthanasia and EOL services bag: • Pens, consent forms, and aftercare materials • Medication/syringe/supply box[a] • Cordless clippers and stethoscope • Disposable underpads and baby wipes • Facial tissue • Basket for small dogs and cats • Stretcher for large dogs
Methods of taking payment: • Pouch for storing check/cash payments • Tablet or mobile phone • Mobile credit card reader	Additional considerations and materials: • Will nurse assistance be needed? • Muzzles/restraint devices • Towels, sheets and blankets

[a] All applicable US Drug Enforcement Administration regulations for controlled drugs must be followed.

- Pooling of resources
  - Additional clinic resources, such as office space and equipment
  - Feasibility of additional staff and assistance, such as receptionist/assistant, nurse
  - Division of business management duties, such as payroll, accounting, inventory, community outreach
- Availability for appointments and emergencies
  - Better able to accommodate emergency and urgent care appointments, helping pets stay at home and avoid emergency clinic visits (especially for euthanasia)
  - Additional options for families with specific doctor preferences
  - Shared on-call time for after-hours patient emergencies
    - One of the hardest parts of this type of care to provide
    - One of the most valued parts of this type of care to families
- Better opportunities for adequate self-care
  - Opportunity for debriefing sessions about difficult cases
  - Ability to have a regular weekday and every other weekend off
  - Easier for doctors to go out of town and/or take vacation time
  - Reduced burnout and/or compassion fatigue

RETROSPECTIVE REPORT OF OUR PATIENT POPULATION
Overview

Presented here are defining characteristics of the care provided to our patient population who died over a 1-year time period (June 1, 2017 to May 31, 2018). The patient population of this practice can offer special insight into provision of veterinary services focused on HPM because, unlike general practice clinics (brick and mortar or mobile), where there is a great diversity of patients and services offered, or mobile euthanasia practices that provide single-visit services only, we provide only HPM services (including EOL/euthanasia) and we see a large number of patients. It is important to state that most of our appointments are for patients receiving HPM services other than EOL. Appointment demographics are summarized in **Fig. 4**. Of the 999 total appointments seen over the course of the year, 61% (609) were for HPM services and 39% (390) were for EOL services. Of the appointments for HPM, 509 (83.6% of HPM appointments and 51% of all appointments) were for ongoing care and treatment/service visits for HPM patients. Of the EOL services appointments, 103 (26.4%) were for current patients, meaning that the patients were already enrolled in HPM services with this clinic. Therefore, only 28.7% (287) of our appointments overall were for new patients requesting EOL services only (this includes in-home euthanasia and deceased pet services where the patient had already died before our arrival).

Patient demographics are summarized in **Fig. 5** based on species, sex, cause of death, and age group. One patient (canine) was excluded because of insufficient data. Of the 394 total patients included, most were canine (310) and the rest were feline (84). This finding is expected but does highlight the common issue in veterinary medicine that cats are often grossly underrepresented in clinic patient populations. Sex was not found to a differentiating factor, because percentages of male and female patients were approximately the same between species. Euthanasia was clearly the predominant cause of death, with only a small percentage of patients (7 total, 1.8%) who died of other causes. Of these 7 patients, 6 died acutely/unexpectedly and 1 had a planned hospice-assisted death without euthanasia. As a side note, although many families express interest in avoiding euthanasia and instead want to plan for a hospice-assisted death without euthanasia for their pets, we have had very few

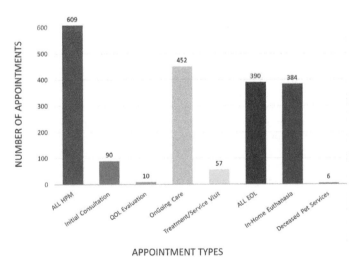

APPOINTMENT TYPES

Fig. 4. Appointment demographics.

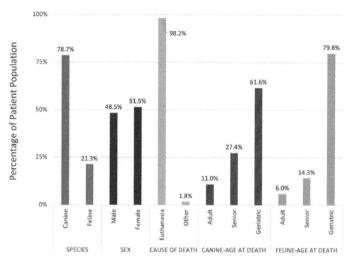

Fig. 5. Patient demographics.

families follow through with this choice because most animals experience significant compromise of QOL before death.

The patient population was divided into 4 age groups based on age at time of death: juvenile (0–1 years), adult (2–8 years), senior (9–12 years), and geriatric (≥13 years). No patients from the juvenile age group were seen, and, as might be predicted, most patients were in the geriatric age group. Note that we are aware of limitations of these age group definitions because species and breed differences were not taken into account. It is encouraging though, that almost all patients were in the geriatric age group, indicating that our pets are leading longer lives. A last consideration in this overview of our patient population, presented in **Figs. 6** and **7** for dogs and cats respectively, is the percentage of patients by age group who were enrolled in HPM at time of euthanasia or death versus being a new patient at time of euthanasia or death.

- HPM patients include patients in whom euthanasia was elected at the first HPM appointment as well as patients with ongoing care of any duration
- EOL-only patients include new patients seen for in-home euthanasia and deceased pet services

These charts show that most of our new patients, both dog and cat, were seen for EOL services only, but that there is no appreciable difference in this by age group. Also, in addition to the total number of cat patients overall being much lower than the number of dog patients, we also see that, within our feline patient population, cats were less likely to be enrolled in HPM at the time of death than dogs in all age groups. Likewise, there is a higher percentage of cats who received EOL services only compared with dogs in all age groups.

Family-Reported Reason for Euthanasia or Death

At the time of death, each family was asked for the reasons they elected euthanasia to help their pet, or, in the case of death without euthanasia, what their pet's major problems were at the time. They were allowed to report unlimited parameters from each of

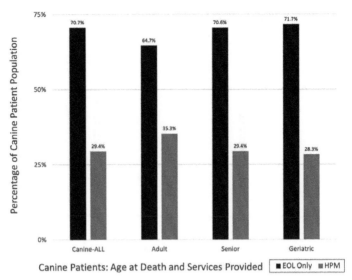

Fig. 6. Canine patient population by age and HPM versus EOL only.

the following groups and subgroups. Based on these responses, a list of family-reported reasons for euthanasia was organized as follows:

- QOL
  - Loss of mobility: includes both acute and chronic mobility issues
  - Incontinence: includes both urinary and fecal incontinence
  - Anorexia: includes both acute anorexia and chronic poor appetite
  - Dyspnea: includes both primary and secondary causes
  - Other: some families stated a general loss of QOL without a specific parameter
- Systemic disease (SDZ)
  - Neoplasia: both confirmed and unconfirmed but with malignant behavior
  - Organ failure: heart, kidney, and liver failure

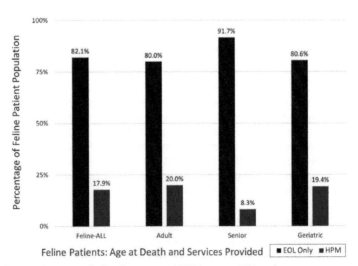

Fig. 7. Feline patient population by age and HPM versus EOL only.

- ○ Cognitive dysfunction syndrome (CDS)
- ○ Other: various systemic disease (eg, endocrine, seizures, immune-mediated disease)
- Behavior: here refers specifically to unmanageable aggression
- Trauma: data not shown; 1 patient (geriatric) was killed in a dog fight

Figs. 8 and **9** summarize corresponding data for dogs and cats respectively based on age at death and the broad categories listed earlier (QOL, SDZ, behavior, trauma). Note that trauma was excluded from charts because it only applied to 1 patient in the geriatric canine group. Important findings include:

- QOL parameters were reported frequently for all canine age groups but trended as more frequent by increasing age. Although a similar trend by age was observed for cats, QOL parameters were reported much less frequently for cats of all age groups than for dogs.
- SDZ parameters were reported with a similar frequency for all canine and feline age groups but were reported at a much higher rate overall for cats versus dogs of all ages.
- Behavioral euthanasia because of unmanageable aggression was only a small subset of all patients and was only reported for dogs. Of these dogs, almost all were in the adult age group, which is expected because dangerous aggression is not something that most families can tolerate for a prolonged period of time.

Our data indicate that families may have a much harder time judging a cat's QOL compared with a dog's, and so may rely more heavily on diagnosis of SDZ to make EOL decisions. These findings may shed some additional light on why cats may be less likely to receive HPM services.

We were also able to study family-reported reasons for euthanasia or death, taking into account the additional parameters defined for QOL and SDZ. We regret that pain is not included here as a QOL parameter, but, as may be expected by the difficulty most families have in evaluating and monitoring their pet's pain, it was not reported as a reason for euthanasia or death by a single family. **Figs. 10** and **11** present the

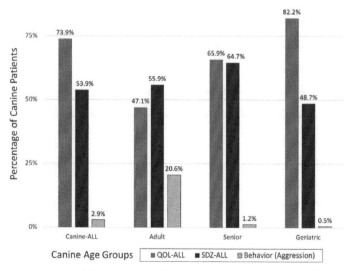

Fig. 8. Canine: overview of family-reported reason for euthanasia or death by age.

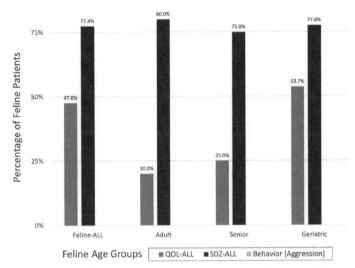

Fig. 9. Feline: overview of family-reported reason for euthanasia or death by age.

specific family-reported reasons for euthanasia or death for dogs and cats respectively. In the feline chart, note that the smaller sample size is a major confounding factor in interpretation. However, several observations and trends are present:

- Besides being reported more frequently for dogs than for cats, specific QOL parameter reporting differed for dogs and cats.

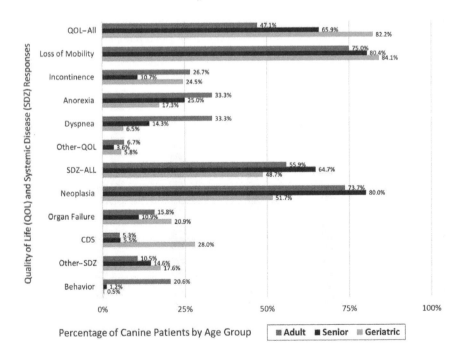

Fig. 10. Canine: specific family-reported reason for euthanasia or death by age.

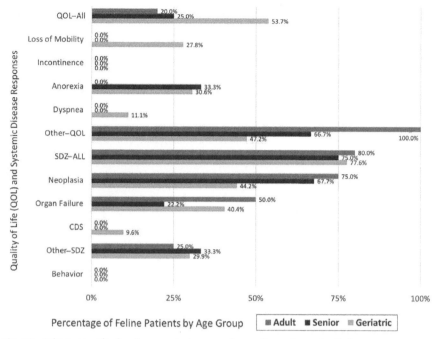

Fig. 11. Feline: specific family-reported reason for euthanasia or death by age.

- ○ Dogs tended to have specific QOL parameters reported, especially loss of mobility, whereas cats were more likely to have the nonspecific other QOL parameter reported.
- Again, cats were overall more likely than dogs to have an SDZ parameter reported, but there are some interesting comparisons in the specific SDZ parameters reported for cats versus dogs:
  - ○ Neoplasia was reported at similar frequencies by species and age but was less likely to be reported for geriatric pets in both species. In our surveyed population, this may indicate that, if dogs and cats live to be geriatric, they are less likely to die from neoplasia.
  - ○ Organ failure was reported at a much higher rate for cats than dogs, likely because of the high rate of chronic kidney disease (CKD) seen in cats versus dogs.
  - ○ CDS was reported at a much lower rate in all age groups of cats versus dogs, and, as might be expected, was reported more frequently in geriatric versus younger dogs.

Duration of Hospice and Palliative Medicine

An additional way that we assessed our patient populations was to focus on our HPM patients, looking at duration of HPM services. Duration of HPM by species is summarized in **Fig. 12**.

- Range: 0 to 1541 days (canine), 0 to 781 days (feline)
  - ○ The overall duration of HPM for dogs and cats was condensed to show only 700 days because of extreme outlier points. The wide duration range observed makes interpretation difficult but also highlights 2 important

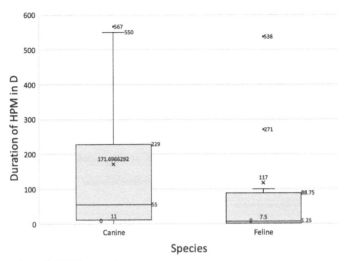

Fig. 12. Duration of HPM by species.

points. First, several patients were unstable at the time of initial consultation or QOL evaluation consultation, and so had a duration of zero or just a few days in HPM. Second, a large number of patients had a prolonged period of HPM. Patients enrolled in HPM for longer periods were often being treated for chronic pain conditions.

- Mean: 171.7 days (canine), 117 days (feline)
  - Despite the range being almost twice as wide for dogs versus cats, the mean duration is more similar between species, amounting to ~6 months for dogs and ~4 months for cats.
- Median: 55 days (canine), 7.5 days (feline)
  - Interpretation of the median is again difficult but is more reflective of the demographics of our patient population because it lessens the influence of the wide range. For dogs, the interquartile range was 11 to 229 days and for cats the interquartile range was 1.25 to 88.75 days.

To round out the discussion of HPM duration, we also studied the influence of age group for each species, summarized in **Figs. 13** and **14**. Similar trends were seen between dogs and cats in terms of range, mean, and median by age group, but, as already discussed, an overall shorter duration across the board for cats. What is interesting is the observation that, with increasing age, duration of time in HPM also increases for dogs and cats. This finding may have various causes, including again that several older patients were being treated for chronic pain conditions, but it also brings up an important observation related to family-reported reasons for euthanasia or death. **Figs. 8** and **9** show that reporting of neoplasia was much lower for dog and cat geriatric groups than it was for adult and senior groups. Therefore, there is the possibility that, if dogs and cats live to be geriatric without a diagnosis of neoplasia, they may be less likely to die from neoplasia. Here again, of the 106 total HPM patients, 84.9% (90) were dogs and 15.1% (16) were cats. Although trends were observed that cats tended to have a shorter duration of HPM and that a smaller percentage of cats versus dogs from the adult and senior

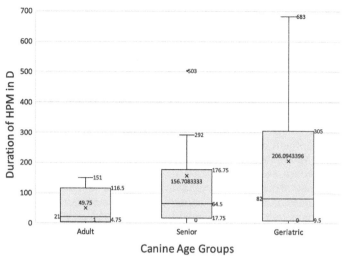

Fig. 13. Canine: duration of HPM by age.

categories were treated, this may only be related to sample size and how the age groups are defined.

FUTURE DIRECTIONS AND AREAS FOR GROWTH AND IMPROVEMENT

Despite veterinary HPM still being limited in terms of availability, and in the early stages of growth and development, demand among families with pets is increasing. In order to support ongoing growth and enable HPM to become more mainstream, it is crucial that the veterinary community becomes more educated on when to implement HPM services or provide a referral. All patients with chronic debilitating conditions and/or serious or terminal illness should be offered HPM services, even if the plan is still to pursue curative therapy. Early referral and implementation of HPM is one of the greatest issues veterinarians face, and it is common for both families and primary or specialty

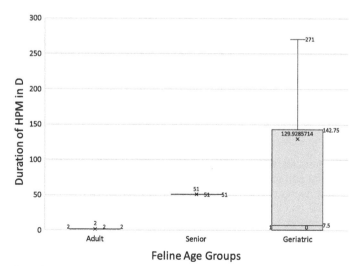

Fig. 14. Feline: duration of HPM by age.

care veterinarians to tell us that they did not know that this type of service existed, and that they wish that they had known sooner. Referral for HPM can strengthen a family's relationship and satisfaction with their primary care veterinarian. By referring patients for care they need, much like referral for specialized surgical services, families recognize the collaborative nature of medical care. Strengthening collaboration between HPM providers and primary/specialty care veterinarians has the potential to streamline patient care and improve convenience for families. Some examples of collaboration are freely sharing medical records and understanding that medical therapies and procedures might be conducted differently for HPM patients.

Further development will necessitate expanding options for the core HPC team, which includes veterinarians, nurses/technicians, the pet's family and additional caregivers, aftercare service providers (such as pet cremation facilities), social workers, other mental health professionals, and spiritual supports such as chaplains. The need for professional emotional support for families cannot be overstated; however, it is important that those providing this support are qualified and licensed in their respective fields. A team approach can also help to delineate the largely medical role of veterinarians, thereby reducing nonmedical activities for veterinarians. This approach could allow improved patient and family care as well as better time management for veterinarians.

Looking to the future, it is hoped that additional research will be conducted, and clinical measures taken to improve available options for veterinary HPM services and also to show the value of HPM in improving patient comfort, QOL, and even survival time. Additional resources for veterinarians could include veterinary school curriculum changes, further growth and development of continuing education opportunities/training programs, novel drug development and administration methods, and additional publications. Some notable considerations for additional retrospective data analysis would be to include a larger sample size and to use a survey with a detailed list of QOL and SDZ parameters to help guide family reporting of reasons for euthanasia/death. Additional resources for families could include increased awareness/greater availability of HPC services and earlier referral for pets with severe illness and/or terminal illness conditions.

CASE REPORT SUMMARY
Background

Tentative diagnosis of serious and/or terminal illness, such as neoplasia, without a definitive diagnosis is common in veterinary medicine. Some of the many factors that may preclude arriving at a definitive diagnosis are:

- Cost, safety, and invasiveness of diagnostics and therapies
- Owner bias, including previous experiences with other pets
- Clinician bias, including lack of information and personal experiences
- Limitations of interspecies communication to understand a pet's wishes

Families are often left with no clear options to help their pet during the precious time that remains. HPM can provide a means for families to continue to support their pet's comfort and QOL without the need for a definitive diagnosis.

To illustrate the use of HPM under these circumstances, this article presents a case summary report for Billy, a 14-year-old, male neutered, mixed-breed dog weighing ~20 kg (**Fig. 15**).

- Past medical history: fairly healthy through life, minor skin masses
- Presenting complaint on emergency: acute lethargy and anorexia

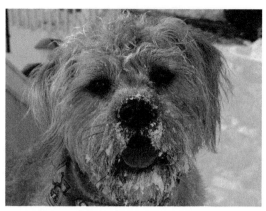

Fig. 15. Billy: enjoying a romp in the snow.

- Emergency visit findings: moderate liver enzyme level increases, mild anemia, mild lymphopenia, hepatic and splenic masses/nodules on ultrasonography

Additional diagnostic options were not elected at the emergency room (ER) visit. Metastatic neoplasia was tentatively diagnosed, and a poor prognosis was given. As is common with emergency clinic visits, all members of Billy's family were not present, so his family elected to bring him home pending further discussion. His family requested medications to help improve comfort, and prednisone, tramadol, and mirtazapine were dispensed. In the days following his emergency visit, Billy's family decided not to pursue any further diagnostics or invasive therapies but were not ready to consider euthanasia, so sought out HPM services 10 days after his emergency clinic visit.

Billy's energy and appetite had already improved at the time of his initial consultation for HPM, which allowed a more relaxed review of his open diagnosis, discussion of goals, and implementation of an initial care plan. His family affirmed that they did not want to pursue any further diagnostics or invasive procedures and wanted to focus on comfort care. Managing his undertreated/uncontrolled joint pain was the initial priority. Over the course of his care (summarized in **Table 4**), Billy and his family experienced many of the most common hurdles seen in HPM:

- Patient compliance:
  - Billy's ongoing finicky appetite (even for treats) and aversion to injections made it difficult to reliably give all recommended medications
- Dynamic nature of pain management:
  - Billy's level of joint pain both waxed/waned and progressed over time, requiring frequent medication adjustments
- Behavior changes with progressive disease:
  - Symptoms of anxiety and insomnia often worsen with progressive disease
  - Therapies of lorazepam and cannabidiol oil were added over time
- Changes in patient status may alter decisions for care and diagnostics:
  - Billy's hyporexia worsened ~6 months into his HPM services, and his family elected to recheck bloodwork, revealing International Renal Interest Society stage 2 CKD
  - Diagnosis of CKD did not necessarily change recommended/possible therapies, but it did help Billy's family better understand his condition

Table 4
A summary of Billy's time in hospice and palliative medicine

Time	Level of Care	Problem List
Day 1	Early hospice	• New finding of abdominal masses • Chronic DJD/osteoarthritis: uncontrolled pain

Medications and therapies:
1. Gabapentin: 5 mg/kg PO q 24 h, with incremental increase
2. Supplements: fish oil, antioxidant
3. Acupuncture: dry needling

| Day 22 | Palliative care | • Abdominal masses: no known change
• Chronic DJD/osteoarthritis: worsening pain
• GI issues: hyporexia; soft stools
• Lethargic: mild/intermittent
• Behavior: anxiety, restless at night |

Medications and therapies:
1. Gabapentin: 15 mg/kg PO q 12 h
2. NSAID (standard dosing): carprofen, then meloxicam, then grapiprant
3. Famotidine: 0.5 mg/kg PO q 24 h
4. Maropitant: 2 mg/kg PO q 24 PRN
5. Metronidazole: 10 mg/kg PO q 12–24 h
6. Pro-Pectalin: standard dosing PRN
7. Lorazepam: 0.05 mg/kg PO q 12 h
8. HempRx (CBD oil): 0.1 mg/kg PO q 12 h
9. Supplements: fish oil, antioxidant, probiotic

| Day 336 | Early hospice | • Abdominal masses: no known change
• Chronic DJD/osteoarthritis: controlled pain
• GI issues: worsening hyporexia, soft stools
• Lethargy: mild to moderate/worsening
• Behavior: anxiety, restless at night |

Medications and therapies:
1. Continued: gabapentin, famotidine, maropitant, metronidazole, Pro-Pectalin
2. NSAID: grapiprant: 3 mg/kg PO q 24 h
3. Lorazepam: 0.1 mg/kg PO q 12 h
4. HempRx (CBD oil): 0.1–0.25 mg/kg PO q 12 h
5. Supplements: probiotic

| Day 378 | Advanced hospice | • Abdominal masses: suspected growth
• Chronic DJD/osteoarthritis: worsening pain
• GI issues: worsening hyporexia
• Lethargy: moderate/worsening
• Behavior: worsening anxiety, insomnia |

Medications and therapies:
1. Gabapentin: 15 mg/kg PO q 24 h
2. NSAID (standard dosing): continued grapiprant, then meloxicam
3. Amantadine: 5 mg/kg PO q 24 h
4. Maropitant: 2 mg/kg PO q 24 h to PRN
5. Pro-Pectalin: standard dosing PRN
6. Lorazepam: 0.15 mg/kg PO q 8–12 h
7. HempRx: 0.25 mg/kg PO q 12 h
8. ER medications for comfort care kit:
    1. Morphine: 0.75 mg/kg TM if needed
    2. Detomidine gel: 0.07 mg/kg TM if needed

| Day 473 | EOL care (in-home euthanasia) | • Family-reported reasons for euthanasia: anorexia, neoplasia |

Abbreviations: CBD, cannabidiol; GI, gastrointestinal; NSAID, nonsteroidal antiinflammatory drug; PO, by mouth; PRN, as needed; q, every; TM, transmucosal.

Billy's story demonstrates several of the difficult decisions that families face when their beloved pet is diagnosed (or tentatively diagnosed) with a serious or terminal illness. His family sought HPM services on their own, knowing that they needed guidance at a time of great uncertainty. Until HPM was implemented, there was no plan for how to best support him or his family. With HPM, he and his family enjoyed more than 15 additional months of good time together.

ACKNOWLEDGMENTS

The authors would like to thank Ron Hazen, MPH, and Sylvia Forman, PhD, for assistance with data analysis.

REFERENCE

1. Villalobos AE. Quality-of-life assessment techniques for veterinarians. Vet Clin North Am Small Anim Pract 2011;41:519–29.

An Objective Exploration of Euthanasia and Adverse Events

Beth Marchitelli, DVM

KEYWORDS

- Euthanasia • Adverse events • Physician-assisted death • Preeuthanasia sedation
- Euthanasia solution

KEY POINTS

- Companion animal euthanasia is an important area for rigorous scientific exploration and study.
- Few studies exist in the current veterinary literature quantifying adverse events during and after the euthanasia process.
- Best practices have yet to be established and scientifically validated for the practice of companion animal euthanasia.
- Literature evaluating human euthanasia and assisted death in countries where such practices are legal can be a useful area of investigation and collaborative inquiry.

INTRODUCTION

The inclusion of euthanasia within the scope of veterinary practice has been well established since the profession's early development.[1] Euthanasia is significant for all animal species; however, euthanasia of companion animal species warrants specific attention in light of their intimate relationships with humans. The potential impact on pet owners of caring for pets who may require euthanasia has far-reaching social, emotional, ethical, financial, and psychological consequences. The cumulative stress on caregivers of seriously ill pets has recently been described.[2] Bioethical literature investigating companion animal euthanasia and ethical decision-making during terminal illness is also expanding.[3–6] The rapid growth of mobile veterinary hospice, palliative care, and in-home euthanasia services has drawn attention to veterinary end-of-life practices on several levels. Although humane standards and methods of euthanasia have improved over time, rigorous studies regarding the incidence of adverse events including physiologic side effects of euthanasia drugs and/or issues

The author has nothing to disclose.
4 Paws Farewell, Mobile Pet Hospice, Palliative Care and Home Euthanasia, Asheville, NC 28806, USA
E-mail address: bmarchitelli@hotmail.com

Vet Clin Small Anim 49 (2019) 553–563
https://doi.org/10.1016/j.cvsm.2019.01.016
0195-5616/19/© 2019 Elsevier Inc. All rights reserved.

with euthanasia completion have been lacking. Similarly, the impact on pet owners of specific physiologic events that may occur during or after the euthanasia process has not been evaluated. In addition, the psychological impact of induction agents, including euthanasia solutions, on animals as they are rendered unconscious has not been elucidated.[7–12] A lack of scientific rigor regarding the former and scientific advances regarding the latter challenge practitioners in establishing best practices. The 2013 American Veterinary Medical Association (AVMA) Guidelines for the Euthanasia of Animals describe methods of euthanasia that are deemed humane and acceptable.[9] Similar guidance on the incidence of adverse events associated with euthanasia methods or agents would be useful. Such information would enable all involved in the euthanasia process to adequately prepare for the procedure and appropriately influence expectations surrounding potentially undesirable events. Adverse event guidelines have the capacity to contribute to best practices. Finally, evaluation of practices and procedures for human euthanasia in countries where such practices are legal and have been used for several decades can provide useful information in establishing a database to guide veterinary practitioners.

INCIDENCE OF ADVERSE EVENTS

Data quantifying the incidence of adverse events, such as agonal respiration, non-productive respiratory effort, and tremors, during companion animal euthanasia, are limited. The heterogeneous nature of the medical conditions of pets being euthanized and the absence of standardized practices regarding the use of sedative medication before euthanasia solution administration contribute to the complexity of this area of study. A pilot study conducted in 2017 quantified the number of adverse events in 94 dogs[13] (Fig. 1). For all dogs included in the study the dose, type, route, and rate of administration of drugs used for presedation and for euthanasia were uniform. Of 94 dogs studied, 52% experienced an adverse event, with 31% experiencing an increase in respiratory rate during euthanasia solution administration.[13]

Although changes in respiratory rate do not necessarily indicate discomfort or distress on the part of the pet, rapid changes in respiratory rate may be perceived by pet owners as distressing. It has been argued that preparing family members for such events is the best and most appropriate defense for alleviating potential distress. It is also possible that evaluation and understanding of such events could lead to their reduction or elimination.

Table 1 includes a list of potential adverse events that have been described both during and after euthanasia solution administration. The diverse nature of euthanasia protocols, variation in disease state, and level of physiologic distress at the time of

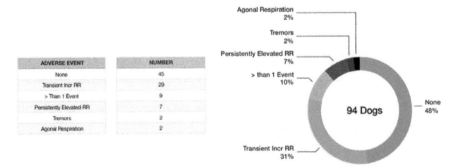

ADVERSE EVENT	NUMBER
None	45
Transient Incr RR	29
> Than 1 Event	9
Persistently Elevated RR	7
Tremors	2
Agonal Respiration	2

Agonal Respiration 2%
Tremors 2%
Persistently Elevated RR 7%
> than 1 Event 10%
None 48%
94 Dogs
Transient Incr RR 31%

Fig. 1. Adverse events in dogs during euthanasia: a study examining 94 dogs.

Table 1			
Potential adverse events during and after euthanasia solution administration			
Seizures	Lip Licking	Tremors	Twitching
Opisthotonus	Transient increase in respiratory rate	Persistently elevated respiratory rate	Panting
Vocalization	Panting	Drooling	Defecation/urination
Dorsal eye position deviation	Pain on intravenous administration	Cheyne-Stokes respiration	Dysphoria
Agonal respiration	Vomiting	Drooling	Lip blowing

euthanasia highlight the challenges in studying these events. Historically, emphasis has not been placed on the existence of adverse events. A reduction in their frequency could reduce potential stressors for veterinary professionals and pet owners during the euthanasia process.

AGONAL RESPIRATION

Evaluation of each adverse event is beyond the scope of this article; however, agonal respiration and its frequency deserves specific mention in light of the distress its presence may cause to human observers.[14] Agonal respiration is thought to be triggered by anoxia, experimentally induced when the Pao_2 is less than 5 mm Hg.[15] This triggers neuronal circuitry in the medulla creating a pronounced respiratory pattern colloquially described as "gasping," which is present in a variety of animal species including human infants.[16] A similar mechanism may also be at play when pets exhibit acute transient elevations in respiratory rate in response to administration of a euthanasia solution.[17] Most studies in human medicine have focused on agonal respiration's positive predictive survival value after cardiopulmonary resuscitation.[15,17–20] Agonal respiration has been shown to have several beneficial effects including increased cardiac output, decreased intracranial pressure, and improved gas exchange.[18] Despite its positive effects on survival in humans undergoing cardiac arrest, agonal respiration is an unwelcome event during companion animal euthanasia.

It is difficult to accurately evaluate the incidence of agonal respiration in veterinary patients. Reference to agonal respiration during euthanasia is seen in a letter to the editor of the Veterinary Record in 1971. KL Vaughan alludes to a discussion regarding "gasps given by dogs destroyed with pentobarbitone sodium" and suggests the addition of the muscle relaxant gallamine as a solution.[21] Several studies report agonal respiration in their findings.[22–30] The Center for Veterinary Medicine (CVM) is the branch of the Federal Drug Administration (FDA) responsible for veterinary drug approval. Most Freedom of Information Summaries provided for euthanasia solutions that have gone through the CVM process of drug approval do not report the incidence of agonal respiration.[31–33] One exception is the Freedom of Information Summary for the drug Tributame, which reported the incidence of adverse events including agonal respiration.[34] Of 81 dogs in the summary, 20 (24.6%) were reported to have agonal respiration[34] (see **Table 1**).

A study conducted by Evans and colleagues[25] in 1993 looked at the effects of augmenting sodium pentobarbital with various concentrations of lidocaine. This study reported fewer incidences of agonal respiration in the 2% and 3% lidocaine groups versus the 1% lidocaine group and the group given sodium pentobarbital alone. In the 1993 publication, Evans and colleagues[25] reference unpublished data that describe the incidence of agonal respiration to be 6.7% (~136) of 2041 dogs euthanized with sodium pentobarbital + 2% lidocaine. In analyzing the unpublished data above, the authors may have more accurately determined the incidence of agonal respiration by controlling for the dose, rate, and route of pentobarbital + lidocaine 2%, and the presence or absence of premedication.

The pilot study of 94 dogs conducted in 2017 (see **Fig. 1**) found the incidence of agonal respiration with sodium pentobarbital alone to be 2% (2 of 94 dogs).[13] As mentioned previously, all dogs received the same premedication and dose, route, and rate of delivery of sodium pentobarbital. The potential impact of 2% lidocaine on the incidence of agonal respiration suggested by Evans and colleagues is worthy of further investigation because lidocaine may have secondary effects on the brain stem and, by extension, dampen this mechanism. In any future study, the variation in underlying disease states, use and type of premedication, type of euthanasia solution, and rate and route of all administered medications are important variables for consideration. There are currently no studies comparing effects of the rate of euthanasia solution administration on the incidence of agonal respiration. Although the incidence of agonal respiration may be small, its effects on family members should not be overlooked.[14] Given the potential negative consequences for family members and by extension their pets, understanding predisposing or mitigating factors in the occurrence of agonal respiration during companion animal euthanasia warrants further study.

THE EFFECTS OF PREMEDICATION BEFORE EUTHANASIA

Two studies have evaluated the effects of oral premedication before administration of euthanasia solution[35,36] and 1 study evaluated the injectable hypnotic anesthetic propofol.[22] There are currently no other studies evaluating administration of premedication before euthanasia. The 2013 AVMA Guidelines for the Euthanasia of Animals strongly encourage premedication, "…with the intent of providing anxiolysis, analgesia, somnolence for easier and safer IV access, and reduction of stage II or postmortem activity that could be distressing to personnel."[9] Administering premedication before euthanasia solution is at the discretion of the veterinary practitioner. The diverse nature of physiologic state and clinical status of pets being euthanized, numerous choices for drug premedication, and the variety of settings in which pets are currently euthanized make this a robust area for further study. Administering specific types of premedication under certain circumstances could elicit unwanted side effects such as nausea, dysphoria, or excitation. Optimal sedative medication for a dyspneic pet with poor cardiac function may be quite different than for a pet actively seizing from a brain tumor at the time of euthanasia. Understanding which premedications work best under which circumstances and disease states may help to maximize the benefits of these drugs. Scientific evaluation of the potential benefits of premedication related to specific disease states would provide data to support best practices in their use for veterinary euthanasia.

EUTHANASIA DRUG APPROVAL

The current CVM/FDA drug approval process does not include the incidence of adverse events as criteria for drug approval. This is a legal issue and not the CVM's preference. CVM "would prefer that animals euthanized not exhibit post injection adverse reactions such as muscle fasciculations (MF), non-productive respiratory effort (NPRE) and terminal gasps after the animal is clinically dead, but cannot legally prevent a drug from being approved because of these adverse events."[34] Tributame (embutramide + chloroquine + lidocaine) is a drug that was officially approved by the CVM/FDA but has not been marketed. Of 81 dogs, 35.8% experienced at least one adverse event: incidence of agonal respiration reported as 24.6%(20) (**Table 2**). The incidence of agonal respiration with this drug may be as high as 60% to 70%,[9,37] making Tributame's adverse event profile significant. Despite this, the drug is approved by the CVM and labeled as an acceptable euthanasia agent in dogs according to the AVMA's 2013 Guidelines for the Euthanasia of Animals.[9]

Table 3 lists euthanasia solutions that have been officially approved by the CVM. Each of these drugs has an associated Freedom of Information Summary, available to the public by request from the CVM/FDA.

T-61 (embutramide + tetracaine + mebezonium), is similar in composition to Tributame with the inclusion of embutramide an opioid/anesthetic medication. T-61 stands apart from other euthanasia solutions approved by the CVM as it contains the neuro-muscular blocking agent mebezonium. T-61 was voluntarily removed from the market in the United States in 1989 due to concern that the paralytic action of mebezonium took effect before complete loss of consciousness. In a study of rabbits and dogs, Hellebrekers and colleagues (1990)[38] concluded that unconsciousness and muscle paralysis occurred simultaneously, refuting the above concern regarding onset of action. This study also reported vocalization and the presence of muscle activity, which, although thought to be occurring when the animals were unconscious, did highlight negative potential emotional and physiologic effects on observers. The Hellebrekers study evaluated the effects of T-61 via the intravenous route only. As such, information regarding alternate routes and corresponding time to flatline electroencephalogram (EEG) is lacking. T-61 is not available in the United States, but is available in Canada and may be available in other countries. Repose, the euthanasia solution containing secobarbital and dibucaine is no longer manufactured.

Single-agent sodium pentobarbital products such as Fatal-Plus did not undergo an official CVM/FDA drug approval process for the indication of euthanasia. Such drugs, therefore, do not have associated Freedom of Information Summaries. Sodium pentobarbital is designated "Generally Recognized As Safe" by the CVM/FDA; therefore, it is officially recognized by the CVM/FDA, but efficacy and/or safety studies are not available through this organization. **Box 1** lists currently available single-agent sodium pentobarbital products.

Vortech Pharmaceuticals is in the process of CVM/FDA drug approval for a combination product of sodium pentobarbital and 2% lidocaine. The addition of lidocaine to the original Fatal-Plus solution is purported to reduce local injection site irritation and may reduce adverse events such as agonal respiration.[25]

Table 2	
Tributame adverse events in 29 of 81 dogs	
Agonal respiration	20 (24.6%)
Vocalization	8 (9.9%)
Muscle twitching	4 (4.9%)
Opisthotonus	1 (1.2%)
Anxious	1 (1.2%)
Swallow reflex	1 (1.2%)
Attempt to stand	1 (1.2%)
Front limb extension	1 (1.2%)
Excitability	1 (1.2%)

Data from FDA/CVM FOIA NADA-141-245 Tributame – Obtained 5/10/18.

Table 3
Euthanasia solutions that have been officially approved by the Center for Veterinary Medicine

NADA/ANADA				
119–807		Beuthanasia-D	Sodium pentobarbital + phenytoin	1981
200–271		Euthasol	Sodium pentobarbital + phenytoin	1994
200–280		Euthanasia III Somnasol	Sodium pentobarbital + phenytoin	2005
128–976	Repose	Secobarbital + dibucaine	1983	No longer manufactured
100–809	T-61	Embutramide + tetracaine + mebezonium	1976	Voluntarily removed from the market
141–245	Tributame	Embutramide + chloroquine + lidocaine	2005	Approved but Never Manufactured

Abbreviations: ANADA, abbreviated new animal drug application; NADA, new animal drug application.

FLAT LINE ELECTROENCEPHALOGRAM AND BRAIN DEATH

Consensus on what physiologic parameters constitute brain death in human medicine has been elusive.[24,39–42] Historically, diagnostic tests such as serial EEG, angiography, computed tomography angiography, and transcranial Doppler in conjunction with clinical neurologic examination have been used as criteria.[39–42] Flatline EEG can be broadly understood to be correlated with a lack of conscious awareness. Unequivocally equating a flatline EEG resulting from administration of sodium pentobarbital euthanasia solution with the term "brain death" may prove more difficult. Administering euthanasia solutions containing sodium pentobarbital intravenously does induce a flatline EEG in roughly 30 seconds.[25] It is fair to say that a pet which has received euthanasia solution and develops a flatline EEG is in an unconscious state.[10,11,43,44] Inferring that a flatline EEG constitutes cerebral death, as stated in the drug insert information for specific euthanasia solutions, may be less accurate. This can be perceived as a matter of importance only semantically; however, understanding exactly what events take place physiologically and temporally allows for a more accurate depiction of events. Methods to understand the potential stress and/ or discomfort that may occur when animals move from the conscious to the unconscious state when under the influence of certain medications have yet to be concretely

Box 1
Single agent sodium pentobarbital products

Fatal-Plus/Fatal-Plus Powder

Pentasol SP Powder

Socumb

Somlethol (no longer manufactured)

Sleepaway (no longer manufactured)

understood and quantified.[7] Scientific advances in brain imaging techniques may illustrate more subtle levels of perception and conscious experience before flatline EEG. Several studies have suggested that arousal may not be equated with perception, further confounding our understanding.[12,45–49] Additional scientific study may provide more precise information regarding the influence of specific medications on states of consciousness. Such information may elucidate opportunities for therapeutic intervention aimed at reducing stress and anxiety in pets being euthanized.

HUMAN EUTHANASIA AND PHYSICIAN-ASSISTED DEATH

Clinical literature does not exist comparing the technical aspects of human and animal euthanasia. Complex cultural, ethical, moral, legal, psychological, and procedural dynamics make human euthanasia and animal euthanasia quite distinct. However, this distinction does not preclude technical comparison or collaborative evaluation. It can be argued that similarities in drug protocols and techniques for medically assisted dying may lend to comparison more readily than other aspects of veterinary and human medicine. Veterinary euthanasia practices are often referenced in discussions of lethal injection practices in the United States but not in comparison with human euthanasia or assisted death in which such practices are legal.[50] Although several scholarly studies do exist in the human medical and veterinary literature, respectively, a direct comparison between human and animal euthanasia practices and procedures does not. In addition, the number of studies on assisted dying and euthanasia is small, relative to studies focused on disease treatment and prevention in both human and veterinary medicine. Animal models of disease are used frequently in human medicine to improve understanding and treatment of disease in humans. Veterinary medicine also looks to advances in human medicine for guidance in the treatment of veterinary patients. Anecdotally, many pet owners report that they are grateful for the option of assisted death via euthanasia if suffering is relentless. Further investigation into the complex social, ethical, and psychological framework within which such decision-making occurs both for humans and animals adds another layer for comparison and scientific understanding.

In the United States, physician assisted-death is legal in six states and the District of Columbia (**Box 2**).

The method of physician-assisted dying in the United States is restricted to medication taken by mouth. Because pets are euthanized predominately by injectable medication given intravenously, comparison between assisted dying practices for humans and animals in the United States provides minimal technical insight. In the Netherlands, however, the practice of human euthanasia via intravenous medication has been legal since 2002. Unlike veterinary medicine in the United States, where there is no standard or best-practice protocol, the procedure for human euthanasia

---

Box 2
States where physician-assisted death is legal

ORAL ONLY
  Oregon 1997
  Vermont 2009
  Washington State 2009
  California 2015
  Colorado 2016
  District of Columbia 2017
  Hawaii 2018

Table 4	
KNMG/KNMP Guidelines for the Practice of Euthanasia and Physician-Assisted Suicide	
1. Coma induction:	Thiopental or pentobarbital 2 g given intravenously (IV) in less than 5 min
2. Neuromuscular blocking:	Rocuronium bromide 150 mg IV

in the Netherlands is described in detail, including type of medication, dose, and rate of administration. According to the 2012 KNMG/KNMP (Koninklijke Nederlandsche Maatschappij tot bevordering der Geneeskunst [Royal Dutch Association of Physicians]/Koninklijke Nederlandse Maatschappij ter bevordering der Pharmacie [Royal Dutch Association of Pharmacists]) Guidelines for the Practice of Euthanasia and Physician-Assisted Suicide, a coma induction agent in the form of thiopental or propofol is given until a medical coma is induced.[51] This is then followed by a neuro-muscular blocking agent (**Table 4**).

The neuromuscular blocking agent is to be given even if death ensues from the coma induction agent alone. Inclusion of a neuromuscular blocking agent is in contrast with veterinary euthanasia protocols in the United States, which historically have not included these agents. The 2013 AVMA Guidelines for the Euthanasia of Animals do not recommend the use of neuromuscular blocking agents in lieu of sodium pentobar-bital, nor that they be administered in the same syringe as sodium pentobarbital.[9] In addition, several states in the United States ban the use of neuromuscular blocking agents in animal euthanasia.[50] This occurs via state law, separate from veterinary practice acts.

The Netherlands' inclusion of a neuromuscular blocking agent as part of a standard of care serves several purposes. It prevents unwanted side effects such as terminal gasping and muscle fasciculations and assures completion of the euthanasia process. It also serves to avoid the side effects of high doses of coma-induction agents such as venous discoloration, in the case of sodium pentobarbital, when given alone.

Much of the current literature in human medicine related to medical aid in dying focuses on the ethical, legal, and epidemiologic aspects of physician-assisted death.[52–55] Data evaluating the technical aspects of drug delivery and potential nega-tive side effects are few and far between.[56–59] In contrast, standardization of drug pro-tocols for human euthanasia in the Netherlands reduces confounding variables in assessment of unwanted side effects or problems with the procedure itself.

SUMMARY

The effects of euthanasia on patients—animal or human—and their families are pro-found. No other medical intervention is as permanent, irreversible, and far reaching in its consequences. Rigorous scientific investigation and debate create the founda-tion for practices that are solidly evidence based, yet malleable in the face of scientific advance. Veterinary medicine stands to benefit from expanded scientific inquiry into the euthanasia process and associated adverse events to establish best practices. May we dedicate ourselves to expanding our knowledge base in this area and continue to honor and respect the significance of the bond between patient and family.

REFERENCES

1. Binois A. Excavating the history of ancient veterinary practices. Vet Rec 2015; 172(22):564–9.

2. Spitznagel MB, Jacobson DM, Cox MD, et al. Caregiver burden in owners of a sick companion animal: a cross-sectional observational study. Vet Rec 2017; 181(12):321.
3. Pierce J. The last walk: reflections on our pets at the end of their lives. Chicago: University of Chicago Press; 2012.
4. Pierce J. The dying animal. J Bioeth Inq 2013;10(4):469–78.
5. Rollin BE. Euthanasia, moral stress, and chronic illness in veterinary medicine. Vet Clin North Am Small Anim Pract 2011;41(3):651–9.
6. Yeates J. Ethical aspects of euthanasia of owned animals. Practice 2010;32:70–3.
7. Meyer RE. Physiologic measures of animal stress during transitional states of consciousness. Animals (Basel) 2015;5:702–16.
8. Alkire MT, Hudetz AG, Tononi G. Consciousness and anesthesia. Science 2008; 322:876–80.
9. AVMA guidelines for the Euthanasia of Animals: 2013 edition. Available at: https://www.avma.org/KB/Policies/Documents/euthanasia.pdf. Accessed May 22, 2018.
10. Mayevsky A, Barbiro-Michaely E, Ligeti L, et al. Effects of euthanasia on the brain physiological activities monitored in real-time. Neurol Res 2002;24:647–51.
11. Jugovac I, Imas O, Hudetz A. Behavioral and electroencephalographic effects of intracerebroventricularly infused pentobarbital, propofol, fentanyl and midazolam. Anesthesiology 2006;105:764–78.
12. Sarasso S, Boly M, Napolitani M, et al. Consciousness and complexity during unresponsiveness induced by propofol, xenon and ketamine. Curr Biol 2015;25(23): 3099–105.
13. Marchitelli, B. Pilot study: adverse events during euthanasia - 94 dogs. Unpublished data. 2017.
14. Perkin RM, Resnik DB. The agony of agonal respiration is the last gasp necessary? J Med Ethics 2002;28:164–9.
15. Ristagno G, Tang W, Sun S, et al. Experimental paper spontaneous gasping produces carotid blood flow during untreated cardiac arrest. Resuscitation 2007; 75(2):366–71.
16. St-John W, Paton JF. Respiratory-modulated activities of the rostral medulla which may generate gasping. Respir Physiol Neurobiol 2003;135(1):97–101.
17. Chang YT, Tang W, Ristagno G, et al. The effects of gasping during cardiac arrest and cardiopulmonary resuscitation. In: Gullo A, Berlot G, editors. Perioperative and critical care medicine. Milano (Italy): Springer; 2006. p. 131–41.
18. Manole MD, Hickey RW. Preterminal gasping and effects on the cardiac function. Crit Care Med 2006;34(12 Suppl):S438–41.
19. Berger S. Gasping, survival and the science of resuscitation. Circulation 2008; 118:2495–7.
20. Krause A, Nowak Z, Srbu R, et al. Respiratory autoresuscitation following severe acute hypoxemia in anesthetized adult rats. Respir Physiol Neurobiol 2016;232: 43–53.
21. Vaughan KL. The last gasp. Vet Rec 1971;88(2):56.
22. Bullock J, Lanaux T, Buckley G. Comparison of euthanasia methods 343 client-owned dogs: pentobarbital/phenytoin alone vs propofol and pentobarbital/phenytoin combination. Abstract IVECCS Conference. 2016. Available at: http://2016.iveccs.org/twocol.aspx?page=Small+Animal+Abstract. Accessed May 22, 2018.
23. Buhl R, Anderson LO, Karlshoj M, et al. Evaluation of clinical and electrocardiographic changes during euthanasia of horses. Vet J 2013;196(3):483–91.

24. Aleman M, Williams DC, Guedes A, et al. Cerebral and brainstem electrophysiologic activity during euthanasia with pentobarbital sodium in horses. J Vet Intern Med 2015;29:663–72.

25. Evans AT, Broadstone R, Stapleton J, et al. Comparison of pentobarbital alone and pentobarbital in combination with lidocaine for euthanasia in dogs. J Am Vet Med Assoc 1993;203(5):664–6.

26. Wallach MB, Peterson KE, Richards RK. Electrophysiologic studies of a combination of secobarbital and dibucaine for euthanasia of dogs. Am J Vet Res 1981; 42(5):850–3.

27. Lumb WV, Doshi J, Scott RJ. A comparative study of T-61 pentobarbital for euthanasia of dogs. J Am Vet Med Assoc 1978;172(2):149–52.

28. Rowan AN. T-61 use in the euthanasia of domestic animals: a survey. In: Fox MW, Mickley LD, editors. Advances in animal welfare science. Washington, DC: Humane Society of the US; 1985. p. 79–86.

29. Barocio LD. Review of literature on use of T-61 as an euthanasic agent. Int J Study Anim Probl 1983;4(4):336–42.

30. Chalifoux A, Dallaire A. Physiologic and behavioral evaluation of CO euthanasia of adult dogs. Am J Vet Res 1983;44(12):2412–7.

31. FDA/CVM FOIA-NADA-128-967-Repose-Obtained 6/19/15. Available at https://www.fda.gov/AnimalVeterinary/Products/ApprovedAnimalDrugProducts/ucm2006466.htm. Acessed February 27, 2019.

32. FDA/CVM FOIA-NADA-100-809-T-61-Obtained 6/19/15. Available at https://www.fda.gov/AnimalVeterinary/Products/ApprovedAnimalDrugProducts/ucm2006466.htm. Acessed February 27, 2019.

33. FDA/CVM FOIA NADA-119-807-Beuthanasia D-Obtained 11/2/17. Available at https://www.fda.gov/AnimalVeterinary/Products/ApprovedAnimalDrugProducts/ucm2006466.htm. Acessed February 27, 2019.

34. FDA/CVM FOIA NADA-141-245 Tributame-Obtained 5/10/18. Available at https://www.fda.gov/AnimalVeterinary/Products/ApprovedAnimalDrugProducts/ucm2006466.htm. Acessed February 27, 2019.

35. Ramsay EC, Wetzel RW. Comparison of five regimes for oral administration of medication to induce sedation in dogs prior to euthanasia. J Am Vet Med Assoc 1998;213(2):240–2.

36. Wetzel RW, EC Ramsay EC. Comparison of four regimes for intraoral administration of medication to induce sedation in cats prior to euthanasia. J Am Vet Med Assoc 1998;213(2):243–5.

37. Webb AI. Euthanizing agents. In: Reviere JE, Papich MG, editors. Veterinary pharmacology and therapeutics. 9th edition. Ames (IA): Wiley Blackwell; 2009. p. 401–8.

38. Hellebrekers LJ, Baumans V, Bertens AP, et al. On the use of T61 for euthanasia of domestic and laboratory animals; an ethical evaluation. Lab Anim 1990;24:200–4.

39. Brasil S, Bor-Seng-Shu E, de-Lima-Oliveira M, et al. Role of computed tomography angiography and perfusion tomography in diagnosing brain death: a systematic review. J Neuroradiol 2016;43(2):133–40.

40. Frampas E, Videcoq M, de Kerviler E, et al. CT angiography for brain death diagnosis. AJNR Am J Neuroradiol 2009;30:1566–70.

41. Poularas J, Karakitsos D, Kostakis A, et al. Comparison between transcranial color Doppler ultrasonography and angiography in the confirmation of brain death. Transplant Proc 2006;38:1213–7.

42. Chen Z, Cao J, Cao Y, et al. An empirical EEG analysis in brain death diagnosis for adults. Cogn Neurodyn 2008;2:257–71.

43. Bird TD, Plum F. Recovery from barbiturate overdose coma with a prolonged iso-electric electroencephalogram. Neurology 1968;18(5):456–60.
44. Saito T, Takeichi S, Tokunaga I, et al. Experimental studies on effects of barbiturate on electroencephalogram and auditory brain-stem responses. Nihon Hoigaku Zasshi 1997;51(5):388–95.
45. Rady MY, Verheijede JL. Awareness in the dying human brain: implications for organ donation practices. J Crit Care 2016;34:121–3.
46. Parnia S. Death and consciousness-an overview of the mental and cognitive experience of death. Ann N Y Acad Sci 2014;1330(1):75–93.
47. Pana R, Hornby MS, Shemie SK, et al. Time to loss of brain function and activity during circulatory arrest. J Crit Care 2016;34:77–83.
48. Bruno MA, Gosseries O, Ledoux D, et al. Assessment of consciousness with electrophysiological and neurologic imaging techniques. Curr Opin Crit Care 2011; 17(2):146–51.
49. Kroeger D, Florea B, Amzica F. Human brain activity patterns beyond the isoelectric line of extreme deep coma. PLoS One 2013;8(9):e75257.
50. Alper T. Anesthetizing the public conscience: lethal injection and animal euthanasia, 35 Fordham Urb. L.J. 817. 2008. Available at: https://scholarship.law.berkeley.edu/facpubs/835/. Accessed May 22, 2018.
51. KNMG/KNMP Guidelines for the Practice of Euthanasia and Physician-Assisted Suicide August 2012. Available at: https://www.knmp.nl/downloads/guidelines-for-the-practice-of-euthanasia.pdf. Accessed May 22, 2018.
52. Rietjens JA, van der Maas PJ, Onwuteaka-Philipsen BD, et al. Two decades of research on euthanasia from the Netherlands. What have we learnt and what questions remain? J Bioeth Inq 2009;6(3):271–83.
53. Steck N, Egger M, Maessen M, et al. Euthanasia and assisted suicide in selected European Countries and US states systematic literature review. Med Care 2013; 51(10):938–44.
54. van der Heide A, Onwuteaka-Philipsen BD, Rurup ML, et al. End-of-life practices in the Netherlands under the euthanasia act. N Engl J Med 2007;356:1957–65.
55. Onwuteaka-Philipsen BD, Brinkman-Stoppelenburg A, Penning C, et al. Trends in end-of-life practices before and after the enactment of the euthanasia law in the Netherlands from 1990 to 2010: a repeated cross-sectional survey. Lancet 2012; 380:908–15.
56. Groenewoud JH, Van der Heide A, Onwuteaka-Philipsen BD, et al. Clinical problems with the performance of euthanasia and physician-assisted suicide in the Netherlands. N Engl J Med 2000;342(8):551–6.
57. Horikx A, Admiraal PV. Utilization of euthanatic agents; experience of physicians with 227 patients, 1998-2000. Ned Tijdschr Geneeskd 2000;144(52):2497–500.
58. Vander Stichele RH, Bilsen JJ, Bernhein JL, et al. Drugs used for euthanasia in Flanders, Belguim. Pharmacoepidemiol Drug Saf 2004;3:89–95.
59. Sprij B. Could it be a little less? Let the dose of thiopental in euthanasia depend on body weight. Ned Tijdschr Geneeskd 2010;154:A1983.

The Social Worker
An Essential Hospice and Palliative Team Member

Sandra Brackenridge, LCSW, BCD[a,b,c,d,*]

KEYWORDS

- Hospice • Veterinary hospice • Social work • Palliative care • Field placement
- Veterinary social work • Animal hospice team

KEY POINTS

- Hospice social workers are required by Medicare as team members. A brief history of social work in hospice is covered to explain how this came to be.
- The unique education to obtain a social work degree is outlined so that readers can understand social work skills, knowledge, and perspective as compatible with hospice work.
- The responsibilities of a human hospice social worker are described.
- The responsibilities of a social worker in veterinary hospice and palliative care are described through a sample case.

A BRIEF HISTORY OF SOCIAL WORKERS IN HOSPICE AND PALLIATIVE CARE

Dame Cicely Saunders is credited with the contemporary human hospice model when she founded St. Christopher's Hospice in London, England in 1967, which continues to operate today. Dame Saunders was a social worker, nurse, doctor, teacher, and writer who had worked with dying individuals and their families throughout her practice. She promoted the possibility of pain management versus curative care, and she introduced her view that pain happens on all levels of human existence: physical, psychological, social, and spiritual. Dame Saunders wrote that social workers who were doing case management in the medical field in the 1940s were laying the foundation for hospice.[1] In fact, there were other hospices even before St. Christopher's was founded. Crusaders in the eleventh century began opening accommodations for the sick and dying, and during the nineteenth century homes were opened in Paris,

The author is sole proprietor of Social Work Consulting and Counseling for Veterinary Practices www.sbrackenridgelcsw.com.

[a] Texas Woman's University, Denton, TX, USA; [b] Idaho State University, Pocatello, ID, USA; [c] Center for Veterinary Specialty & Emergency Care, Lewisville, TX, USA; [d] Consulting and Counseling, Veterinary Practices, Corinth, TX, USA
* 4206 Creek Falls Drive, Corinth, TX 76208.
E-mail address: SANDRA@SBRACKENRIDGELCSW.COM

Dublin, Sydney, Melbourne, and New York for the poor who needed what is now referred to as palliative care. All of the homes at this time were connected to or operated by nuns of the Catholic Church. Also, during the nineteenth century and the first half of the twentieth century, medical professionals became more involved with the process of dying, and there was some focus on disease-specific dying.[2]

Another pioneer in death and dying, Elisabeth Kubler-Ross, was studying dying individuals and their dying process at the same time that Dame Saunders' concepts were gaining notice and momentum. Kubler-Ross published her first book *On Death and Dying* in 1969,[3] in which she described five stages of the dying process and associated emotional experiences. The book was the first of its kind, and it gained the attention of the medical community around the world. Heretofore, medical professionals largely ignored patients once they had determined that they could not be cured. The book was a worldwide bestseller, and Kubler-Ross was a much sought-after speaker around the world. She argued publicly and in her writings for patients to be allowed to participate in end-of-life decision making, and she argued for deinstitutionalized dying. In 1972, Kubler-Ross testified before the United States Senate Special Committee on Aging, and her testimony encouraged the first legislation proposed in 1974 for hospice funding. However, the legislation was not enacted. The country would wait until 1982 for Congress to introduce a Medicare Hospice Benefit, which was made permanent in 1984.[4]

The Medicare Hospice Benefit Amendment to the Social Security Act (Title 18, Section 1861, Subsection dd) defines hospice care, and it defines what characteristics qualify an individual for services. Furthermore, the law requires involvement of a doctor, nurse, pastoral or other counselor, and a social worker on the interdisciplinary care team.[4] An explanation as to the reason Medicare specified a social worker rather than any licensed mental health profession is discussed in this article, delineating their unique and explicit training, which is standardized internationally.

There are many similarities between human and animal hospice and palliative care. They are similar in the philosophic approach of: (1) having choices about end-of-life care; (2) valuing palliative versus curative treatment; (3) treating the whole patient and family as a unit of care, including psychological, social, and spiritual needs; and (4) recognizing the emotional burden placed on the interdisciplinary care team. Several organizations have established guidelines and/or position statements regarding veterinary hospice and palliative care, including the American Veterinary Medical Association. Their Guidelines for Hospice Care state that treatment should involve contact with "licensed mental health professionals who are trained and experienced in grief and bereavement."[5]

INTERNALLY STANDARDIZED TRAINING OF SOCIAL WORKERS

Perhaps one reason that Medicare selected the social worker as the only mental health professional for the interdisciplinary hospice team is the long history that social workers have had in working with the dying. This author is of the opinion that social work was selected by Medicare because it is the only mental health discipline with a standardized, mandatory educational curriculum, which must be accredited by the Council on Social Work Education (CSWE) for the social worker to become licensed in any state.[6] Many states license "counselors," but one cannot assume details of their training from the licensure. The title "social worker" is regulated by laws in each state in the United States and internationally. The National Association of Social Workers Code of Ethics, first written in 1960 and amended every 3 years, sets the standards in the United States for each state board's regulations about ethics, values, and conduct.[7] The International Federation of Social Workers includes social workers from all continents and 80 countries, and this organization has also developed ethical standards.[8]

University-level instruction in social work and clinical social work has existed since 1898 and 1904, respectively. The National Council on Social Work Education was formed in 1946, followed by the creation of the CSWE in 1952.[9] CSWE accredits programs in the United States and Canada, and also collaborates with other countries. Many accredited programs in the United States work with other countries' university programs to ensure that all students receive the same education. This author was an Associate Professor of Social Work at two universities for a total of 23 years, participated in reaccreditation several times, and is familiar with the accreditation requirements of the CSWE.

Within a bachelor-level accredited social work program, undergraduate students are required to take core courses that include instruction in work with individuals, families, and communities. Students are required to learn psychosocial assessment of individuals and families, and to become adept at forming, facilitating, and evaluating groups of all kinds, such as support groups or focus groups. They must develop a foundation in human behavior and development throughout the life span. Additionally, they learn how to conduct scientific research and develop policy for organizations and communities. They must have a good foundation in cultural competence. Undergraduate-level social workers earn the bachelor of social work (BSW).

Graduates of bachelor-level social work programs and individuals with other undergraduate backgrounds may work toward a masters-level social work degree, the Master of Social Work (MSW). Depending on curricular offerings in their MSW programs, students may specialize in a track that is clinically focused, such as mental health, or health care focused, such as medical social work or hospice. They may choose a broader, "macro" focus on community, policy and administrative practice. Some schools offer additional tracks or certificates of advanced study in such topics as palliative care, gerontology, or trauma, and dual degrees, such as an MSW and a Doctor of Law. Some social work schools offer the "generalist" MSW, which means that graduates should have good proficiency in all areas without specialization.

A cornerstone of social work education and training is "field placement" or internship hours spent in the social work field. A minimum of 900 hours is required by CSWE for completion of the MSW degree; some MSW programs require as many as 1920 hours. BSW students complete fewer field placement hours, typically ranging from 400 to 600 hours in various human service organizations. It is during these field placement experiences that students learn to practice their skills, and they become more confident and proficient.

All social work students are trained to use a strengths perspective when working with any client: individual, family, group, or community. Social workers do not focus on pathology or deficiencies; they assess a client's strengths with goals of empowerment. All social work students are taught to use the ecosystems theoretic orientation to assess not only the individual but also the larger systems influencing the individual: the family; the neighborhood; other community systems; and larger governmental systems, such as legislation or public policy. Following assessment, the social worker is able to explore and possibly facilitate changes in any system that might benefit the client's well-being.

Importantly, all levels of social workers receive instruction about the National Association of Social Workers Code of Ethics, which is infused throughout BSW and MSW curricula. This Code of Ethics is well known to be the most stringent of any group of helping professionals in terms of ethical behavior with clients, colleagues, employers, and the broader society. Finally, self-care is a topic that is mandated by the Code of Ethics, and it is taught and infused throughout any program. An experienced and efficient social worker should be aware of themselves so that they are aware of boundaries, the need to combat compassion fatigue, and they should be able to implement strategies for coping and management to ensure longevity and objectivity in practice.

A clinically trained social worker has more coursework and field placement or work experience in a setting focused on mental illnesses and diagnosis, substance use disorders, and medical conditions that affect cognition (eg, dementia, traumatic brain injury, intellectual disability). Licensed Clinical Social Workers (LCSW) are able to practice independently, without supervision, and to diagnose and treat people with these disorders. LCSWs often function as an individual psychotherapist in this regard, whereas Licensed Masters Social Workers (LMSW) do not. Relevant for social work practice in end-of-life settings, grief and bereavement have long been considered a normal response to loss, anticipated loss, and to transitions during the life span, and there is no psychiatric diagnosis of grief or bereavement. One need not be an LCSW to appropriately support people through grief and loss.

Social workers work cooperatively with other mental health professionals, such as psychologists and psychiatrists, when their assessment of clients warrants that they should, such as a situation in which clients would benefit from either psychological testing or psychiatric medication. Social workers work within interdisciplinary teams in most areas of practice, and when a social worker is not formally a member of an interdisciplinary team, they frequently refer to and consult with other professionals as needed. The other professionals may include nurses, physicians, lawyers, probation officers, teachers, or administrators of any system that influences the client.

Social workers are uniquely trained to "meet clients where they are." Historically, social workers have done much of their work in the field, away from an office. They are comfortable going to the client's home environment, which fits with palliative and hospice care and differentiates the profession from other mental health providers. This principle of meeting the client where she or he is also applies to the problem-solving process and therapeutic alliance, regardless of physical location.

SOCIAL WORK RESPONSIBILITIES WITHIN HUMAN HOSPICE AND PALLIATIVE CARE

Social workers support human clients within a variety of settings whether these clients are terminally ill patients on a hospice census or chronically ill patients receiving palliative care. For humans, delivery of services may occur within the home of the patient, residential hospice centers, or within palliative care departments of hospitals. A distinction made between social work within hospice and social work with palliative care is that "social workers who work in hospice care by necessity work in palliative care, while palliative care social workers may not work in hospice settings."[10]

An important responsibility of the social work team member is to complete a psychosocial assessment in the beginning of their work with the patient and the family. This initial assessment is required documentation by Medicare and other insurers. It includes history of past and present medical conditions, previous and current treatment plans, and considers the mental and emotional health of the patient and all family members. Any past or present mental illnesses, substance use, and behavioral conditions that may affect the patient or the patient's care are assessed. Finally, a psychosocial assessment provides documentation of "social, cultural, financial, or familial" factors that may affect patient care, "including socioeconomic hardships, family conflicts, engagement and/or disengagement with friends and the community in general, etc."[10] The psychosocial assessment is instrumental in preparation for recommendations that the social worker will make regarding psychological and social support for the patient and their family. It is also instrumental in determining risks, such as substance use history in the context of prescribed medications. Assessing risks and planning accordingly increases the likelihood of a positive outcome.

Social workers in all hospice and palliative care settings improve coordinated care of the patient through communication with the interdisciplinary team of physicians, nurses, chaplains and the patient's family. Social workers may hold family meetings to assess needs and concerns, and provide individual counseling for struggling individuals. Psychotherapy is provided, and conflict mediation when family members disagree. Social workers may help the family complete a power of attorney for medical care, a living will, or a do-not-resuscitate order. They may help family members navigate insurance, or recommend specific equipment for the home. Logistics of caregiving are a major concern for some families, whereas other families are overwhelmed with anticipatory grief or with funeral planning.[10,11] Social workers can help with all of these concerns.

Human patients and their families receiving hospice care often benefit from respite care, or a break from the demands of caregiving. Hospice staff members do not provide round the clock care, and a significant amount of patient care is provided by family members. A hospice nurse may visit once per week, depending on the assigned level of care; an aide may visit several times per week to provide hygienic and nutritional services. The social worker and the chaplain typically visit once per month unless their services have been declined, but when needed they visit more frequently. Thus, family and friends are depended on greatly, and these caregivers often suffer from enormous emotional and physical stress. The social worker or the nurse may recommend and arrange for a time of respite, and arrange that the patient is placed in a facility for the family to rest, if respite care cannot occur in-home. Volunteer hours are part of Medicare requirements for hospice organizations; a significant proportion of volunteer hours are spent providing respite care for caregivers. Often, families are temporarily relieved from caregiving to be able to run errands or engage in activities of normal life.

For the patient, the social worker may provide counseling aimed at addressing fears of dying, other sources of existential suffering, or navigating the emotional experiences of chronic pain or other physical symptoms. The patient's goals for their care and their life are ascertained and treatment planning is adjusted accordingly. Social workers may assist the patient in resolution of unfinished business or regrets through counseling, or through facilitating conversations or reunions. Such issues as estrangement from family members or friends who are important to the patient may be addressed. Many social workers work with patients as they are struggling with their life review during the dying process. Through use of many skills, the social worker may help the patient find meaning in their life story.[10]

Following a death, bereavement services, such as counseling, grief support groups, and memorial/remembrance events, are part of the Medicare Hospice Benefit for 1 year. Some families decline these services, but many welcome them. Although social workers are trained to provide these services, some hospices use the chaplains in this capacity.

Finally, although it is not usually listed within a social worker's job description, many human hospice and palliative care social workers serve as a support for the professional team. Burnout and compassion fatigue are serious risks for people who work in hospice care, because caring for patients and families around death may awaken unresolved, accumulated grief in these professionals. In addition, the professionals themselves may experience their own grief response when a patient for whom they have cared, dies. The social worker may arrange for individual counseling of staff, organize monthly debriefing or provide group counseling. In this way, the presence of a social worker also helps to lessen compassion fatigue among the professional team.[12–14]

In summary, social workers perform all of the responsibilities listed in **Table 1** when they are working in human hospice and palliative care. This is not intended as an exhaustive list, but these are common activities of the social worker.

SOCIAL WORK RESPONSIBILITIES WITHIN VETERINARY HOSPICE AND PALLIATIVE CARE

The most remarkable difference between human hospice and palliative care and its veterinary counterpart is of course the patient. Animal patients receiving care cannot make choices regarding their disease process, chronic debilitating condition, or when they are ready to die. These choices are a grave responsibility for the humans that love them: their family. The human-animal relationship is much different than it was 30 years ago. People proudly revere their pets as family members, and the relationships they have with them are beneficial, mutually dependent, and sometimes decades long.[15–19] As such, many human family members consider choices for their beloved animal seriously, and with much ambivalence. They may also underestimate the burden that caregiving can have on the entire family system. Humans who commit to the tremendous task of caring for a chronically ill or disabled pet, and those who struggle with how and when to make a decision for euthanasia, can benefit from a social worker's therapeutic and supportive guidance. Often there is not one clear medical option, and social workers are trained to guide people through the many concerns that arise, consciously or subconsciously, in decision making.

One goal of this article is to help practitioners who are providing palliative care in the hospital or at home to understand what social workers can do to help the family, the team, and improve care. The following is a hypothetical case example that illustrates a social worker's role and responsibilities in veterinary hospice and palliative care, and demonstrates commonly used types of intervention. There is not a "typical case" in this type of care. Every family is unique, and the disease processes treated are varied and numerous. However, there are common themes and needs that social workers are uniquely equipped to address. Readers are encouraged to recognize these in the following case study, and consider implementing some of the supports described to optimize care in their own veterinary settings for seriously ill patients and their families.

Table 1
Responsibilities of a social worker within a human hospice or palliative care practice

Psychosocial Assessments	Counseling and Psychotherapy	Mediation Between Family Members
Regular visits with patient and/or family	Goals of care conversations	Documentation
Resource acquisition, education, assistance	Participation in interdisciplinary team meetings	Assistance with paperwork, funeral planning
Advocating for the family/patient with systems to provide support	Support, counseling, debriefing for the team members	Life review/finding meaning/acceptance with life story
Arrangements for respite	Facilitation of last wishes	Grief support groups

Sample Case

Seapaws, a 12-year-old neutered male Newfoundland, presents to the emergency department of a large multispecialty referral hospital for inappetence and vomiting. He has a history of poor mobility and lethargy, and diarrhea. After an initial suspicion of mesenteric torsion, and assessment by multiple veterinary facilities, megaesophagus without aspiration pneumonia was diagnosed, with myasthenia gravis strongly suspected. The owner indicates an interest in hospice care for Seapaws rather than extensive hospitalization. The owner enlists the help of a veterinary practice that advertises in-home hospice and palliative care, and Seapaws is discharged from the hospital. The discharge instructions include detailed instructions for feeding, and administration of oral and injectable medications. The hospice/palliative care veterinarian, nurse, and social worker arrive the next morning for intake and treatment planning.

While the nurse and veterinarian examine Seapaws, the social worker begins her assessment with the owner and her husband. She notes the owner's long history with the breed, the owner's type 1 diabetes (which has resulted in comfort with injections), and her dogs' ability to alert for blood sugar changes. Following the initial physical examination, the team initiates a goals of care conversation with the clients, using the Serious Veterinary Illness Conversation Guide.[20] (Additional information about this conversation guide is found in Katherine Goldberg's article, "Goals of Care: Development and Use of the Serious Veterinary Illness Conversation Guide," in this issue.) Each of the seven areas for conversation are led by the veterinarian, and the social worker uses clarification and reflection skills to hone mutual understanding and thorough communication.

It is ascertained that the owner and her husband have a good understanding of Seapaws' illness, probable course, and prognosis. Their goals are to have him at home, easing the separation anxiety of all, including their other dog. Their fears are of Seapaws suffering dramatically or suddenly, and of helplessness in comforting him. The social worker uses a technique called implosion, in which the couple are asked to describe their imagined worse-case scenarios. As they respond, the veterinarian comments about what is unlikely and what is realistic in each scenario, and then possible action steps and outcomes are suggested should the realistic scenarios occur.

The social worker gently asks the owners how they know that Seapaws is still strong, and what of his abilities, if diminished or absent, might make them think he is willing to die. In describing Seapaws' strengths, the owner begins to weep, and the social worker offers tissue and water. The owner describes his love of swimming, and how she knows he may never swim again. She talks about how nurturing he is, and she says that she would begin to think about euthanasia if he "lost the light in his eyes" or lost interest in his family members. She remembers the euthanasia of a previous dog, and says she knows the process is peaceful. She says that although she prefers "natural death," she is prepared to euthanize if necessary. The social worker asks about the husband's feelings and impressions and addresses his fear about providing support for his wife. She describes the care team's dual purpose in providing physical aspects of medical care for Seapaws and emotional support for him and his wife. She explains the bereavement services offered after death, available for a year or until no longer needed.

The veterinarian reflects what has been communicated and outlines a treatment plan that includes medications, biweekly nurse visits, and daily nurse check-ins by telephone. Equipment, such as a harness to help Seapaws ambulate, is chosen from available inventory. Financial estimates are presented and negotiated, and the veterinarian and nurse depart. The social worker begins the in-depth psychosocial history by explaining that she needs a bit more information and history to ensure success of the plan. She asks questions about the history of the family, ages of each household member (including pets), length of the marriage, and names and ages of other family members or friends who would be coming into the home. She inquiries about the physical health of each person who would be caring for Seapaws and helping with ambulation, hygiene, and so forth. The owner's diabetes is discussed thoroughly as potentially impacting care of Seapaws. The social worker also gathers information about family mental health history, including substance use. The clients mention that their 20-year-old son, away at college at this time, is in recovery from an opioid addiction. The social worker discusses preparation and securing medication, in the event that their son visits during Seapaws' care.

The social worker explores other losses experienced by each owner, and of particular interest to the social worker is how they experienced grief. The deaths of their parents are noted, and the couple reports that they have not lived near their parents for many years. They both express guilt about their grief being somewhat truncated because of the distance. The social worker normalizes their feelings and shares psychoeducational information about grief responses.

The social worker asks about past losses of dogs and other pets. They describe how each died, including experiences of euthanasia. Feelings associated with euthanasia as a treatment choice are explored, and the social worker learns that both individuals value the choice to prevent further suffering. The social worker says, "Sometimes a family needs time to think about these choices," and she provides a list of resources including local crematoriums, pet cemeteries, and an article about memorializing pets that includes unique options, such as plantings, rocks, jewelry, and fireworks made from cremains. Finally, spiritual beliefs are explored, and both owners relay confidence in their belief of an afterlife for animals.

Finally, to gain a sense of the degree of attachment to Seapaws that will help her to prepare and assist the owners in their grief, the social worker says, "Tell me about how you came to live a life with Seapaws." The owner shares her story about selecting him from the breeder, earning his unique name, and working toward his championship in the show ring. The social worker also explores dependency between the owner and the dog, especially because he alerts her regarding blood sugar. The social worker concludes that attachment is in the highest range, and therefore the owner's grief response will be intense. Consequently, the social worker provides written and verbal education about grief, and in particular, anticipatory grief. They talk about the emotions of grief, reactions that are commonly experienced, and the stressful nature of the entire experience. An appointment is made for the following week for the social worker to return, but she says that she is available by telephone or as per need in the interim. Before departing, the social worker kneels and pets Seapaws, saying to him, "You have been a very good dog, Seapaws. Thank you for loving these nice people."

During a regular weekly interdisciplinary team meeting at the veterinary practice office, the social worker is informed that Seapaws has markedly declined, aspiration pneumonia is suspected, and the family is requesting a visit from her. The social worker returns for a home visit, during which the owners ask for help in determining when or if they should euthanize. They express diminished hope that Seapaws will maintain an acceptable quality of life, and they express fear that they are asking for "too much from him." The social worker reminds them of their first conversation, and what the owner said about the light in Seapaws' eyes. Both owners tearfully reflect about how "he is not himself." They state their other dog now avoids Seapaws. The social worker explains that they may take some time to decide, and she says, "Whatever decision you make out of your love for Seapaws, with the motivation to do best by him, will be a good decision." Before leaving, the social worker suggests a video chat with their son for him to say goodbye.

The owner arranges for an in-home euthanasia the following day with specific requests around timing, location, and so forth. During euthanasia, the social worker is present to provide emotional support to the family, and to coordinate aftercare with a crematorium. Everyone present reminisces about the special dog Seapaws.

Following Seapaws' death, the social worker debriefs the veterinary care team so that they can process their own grief. Team members are relieved to know that social work services will continue with the family. The team also decides to memorialize Seapaws on the practice Web site. The social worker continues to make home visits for grief counseling with the owners, and the visits decrease over time.

SUMMARY

The social worker's interventions and job responsibilities in the hypothetical case of Seapaws are modeled after the social work role within human hospice and palliative care (see **Table 1**). Many of these same responsibilities may be performed by a social worker within an animal hospice or palliative care setting. Social workers in any veterinary setting should be educated in an accredited social work program as described previously, and have some training in grief counseling and the dying process, family dynamics, and the role of animals in family systems. They should be licensed, working within their scope of practice, and supervised appropriately as determined by the state.

Ideally, the animal hospice/palliative care social worker should be exposed to veterinary settings, such as emergency and critical care; familiarized with various medical procedures; and educated about the human-animal bond. They should also be familiar with human hospice either as a hospice social worker, medical social worker, or even a volunteer. Social workers should never engage in the handling of animals for treatment, because it is beyond their scope of practice. However, they are uniquely trained to help every human, team members and patient caregivers, to increase positive outcomes and to reduce risks.

This author realizes that human hospice/palliative care work is not completely transferable or translatable to veterinary settings because of some barriers. One barrier is that of money. Whereas the social worker's time and work in human hospice is reimbursed by Medicare or insurance, there is no such mechanism in veterinary hospice. The responsibilities of a social worker must be covered in fees charged to veterinary clients.

Most importantly, because of their unique training and capabilities, social workers are indispensable in this highly emotional and intimate form of veterinary practice. Practitioners of animal hospice and palliative care may be able to contract with or employ a social worker fairly inexpensively. The cost for their services could be reimbursed with an estimate for higher level of care presented to clients. Alternatively, and at the very least, a social worker could be enlisted to attend one interdisciplinary team meeting every 4 to 6 weeks, to debrief with staff and to consult about cases. Clients and staff can benefit enormously from their participation in this area of veterinary practice.

REFERENCES

1. Saunders D. Social work and palliative care—the early history. Br J Soc Work 2001;31(5):791–9.
2. Marocchino K. In the shadow of a rainbow: the history of animal hospice. Vet Clin North Am Small Anim Pract 2011;41(3):477–98.

3. Kübler-Ross E. On death and dying. New York: Scribner; 1969.
4. Hospice social work: linking policy, practice, and research. Washington, DC: Social Work Policy Institute; 2010. p. 3.
5. American Veterinary Medical Association. American Veterinary Medical Association hospice guidelines. Available at: https://www.avma.org/KB/Policies/Pages/Veterinary-End-of-Life-Care.aspx. Accessed February 15, 2019.
6. Gibbs P. Accreditation of BSW programs. J Soc Work Educ 1995. https://doi.org/10.1080/10437797.1995.10778834.
7. National Association of Social Workers. Code of ethics. Washington, DC: National Association of Social Work; 2008.
8. Council on Social Work Education. No Title. Katherine A. Kendall Institute for International Social Work Education. 2018. Available at: https://www.cswe.org/Centers-Initiatives/Centers/International-KAKI/About/History-and-Goals. Accessed February 15, 2019.
9. Council on Social Work Education. CSWE a brief history. Available at: CSWE.org https://www.cswe.org/About-CSWE/CSWE-A-Brief-History. Accessed February 15, 2019.
10. Louie K. Introductory guide to hospice and palliative care social work 2018. Available at: https://www.onlinemswprograms.com/features/guide-to-hospice-palliative-care-social-work.html. Accessed June 8, 2018.
11. A day in the life of a social worker. Vitas Healthcare. Available at: www.vitas.com/resources/hospice-care/a-day-in-the-life-of -a-social-worker. Accessed June 8, 2018.
12. Slocum-Gori S, Hemsworth D, Chan WWY, et al. Understanding compassion satisfaction, compassion fatigue and burnout: a survey of the hospice palliative care workforce. Palliat Med 2013. https://doi.org/10.1177/0269216311431311.
13. Alkema K, Linton JM, Davies R. A study of the relationship between self-care, compassion satisfaction, compassion fatigue, and burnout among hospice professionals. J Soc Work End Life Palliat Care 2008. https://doi.org/10.1080/15524250802353934.
14. Keidel GC. Burnout and compassion fatigue among hospice caregivers. Am J Hosp Palliat Care 2002. https://doi.org/10.1177/104990910201900312.
15. Sable P. Pets, attachment, and well-being across the life cycle. Soc Work 1995; 40(3):334–41.
16. Sable P. The pet connection: an attachment perspective. Clin Soc Work J 2012; 41(1):93–9.
17. Friedmann E, Son H. The human-companion animal bond: how humans benefit. Vet Clin North Am Small Anim Pract 2009;39(2):293–326.
18. Zilcha-Mano S, Mikulincer M, Shaver PR. An attachment perspective on human-pet relationships: conceptualization and assessment of pet attachment orientations. J Res Pers 2011;45(4):345–57.
19. Walsh F. Human-animal bonds II: the role of pets in family systems and family therapy. Fam Process 2009;48(4):481–99.
20. Goldberg KJ. Serious veterinary illness conversation guide. 2015. Adapted from the Serious Illness Conversation Guide Ariadne Labs: A Joint Center for Health Systems Innovation (www.ariadnelabs.org) at Brigham and Women's Hospital and the Harvard T. H. Chan School of Public Health, in collaboration with Dana-Farber Cancer Institute. Licensed under the Creative Commons Attribution-NonCommercial-ShareAlike 4.0 International License. Available at: http://creativecommons.org/licenses/by-nc-sa/4.0/. Accessed February 15, 2019.

Brain Awareness and Conflict in Veterinary Medical Practice

What Happens and How to Deal with It

Elizabeth B. Strand, PhD, MSSW

KEYWORDS

- Conflict • Emotional brain • Interpersonal neurobiology • Conflict management
- Compassion-focused therapy • Polyvagal theory

KEY POINTS

- Human beings alternate between higher and lower brain states throughout each day.
- Lower brain states are associated with negative emotions and rigid thought processes.
- Conflict triggers lower brain states.
- Recognizing lower brain states and creating "safe environments" aids in conflict resolution.

 Video content accompanies this article at http://www.vetsmall.theclinics.com.

INTRODUCTION

Interpersonal conflicts in veterinary medical environments can cause both harm and benefit, depending on how they are addressed. If handled poorly, they negatively affect a veterinary professional's well-being, patient safety, and client satisfaction. If handled well, they create strong interpersonal relationships between veterinary professionals and clients. When veterinary care requires palliative and end-of-life decisions, conflict issues are value laden, emotionally driven, and require expert skill to shepherd the end of life process with honesty, compassion, and strength. Creating "safe environments" for hard discussions is essential. This article explores conflicts through a brain awareness lens and offers tools for successfully managing conflicts in veterinary practice.

Disclosure: The author has nothing to disclose.
Veterinary Social Work Program, University of Tennessee, College of Veterinary Medicine, College of Social Work, Knoxville, TN 37996, USA
E-mail address: estrand@utk.edu

Vet Clin Small Anim 49 (2019) 575–586
https://doi.org/10.1016/j.cvsm.2019.01.017
0195-5616/19/© 2019 Elsevier Inc. All rights reserved.
vetsmall.theclinics.com

CONFLICT IN THE MEDICAL ENVIRONMENT

Competently managing conflict in the medical environment is a growing expectation in medical education and practice.[1,2] This expectation is warranted given that malpractice claims and adverse patient safety events are often associated with a breakdown in communication among medical personnel.[3–5] The presence of conflict in the medical environment is well documented both in standard care[6] and during end-of-life care.[7] For instance, 31% of medical team members across 5 human teaching hospitals reported experiencing rude, dismissive, and aggressive (RDA) behavior; 41% of those surveyed stated that the RDA behavior significantly affected their workday and home life. Factors associated with RDA include feeling powerless to make impactful decisions, patient safety concerns, and high workload with lack of perceived support.[8] Skills such as reflective listening are more often used among palliative care professionals; these communication skills are often associated with environments where people feel safe to express their concerns.

In the veterinary field, toxic attitudes and toxic work environments contribute to conflict in the medical environment.[9] Toxic attitudes among team members include chronically negative moods that affect others, an inability to take responsibility, and being the constant "go-to" person for decisions and information. Toxic environments include settings where leadership fails to enforce consequences for poor work behavior, employees feel unappreciated, and work expectations are unclear.[9] Moreover, moral dilemmas in the veterinary setting can create conflict, especially when team members have opposing values regarding patient care.[10]

RDA in the medical environment is associated with decreased well-being among medical professionals and reduced helpfulness among team members.[11] RDA also negatively affects cognitive performance, memory recall,[11,12] and, most importantly, patient care. For instance, Riskin and colleagues[13] randomized medical team members into 2 groups. One group had an RDA team member and the other control group did not. Findings indicated that diagnostic and procedural performance was significantly impaired in the RDA group compared with the control group. Factors associated with poor performance included less information sharing or seeking help from team members in the RDA group.[13] Sharing information and seeking help are essential to working successfully in a medical environment. This research suggests that, in the presence of an RDA team member, healthy patient care behaviors were compromised.

Research asserts that conflict causes undue stress. When stressed, people experience the fight, flight, or freeze response. However, humans have "tricky" brains, as psychologist and compassion-focused therapy founder Paul Gilbert[14] calls it. Humans are intelligent beings with large cortical brains capable of complex creative and abstract thought. Oftentimes, this cortical capacity produces accurate diagnoses and innovative treatment plans, but, when in conflict, the cortical capacity is often immobilized, imagining and remembering the worst-case scenarios within a conflict. With regard to patient care, medical team members ought to "rise above" the tricky brain, prioritizing patient care. However, the natural mammalian stress response overrides humans' ability to use their cortical brains. Although veterinarians know that patient care is more important than RDA comments, the mammalian drive to fight, flight, or freeze in times of stress "tricks" the reasonable and compassionate part of the brain to defer to the part driven by biological safety and survival. Given this glitch, it is important to understand brain awareness through the concepts of polyvagal theory, compassion-focused therapy, interpersonal neurobiology, and emotional-brain training.

BRAIN AWARENESS LENS

It is helpful for people to examine their conflict experiences in terms of the brain and couch their experiences as brain states instead of personality defects. The brain state lens can cultivate a sense of understanding, whereas the latter generates blame and accusation toward others or self. Understanding that everyone experiences brain glitches because of tricky brain enables us to remain "compassionately curious"[15] when conflict arises.

BRAIN STATES

Emotional-brain training, founded by health psychologist Dr Laurel Mellin, offers a useful model of 5 human brain states. Brain state 1 is the highest brain state, in which people feel connected to themselves, others, their purpose, and experience well-being and peace. Alternatively, brain state 5 is the lowest brain state, in which people feel disconnected from others and themselves; life feels meaningless; and thoughts, words, and actions are uncompromising and hostile. Furthermore, people in brain state 5 are completely numb, without feeling. The other states include brain state 2, in which people feel connected but are aware of some painful feelings appropriate to the situation. In brain state 3 there are slight feelings of stress from multiple sources. In brain state 4 there is definite stress from a specific, identifiable source with strong reactions disproportionate to the situation (ie, breaking a coffee cup and bursting into tears). Brain states 1 and 2 are considered "connected brain states." Brain states 4 and 5 are "disconnected brain states." Brain state 3 is the cusp between connected and disconnected (**Table 1**).

In addition, emotional-brain training posits that there are emotional set points, or the tendency for the brain state to maintain a homeostatic level unique to each individual's neural wiring. Some tend to have higher emotional set points, generally homeostatic at brain states 1 or 2, occasionally dipping into brain states 3 to 5. Others may have emotional set points at brain states 4 or 5, occasionally having moments of joy in brain state 1. Factors establishing emotional set point are genetics; early childhood experiences, such as adverse events; and temperament. Being in brain states that are connected or disconnected also correlates with neural integration,[16] a construct coined by Dan Siegel, MD.

Table 1 Brain states				
	Cognitive	Emotional	Relational	Behavioral
1	Abstract	Joyous	Intimate	Optimal
2	Concrete	Balanced	Companionable	Healthy
3	Rigid	Mixed	Social	Moderate
4	Reactive	Unbalanced	Needy/distant	Unhealthy
5	Irrational	Terrified	Merged/disengaged	Destructive

As stress increases, brain states decrease. At higher brain states people are able to use creative thinking, positive emotions, social bonds, and effective behavior to solve conflicts. As the brain state lowers, people default to more primitive and rigid techniques for management and self-soothing.

From Mellin L. Wired for joy!: a revolutionary method for creating happiness from within (1st edition). Carlsbad (CA): Hay House; 2010; with permission.

INTERPERSONAL NEUROBIOLOGY

Interpersonal neurobiology is an interdisciplinary field that explores how nervous systems relate to each other. A core founder of the interpersonal neurobiology field is Dan Siegel, MD, who coined the term. Two contributions of Dr Siegel's work are the 9 domains of neural integration and the hand or upstairs/downstairs model of the brain (**Fig. 1**).

Integration is defined through 2 components: differentiation, or respecting differences between people, things, and ideas; and connection, or observing how these differences connect in significant ways.[16] This concept is broad and applies to all forms of science and life. For example, a veterinary nurse changing a client's appointment without notifying the front desk associate who manages appointments, resulting in a conflict between the nurse and the associate. The conflict's cause is a lack of differentiation between roles and a lack of proper communication. Ultimately, this lack of differentiation or connection resulted in ineffectual team performance, because the client arrived despite not being in the appointment book.

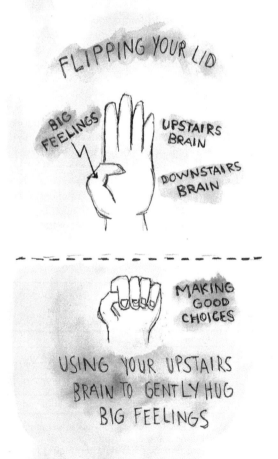

Fig. 1. Hand model of the brain.

Integration can be applied to brain function as well. Neural integration is defined as all 3 differentiated parts of the brain connected and working together. The brain regions can be understood by Dr Siegel's model describing brain regions. The hand model is a tool to describe large areas of the brain associated with the so-called survival center, the limbic system, and the cortical brain. The premise is that the survival center, the most developmentally ancient part of the brain, is associated with the brain stem and controls bodily processes, such as heartbeat and breathing. The limbic brain is associated with emotional experience. The cortical brain is associated with thinking, planning, and inhibiting the impulses of the lower brain stem and limbic brain regions. The hand model is effective at showing how the subcortical responses and limbic system can become aroused, disabling the inhibitory function of the cortical brain, particularly the prefrontal cortex, causing a volatile outburst. Another aspect of this model understands the brain as having upstairs and downstairs areas. The upstairs brain is responsible for thinking, planning, and controlling the body, whereas the downstairs brain is associated with emotions; bodily processes, such as heart rate; and the center for the fight, flight, and freeze responses. Although the hand model of the brain is easy to understand, explain, and experience, another clinically accurate brain model is the large brain network model.

Brain Network Model

A widely accepted understanding of brain functionality is the recognition that there are many complex, interconnected networks that create human life. Although the hand model differentiates between the cortical and subcortical functions, it fails to show the complexity of the brain. Moreover, it has been criticized for creating "good" and "bad" parts of the brain, which is unhelpful because all parts have important functions.[17] Recently, there has been some agreement about the 3 main networks in the brain: the default mode network, the salience network, and the central executive network.

The default network is the aspect of brain functioning occurring when people are at rest, such as mind wandering and habitual thought patterns. The salience network is the aspect of brain functioning identifying important information from the internal world and the external environment. The central executive network is focused on solving problems and/or performing tasks. All of these networks involve many layers of the brain that cross over the old triune model of the brain. In the large brain network model, brain areas specific to the survival center, the limbic brain, and the cortical are all involved in aspects of default, salience, and executive functioning. In addition, the salience network is very powerful because it switches between the default mode and central executive mode of functioning, often occurring subcortically, or beneath people's conscious awareness. What a person assesses as important can be based on previous memories of distress. For instance, a client may hear a veterinarian mention a routine blood test for her dog, creating distress and aggression in the client. Her intense fear reaction was linked to her brother's routine blood test, which resulted in an acute myeloid leukemia diagnosis. The phrase "blood test" becomes very salient, triggering brain regions to react. Because salience network functioning occurs mostly beneath people's conscious awareness, the tricky brain can easily become triggered. Thankfully, humans can become aware of subcortical functioning, helping the tricky brain become manageable, calm, and compassionate in times of conflict and stress.

The hand model of the brain accurately describes cortical and subcortical functioning, which is in keeping with the large network model (see the video of the hand model: https://www.youtube.com/watch?v=f-m2YcdMdFw). This hand model is considered vertical integration, in which the higher cortical regions of the brain are connected to the lower subcortical regions. Dr Siegel calls the connection the stairwell in the upstairs/downstairs brain model. Vertical integration is important because emotions run high in conflict, and a lack of awareness of the subcortical firing of the brainstem and limbic regions (heart racing, sweating, clenched stomach, angry emotions) disables the prefrontal cortical part of the brain. The prefrontal cortical part of the brain uses neural integration, keeping all brain areas connected and working together. When the prefrontal cortex is disabled because of intense subcortical bodily and emotional sensations, people say and do regretful things, inflaming the conflict because there is no management over the interpersonal relationship (**Box 1**).

Polyvagal Theory

Polyvagal theory underlies the brain awareness principles, positing that the autonomic nervous system contains more than just the parasympathetic and sympathetic brain states. Polyvagal theory argues there are 3 states: a state of social engagement (the highest state), a state of mobilization (fight/flight) in response to perceived danger (lower state), and an immobilization or freeze state (the lowest state).[18] The higher aspects of brain function rely on social engagement as a survival tool, in which bonding behaviors through facial expressions and vocal prosodies are used to maintain survival within the social group. The social engagement system is intact when the brain is in a state of neural integration and/or in brain states 1 or 2, which suggests that the most evolutionarily advanced way to handle conflict is to use the social engagement system to ensure continued connection with those important for survival. However, as stress increases, the lower aspects of the brain take over as primary problemsolving methods. The mobilization state triggers the engagement in fight or flight to

---

Box 1
Nine functions of the prefrontal cortex

1. Body regulation: coordinating the bodily stress response.

2. Attuned communication: communicating in a way that connects with the internal state of the other.

3. Emotional balance: the ability to return to a state of balance between being either overwhelmed by or completely disconnected from our emotions.

4. Fear modulation: the ability to experience fear without it becoming overwhelming and creating panic.

5. Response flexibility: the ability to pause before acting and assessing how best to respond to a situation.

6. Insight: the ability to connect our past experience with our present experience and our anticipated future.

7. Empathy: the ability to see the world from another person's perspective. This is more advanced than simply attuning to the emotions of another.

8. Intuition: the ability to be aware of the way the body gives us information; having a "gut feeling."

9. Morality: the ability to sense the emotions and meaning of present circumstances, inhibit impulses, and choose actions for the greater social good.

Adapted from Siegel DJ. Mindsight: the new science of personal transformation. New York: Bantam; 2010; with permission.

secure safety and survival. People start to experience bodily sensations such as heart racing, sweating, and tight muscles. The state also can manifest the fight tendency when blame is placed on others or the self. The immobilization state (brain states 4 and 5) is a form of freezing. The freezing experience can happen when confronted with a person expressing a complaint in a surprising or bold manner.

Dr Paul Gilbert's compassion-focused therapy[14] also shares a model of brain systems that progress from less evolved to more evolved motivational drives (**Fig. 2**). The more recently evolved human brain systems are concerned with social engagement through extended relationship attachments. The mammalian brain systems are driven by caring and status, and the ancient reptilian brain systems are driven by food, sex, and territory. Dr Gilbert also posits 3 basic drives corresponding with less and more evolved motivations: the threat system, the drive system, and the caregiving system (**Table 2**). Understanding experiences and observing conflicts through this lens can help assess what part of the brain takes control during conflict.

CONFLICT ESCALATION AND PREDICTABLE STRATEGIES FOR SURVIVAL

It is useful to examine predictable symptoms of escalating conflict. Pruitt and colleagues[19] identify 5 ways in which human conflict tactics escalate, understanding that not all conflicts exhibit all 5 aspects. Consider the brain states (1–5) and/or systems (social engagement, mobilization, immobilization) that are triggered and in control in these escalation symptoms.

1. Light to heavy tactics: light tactics, such as making requests, saying please, and ingratiating, transform to heavy tactics, such as power plays, threats, and violence.
2. Small to large number of issues: the numbers of issues causing conflict increase as people express more aspects making them annoyed or angry.
3. Specific to general: the original issue causing the disagreement begins to transform into a more general view, from a one-time event to something that always happens.
4. One too many: the original disagreement occurred between 2 people, but, as people begin to gossip and form alliances, more people are drawn into the conflict.
5. Winning to hurt one another: initially, 1 party is interested in winning, but, as the conflict worsens, the person may experience thoughts of negatively affecting the other side.

Conflict escalation might occur like this: there is a disagreement between a veterinary nurse and a front desk associate. The veterinary nurse begins to personalize the disagreement, thinking, "What have I done to deserve that," and "There is something wrong with her!" Then the nurse remembers previous times the front desk associate said similar things that caused similar feelings, thus inflating the disagreement by bringing up the past. The nurse then forms alliances, recounting the story to fellow nurses and establishing an offensive alliance against the front desk associate. At

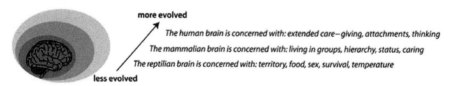

more evolved

The human brain is concerned with: extended care–giving, attachments, thinking

The mammalian brain is concerned with: living in groups, hierarchy, status, caring

The reptilian brain is concerned with: territory, food, sex, survival, temperature

less evolved

Fig. 2. Compassion-focused therapy brain model. Copyright © 2018. Reprinted with permission from Psychology Tools. Whalley, M. G. (2018). What is compassion focused therapy (CFT)? Retrieved from https://www.psychologytools.com/worksheet/what-is-compassion-focused-therapy-cft/. Accessed November 27, 2018.

Table 2
Compassion-focused therapy

Functioning	Threat System	Drive System	Caregiving System
Motivation	Survive	Achieve/win	Look after, soothe
Attention	Threat focused	Goals/advantage	Empathy to distress
Thoughts	About danger	Achieving	Caring, soothing
Emotions	Fear/anxiety	Positive motivated	Safeness
Physiology	Highly aroused	Aroused	Calm
Behavior	Fight or flight	Focused	Look after, soothe

this point, the associate has an enemy image, no longer consisting of both positive and challenging qualities, but rather as an unredeemable enemy. Rumors solidify the enemy image, as more people are pulled into the disagreement. Then there is a moment of open hostility, when the veterinary nurse and the front desk associate speak aloud directly, which often results in separation (leaving the job) or a verbal and/or physical fight. The two may engage in outward arguing, and many in the practice may engage in flight, avoiding the uncomfortable situation. The leaders in the clinic may freeze, not knowing how to respond.

In this scenario, the brain states continue to lower until all flexibility turns into rigid responses, or from high to low neural integration.

WHAT TO DO

Kwame Christian, an attorney and expert negotiation coach, encourages people in conflict to reach for "compassionate curiosity"[15] in understanding the perspective and position of the other person. To accomplish this, it is necessary for people to be compassionately curious about brain state levels in others and themselves. Three useful tools are the triangle of awareness, the circle process, and using interprofessional teams.

Use the Triangle of Awareness

Jon Kabat-Zinn, the founder of the well-renowned mindfulness-based stress reduction program, teaches a tool called the "Triangle of Awareness."[20] This tool helps people respond to conflict and stress rather than react to it. There are 3 processes occurring in human beings all the time: thinking, emotions, and body sensations (**Fig. 3**). Most of these experiences are subcortical, or beneath people's conscious awareness. With practice and self-inquiry, people can pause to assess the physical body, assess current emotions, and assess current thoughts. Using this tool daily can train people to have all aspects of experience inside, instead of outside, the conscious awareness. When people can identify the emotion, body sensation, or thought process, people can catch themselves before they react and say or do something from a state of threat instead of social engagement.

Use a Circle

The need for medical professionals to gain skills in facilitating discussions among family members facing medical decisions for loved ones is growing.[1] The circle process is a tool to help elicit the higher social engagement brain systems in times of conflict. The circle process does this by providing structure and rules that support a sense of

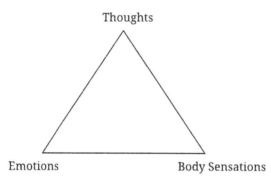

Fig. 3. Triangle of awareness.

predictable safety in the interactions. The circles can be a group of 2 or more people. Circles can be a mixture of family members and work teammates. It can be helpful to have a leader; however, with regular practice and familiarity, circles can be facilitated nonhierarchically.

There are many types of circle processes. A popularly known circle is the Native American talking-stick approach.[21,22] Another indigenous tool is the Hawaiian technique, called ho'oponopono, meaning to make right.[23–25] It is usually facilitated by an elder in the community and is a effective tool for resolving conflicts between parties that have ongoing interdependent relationships. Forgiveness, a higher order emotion associated with the social engagement system,[26] is a major component of ho'oponopono. The process began as a tool for families and close-knit communities but has expanded to secular and business environments.[27] Although the ho'oponopono process is a time investment, it can ultimately save time and financial resources by repairing important work relationships. For a series of videos showing the ho'oponopono process in the veterinary environment, see Videos 1–5.

Another useful tool in a circle process is the Ten Guidelines for Making Conversations with Emotional Charge Productive (**Box 2**). Step 1: invite each person in the circle to read 1 of the guidelines. Step 2: seek agreement that all members of the circle are willing to abide (if they are not willing, a different approach should be used; discussed later). Step 3: invite people to concisely share their opinions, experiences, and thoughts about a situation. Step 4: invite people to acknowledge what they heard from others. Step 5: invite circle members to give and receive "olive branches." Step 6: invite circle members to share any gratitude or personal growth insight they are taking away from the circle. When using this approach, be sure to allow enough uninterrupted time. In addition, each member is invited but not required to share; members can say "pass" as needed.

These approaches are for groups in which relationships are valued and there is a desire to maintain positive connections. These approaches work when people are willing to listen and even forgive transgressions that have occurred in the relationship. However, in conflict, this is not always the case. In situations that are more intractable, it is important to consider adding to the team.

Add to Your Team

Adding members to medical teams with expertise in human communication is gaining attention as an important resource. Interprofessional collaboration can help with navigating the often challenging and value-laden aspects of medical care.[28] By working together across the discipline, the patient's/client's needs can be met by a multitude

Box 2	
Ten guidelines for making conversations with emotional charge productive	
Speak for yourself	Avoid making statements like "I am sure we would all agree." Inevitably there will be someone who does not agree with you who will be offended by your assumption
Do not interrupt	Allow people to fully share their perspectives by not interrupting
Be concise	Be mindful to express your opinion, interest, or position in a manner that is clear and concise. Saying too much without coming to a point can harm people's ability to listen to you
Really listen	Listen completely to what is being said. Listening is compromised when you are mentally focused on your rebuttal instead of the speaker's comments
Acknowledge what has been said	Letting a person know you understand their perspective does not mean that you agree. It is simply a sign of respect, not a show of agreement
Agree where you can	Highlighting the areas in which you do agree makes the places where you differ less difficult
Be courteous	Avoid labels like "That is stupid" or "He's an idiot." These types of labels of person or position inflame emotion and conflict and reduce productivity
Give and receive "olive branches"	Admit your mistakes or misunderstandings and outwardly acknowledge such admissions from others
Keep an open mind	Conversations about topics on which people have differing opinions and positions have the greatest possibility of teaching something new. Allow yourself to be open to the possibility that your perspective may change through participation
Express gratitude and growth	Share the ways your connection with others helps you be grateful and grow in your life

Courtesy of Elizabeth B. Strand, PhD, LCSW.

of professions working together. Although a helpful concept, the application can be a challenge because of the ethics, values, and cultures that differ between professional identities. Thus, one core aspect of interprofessional practice is the development of conflict resolution skills.[29] The application of professionals whose skills lie in the area of social science[30] and mediation[31] can be particularly important when dealing with end-of-life issues. At the time of treatment, emotions run high and people's core values become extremely important to them. Having communication experts whose job is to attend solely to the human species can be supportive for both the veterinary team and the clients, both of whom have the animal's best interest in mind.

SUMMARY

Being in conflict lowers brain states, moving people to engage in behaviors associated with fight, flight, and freeze. In the medical environment, poorly handled conflicts and lower brain states negatively affect patient care and professional well-being. Seeing conflicts through the lens of brain awareness helps use tools and strategies to maintain the social engagement system and solve conflicts peaceably. Everyone can engage in these strategies, and particularly difficult conflicts may benefit by adding interprofessional care.

SUPPLEMENTARY DATA

Supplementary data related to this article can be found online at https://doi.org/10.1016/j.cvsm.2019.01.017.

REFERENCES

1. Hagiwara Y, Ross J, Lee S, et al. Tough conversations: development of a curriculum for medical students to lead family meetings. Am J Hosp Palliat Care 2017; 34(10):907–11.
2. Cochran N, Charlton P, Reed V, et al. Beyond fight or flight: the need for conflict management training in medical education. Conflict Resolution Quarterly 2018; 35(4):393–402.
3. Greenberg CC, Regenbogen SE, Studdert DM, et al. Patterns of communication breakdowns resulting in injury to surgical patients. J Am Coll Surg 2007;204(4): 533–40.
4. Bishop TF, Ryan AM, Casalino LP. Paid malpractice claims for adverse events in inpatient and outpatient settings. JAMA 2011;305(23):2427–31.
5. Morris JA Jr, Carrillo Y, Jenkins JM, et al. Surgical adverse events, risk management, and malpractice outcome: morbidity and mortality review is not enough. Ann Surg 2003;237(6):844–51 [discussion: 851–2].
6. Stecker M, Stecker MM. Disruptive staff interactions: a serious source of interprovider conflict and stress in health care settings. Issues Ment Health Nurs 2014;35(7):533–41.
7. Higginson IJ, Rumble C, Shipman C, et al. The value of uncertainty in critical illness? An ethnographic study of patterns and conflicts in care and decision-making trajectories. BMC Anesthesiol 2016;16:11.
8. Bradley V, Liddle S, Shaw R, et al. Sticks and stones: investigating rude, dismissive and aggressive communication between doctors. Clin Med 2015;15(6): 541–5.
9. Moore IC, Coe JB, Adams CL, et al. Exploring the impact of toxic attitudes and a toxic environment on the veterinary healthcare team. Front Vet Sci 2015;2. https://doi.org/10.3389/fvets.2015.00078.
10. Tannenbaum J. Veterinary medical ethics: a focus of conflicting interests. J Soc Issues 1993;49(1):143–56. Available at: http://onlinelibrary.wiley.com/doi/10.1111/j.1540-4560.1993.tb00914.x/full. Accessed April 12, 2017.
11. Kabat-Farr D, Marchiondo LA, Cortina LM. The emotional aftermath of incivility: anger, guilt, and the role of organizational commitment. Int J Stress Manag 2018;25(2):109–28.
12. Porath CL, Foulk T, Erez A. How incivility hijacks performance: it robs cognitive resources, increases dysfunctional behavior, and infects team dynamics and functioning. Organ Dyn 2015;44(4):258–65.
13. Riskin A, Erez A, Foulk TA, et al. The impact of rudeness on medical team performance: a randomized trial. Pediatrics 2015. https://doi.org/10.1542/peds.2015-1385.
14. Gilbert P. The origins and nature of compassion focused therapy. Br J Clin Psychol 2014;53(1):6–41.
15. TEDx Talks. Finding confidence in conflict | Kwame Christian | TEDxDayton. Youtube 2017. Available at: https://www.youtube.com/watch?v=F6Zg65eK9XU&feature=youtu.be. Accessed November 30, 2018.
16. Siegel DJ. Mindsight: the new science of personal transformation. Reprint edition. Bantam; 2010. Available at: https://www.amazon.com/Mindsight-New-Science-Personal-Transformation/dp/0553386395/ref=sr_1_1?ie=UTF8&qid=1543592743&sr=8-1&keywords=mindsight. Accessed November 27, 2018.

17. The magnificent, mysterious, wild, connected and interconnected brain - mindful. Mindful. Available at: https://www.mindful.org/the-magnificent-mysterious-wild-connected-and-interconnected-brain/. Accessed October 21, 2018.

18. Porges SW. The polyvagal perspective. Biol Psychol 2007;74(2):116–43.

19. Pruitt D, Rubin J, Kim SH. Social conflict: escalation, stalemate, and settlement. 3rd edition. New York: McGraw-Hill Education; 2003. Available at: https://www.amazon.com/gp/product/0072855355/ref=dbs_a_def_rwt_bibl_vppi_i0. Accessed November 27, 2018.

20. Kabat-Zinn J, Hanh TN. Full catastrophe living (revised edition): using the wisdom of your body and mind to face stress, pain, and illness. Rev Upd edition. New York: Bantam; 2013. Available at: https://www.amazon.com/Full-Catastrophe-Living-Revised-Illness-ebook/dp/B00C4BA3UK/ref=sr_1_2?ie=UTF8&qid=1543600071&sr=8-2&keywords=jon+kabat+zinn. Accessed November 27, 2018.

21. Fujioka K. The talking stick: an American Indian tradition in the ESL classroom. The Internet TESL Journal 1998;4(9):1–6. Available at: http://iteslj.org/Techniques/Fujioka-TalkingStick.html. Accessed November 27, 2018.

22. Donaldson LE. Writing the talking stick: alphabetic literacy as colonial technology and postcolonial appropriation. Am Indian Q 1998;22(1/2):46–62. Available at: http://search.ebscohost.com/login.aspx?direct=true&db=a9h&AN=1632204&scope=site. Accessed November 27, 2018.

23. Hurdle D. Native Hawaiian traditional healing: culturally based interventions for social work practice. Soc Work 2002;47(2):183–92.

24. Dragonetti J. Embracing Hawaiian culture: applying traditional Hawaiian values to modern ethical discussions. Am J Geriatr Psychiatry 2018;26(3):S76–7.

25. Wall JA, Callister RR. Ho'oponopono: some lessons from Hawaiian mediation. Negotiation Journal 1995;11(1):45–54.

26. Ricciardi E, Rota G, Sani L, et al. How the brain heals emotional wounds: the functional neuroanatomy of forgiveness. Front Hum Neurosci 2013;7:839.

27. Patten TH Jr. Ho'oponopono: a cross cultural model for organizational development and change. International Journal of Organizational Analysis (1993 - 2002) 1994;2(3):252.

28. Vandergoot S, Sarris A, Kirby N, et al. Exploring undergraduate students' attitudes towards interprofessional learning, motivation-to-learn, and perceived impact of learning conflict resolution skills. J Interprof Care 2018;32(2):211–9.

29. D'Amour D, Ferrada-Videla M, San Martin Rodriguez L, et al. The conceptual basis for interprofessional collaboration: core concepts and theoretical frameworks. J Interprof Care 2005;19(Suppl 1):116–31.

30. Bomba PA, Morrissey MB, Leven DC. Key role of social work in effective communication and conflict resolution process: Medical Orders for Life-Sustaining Treatment (MOLST) program in New York and shared medical decision making at the end of life. J Soc Work End Life Palliat Care 2011;7(1):56–82.

31. Fiester A. Neglected ends: clinical ethics consultation and the prospects for closure. Am J Bioeth 2015;15(1):29–36.

Moving?

Make sure your subscription moves with you!

To notify us of your new address, find your **Clinics Account Number** (located on your mailing label above your name), and contact customer service at:

Email: journalscustomerservice-usa@elsevier.com

800-654-2452 (subscribers in the U.S. & Canada)
314-447-8871 (subscribers outside of the U.S. & Canada)

Fax number: 314-447-8029

Elsevier Health Sciences Division
Subscription Customer Service
3251 Riverport Lane
Maryland Heights, MO 63043

*To ensure uninterrupted delivery of your subscription, please notify us at least 4 weeks in advance of move.

Printed and bound by CPI Group (UK) Ltd, Croydon, CR0 4YY

03/10/2024

01040403-0003